Peritoneal Dialysis
New Concepts and Applications

CONTEMPORARY ISSUES IN NEPHROLOGY

VOLUME 22

Series Editor
Jay H. Stein, M.D.

Series Editors, Vols. 1–21
Barry M. Brenner, M.D.
Jay H. Stein, M.D.

Volumes Already Published

Forthcoming Volume in the Series

Peritoneal Dialysis
New Concepts and Applications

Guest Editors

ZBYLUT J. TWARDOWSKI, M.D.
Professor
Department of Medicine
University of Missouri—Columbia School of Medicine
Director
Continuous Ambulatory Peritoneal Dialysis Program
University of Missouri Health Sciences Center
Columbia, Missouri

KARL D. NOLPH, M.D., F.R.C.P.S. (GLASGOW)
Broaddus and Curators Professor
Department of Medicine
University of Missouri—Columbia School of Medicine
Director
Division of Nephrology
University of Missouri Health Sciences Center, Veterans Administration Hospital,
    and Dalton Research Center
Columbia, Missouri

RAMESH KHANNA, M.D.
Professor
Department of Medicine
University of Missouri—Columbia School of Medicine
Director
Inpatient Peritoneal Dialysis Programs
University of Missouri Health Sciences Center
Columbia, Missouri

Series Editor

JAY H. STEIN, M.D.
Professor and Chairman
Department of Medicine
Dan F. Parman Chair in Medicine
University of Texas Medical School at San Antonio
San Antonio, Texas

CHURCHILL LIVINGSTONE
New York, Edinburgh, London, Melbourne

Library of Congress Cataloging-in-Publication Data

Peritoneal dialysis : new concepts and applications / guest editors,
   Zbylut J. Twardowski, Karl D. Nolph, Ramesh Khanna.
      p. cm. — (Contemporary issues in nephrology ; vol. 22)
   Includes bibliographical references.
   ISBN 0-443-08716-4
   1. Peritoneal dialysis.   I. Twardowski, Zbylut J. II. Nolph,
Karl D.   III. Khanna, Ramesh.   IV. Series.
   [DNLM: 1. Peritoneal Dialysis.   W1 CO769MR v. 22 / WJ 378 P4465]
   RC901.7.P48P475   1990
   617.4′61059—dc20
   DNLM/DLC
   for Library of Congress   89-13919
                                                                    CIP

Distributed in the United Kingdom by Churchill Livingstone, Robert Stevenson
House, 1–3 Baxter's Place, Leith Walk, Edinburgh EH1 3AF, and by associated
companies, branches, and representatives throughout the world.

Accurate indications, adverse reactions, and dosage schedules for drugs are
provided in this book, but it is possible that they may change. The reader is
urged to review the package information data of the manufacturers of the
medications mentioned.

The Publishers have made every effort to trace the copyright holders for
borrowed material. If they have inadvertently overlooked any, they will be
pleased to make the necessary arrangements at the first opportunity.

Acquisitions Editor: *Avé McCracken*
Copy Editor: *Marian Ryan*
Production Designer: *Jill Little*
Production Supervisor: *Christina Hippeli*

Printed in the United States of America

First published in 1990

Dedicated to peritoneal dialysis patients

Contributors

Steven R. Alexander, M.D.
Associate Professor, Department of Pediatrics, University of Texas Southwestern Medical Center at Dallas Southwestern Medical School; Medical Director, Dialysis and Renal Transplantation, Children's Medical Center, Dallas, Texas

Giovanni C. Cancarini, M.D.
Senior Assistant, Division of Nephrology, Civil Hospital, Brescia, Italy

James A. Delmez, M.D.
Associate Professor, Department of Medicine, Washington University School of Medicine; Medical Director, Chromalloy American Dialysis Center; Associate Physician, Barnes Hospital, St. Louis, Missouri

E. Dale Everett, M.D.
Professor, Department of Medicine, University of Missouri—Columbia School of Medicine; Director, Division of Infectious Disease, University of Missouri Health Sciences Center, Columbia, Missouri

Lazaro Gotloib, M.D.
Head, Department of Nephrology, and Director, Kornach Laboratory for Experimental Nephrology, Central Emek Hospital, Afula, Israel

Ramesh Khanna, M.D.
Professor, Department of Medicine, University of Missouri—Columbia School of Medicine; Director, Inpatient Peritoneal Dialysis Programs, University of Missouri Health Sciences Center, Columbia, Missouri

Sunder M. Lal, M.D.
Assistant Professor, Department of Medicine, University of Missouri—Columbia School of Medicine, Columbia, Missouri

Anne S. Lindblad, M.S.
Statistician, The EMMES Corporation, Potomac, Maryland

Robert A. Mactier, M.D., M.R.C.P.
Senior Registrar, Department of Medicine and Renal Unit, Ninewells Hospital, Dundee, Scotland

Rosario Maiorca, M.D.
Chairman, Department of Nephrology, University of Brescia School of Medicine; Chief, Division of Nephrology, Civil Hospital, Brescia, Italy

Karl D. Nolph, M.D., F.R.C.P.S. (Glasgow)
Broaddus and Curators Professor, Department of Medicine, University of Missouri—Columbia School of Medicine; Director, Division of Nephrology, University of Missouri Health Sciences Center, Veterans Administration Hospital, and Dalton Research Center, Columbia, Missouri

Joel W. Novak, M.S.
Statistician, The EMMES Corporation, Potomac, Maryland

Avshalom Shostak, M.D.
Department of Nephrology and Kornach Laboratory for Experimental Nephrology, Central Emek Hospital, Afula, Israel

Zbylut J. Twardowski, M.D.
Professor, Department of Medicine, University of Missouri—Columbia School of Medicine; Director, Continuous Ambulatory Peritoneal Dialysis Program, University of Missouri Health Sciences Center, Columbia, Missouri

Foreword

The tremendous changes that have occurred in peritoneal dialysis in the last 25 years have transformed the technique from a second-class therapy (compared with hemodialysis) to a measure that is the equal of hemodialysis in many respects and even superior to hemodialysis in terms of cost, maintenance of hemoglobin, and independent living.

The revolution began with the introduction of continuous ambulatory peritoneal dialysis (CAPD) by Popovich and Moncrief, who deserve the lion's share of credit for our progress. The introduction of plastic bags and the Toronto Western Hospital technique for CAPD led to the widespread acceptance of this mode of dialysis and to a significant reduction in the frequency of peritonitis from one episode every 3 to 4 patient months to one episode per patient year. In the last few years peritonitis rates fell further after the introduction of the Y-set system by Buoncristiani. Today many centers achieve peritonitis rates of less than one episode per 2 patient years.

The editors of this volume, Twardowski, Nolph, and Khanna, have made important contributions to our knowledge of the physiology of peritoneal dialysis as well as to its various clinical aspects.

Automated peritoneal dialysis, in the form of either continuous cyclic peritoneal dialysis (CCPD), which was proposed and advanced by Suki and Diaz-Buxo, or the more expensive nightly intermittent peritoneal dialysis, (IPD) is gaining ground; thus, we are able to maintain a number of patients who cannot be managed by CAPD and otherwise would be converted to hemodialysis.

CAPD plays a particularly important role in the management of children and diabetics with end-stage renal disease. Maiorca describes the experience of his group in the Y-system chapter, illustrating what CAPD can achieve in adults.

The last few years have witnessed great advances in our understanding of the anatomy and physiology of the peritoneal membrane, the complex function of the mesothelial cells, and the role of lymphatics during peritoneal dialysis. However, despite these advances, major problems remain; all who wield influence should encourage the continued dedication of the pioneers as well as the work of new scientists in the field. We need financial support for scientists from many disciplines, who will contribute their ingenuity to solving the lingering problems. These challenges include prevention of exit-site infection and subsequent peritonitis; malnutrition; and ultrafiltration failure. Of course, all who have worked with CAPD over the years are conscious of the risk of encapsulating sclerosing peritonitis—the precise mechanisms of which have yet to be identified.

Although a significant number of patients have remained on CAPD for 10 years or more, it has not yet been established that CAPD is a true long-term dialysis modality.

Our progress to date gives me the encouragement to believe that we will solve most of the problems and that CAPD will take its place among the genuine kidney-replacement techniques, thus providing the nephrologist with a wide range of alternatives in the management of patients with end-stage renal disease.

D. G. Oreopoulos, M.D., Ph.D., F.R.C.P. (C).
Professor, Department of Medicine
University of Toronto Faculty of Medicine
Director, Peritoneal Dialysis Unit
Toronto Western Hospital
Toronto, Ontario, Canada

Preface

Treatment of uremia by intraperitoneal infusion and drainage of dialysis solution was first reported in 1923 by Georg Ganter, a German physician. Ganter found followers very quickly, and in the next 25 years, more than 100 cases of such treatment were reported. The development of the Tenckhoff catheter in 1968 and, particularly, the introduction of continuous ambulatory peritoneal dialysis (CAPD) in the late 1970s encouraged the use of peritoneal dialysis in the treatment of chronic renal failure. The development of new catheters, automated cycling equipment, variable flow techniques, and many other techniques have yielded both improved results and increased interest in peritoneal dialysis; by the end of 1989 more than 45,000 patients worldwide were on peritoneal dialysis.

Research is intense, with more than 400 papers related to peritoneal dialysis published annually. With such rapid progress, a book devoted to the latest developments in the field cannot be written by a few persons; it must be a multiauthored volume. The authors have written up-to-date, comprehensive, extensively referenced chapters. We have selected for discussion in this volume areas of peritoneal dialysis we believe to be most important and that have been central to the most striking recent progress in the field.

Many contributors have been our colleagues in the Department of Medicine at the University of Missouri; we have followed the work of the other authors for many years, and are pleased to have their contributions. Lazaro Gotloib and Avshalom Shostak, leading students of peritoneal anatomy, have written an excellent chapter on the functional anatomy of the peritoneum as a dialyzing membrane, describing new discoveries relative to fenestrated capillaries, lymph drainage, and the structural basis of transperitoneal transport. Rosario Maiorca and Giovanni C. Cancarini have contributed the chapter on the Y-set, the system that revolutionized peritoneal dialysis connectology and dramatically reduced the rate of peritonitis, the scourge of peritoneal dialysis. Our Italian colleagues have long reported excellent results with this system; now their methods are emulated in other countries. James A. Delmez, a most erudite scholar in the field of bone metabolism and peritoneal dialysis, has authored the chapter on bone and mineral metabolism in CAPD patients. His topics include recent advances in the use of calcium carbonate as a phosphate binder, prevention of hypercalcemia with low calcium dialysis solution, and aluminum toxicity and its treatment. Steven R. Alexander, one of the pioneers of peritoneal dialysis in

children, has coauthored the chapter on CAPD and continuous cyclic peritoneal dialysis results in the United States pediatric population.

E. Dale Everett, Director of the Division of Infectious Diseases in our
department, who has been helping us treat infectious complications since the
beginning of our CAPD program in 1977, has written a chapter on
prevention, diagnosis, and treatment of peritonitis. Robert Mactier has authored the chapter on kinetics of ultrafiltration, a topic he studied during his
fellowship in our department. In addition, Sunder Lal, a current member of
our faculty and our former fellow, has coauthored a chapter on pharmacologic manipulations of peritoneal transport.

Finally, we have prepared chapters in areas of our own research involvement: adequacy of dialysis and newer cycler techniques; peritoneal access;
clinical results with peritoneal dialysis according to experiences of four
registries in three continents; and peritoneal dialysis in diabetics.

We thank the chapter authors for timely delivery of the manuscripts,
allowing the book to be published on schedule. We are proud to have the
contribution of Dimitrios G. Oreopoulos, a pioneer of peritoneal dialysis and
editor of *Peritoneal Dialysis International,* who has written the foreword. We
also thank Jan Leroux for indispensable secrétarial assistance. Finally, we
wish to acknowledge the invaluable help of the Churchill Livingstone staff,
particularly Linda Panzarella, Avé McCracken, and Marian Ryan, without
whose technical assistance publication of the book would not have been
possible.

Zbylut J. Twardowski, M.D.
Karl D. Nolph, M.D., F.R.C.P.S. (Glasgow)
Ramesh Khanna, M.D.

Contents

The Functional Anatomy of the Peritoneum As a Dialyzing Membrane

Lazaro Gotloib
Avshalom Shostak

INTRODUCTION
BLOOD MICROVESSELS
THE INTERSTITIAL SPACE
LYMPHATICS
THE MESOTHELIUM
CONCLUSION

There is not one science of chemistry, another of electricity, another of medicine and so on. There is only one natural world and there is only one knowledge of it.
Sir William Bragg, 1941

INTRODUCTION

The beginning of the 16th century saw the dawn of the peritoneal function as interpreted by Asellius (1581–1626) in the mesentery of dogs.

Since that time, morphologic,[1–4] physiologic,[5–8] and clinical studies[9–13] have given strength and scientific foundation to the idea of using the peritoneum as a dialyzing membrane for long-term care of chronic uremic patients. However, four centuries of intensive, multidisciplinary research failed to completely disclose the way in which nature has solved the blood-tissue contact problem. A rational, analytic approach to the problems of peritoneal permeability should be based on the morphologic and functional analysis of each of the several components of the peritoneal dialysis system.[8] Consequently, in this review the peritoneal membrane is conceived as the embodiment of several biologic membranes, each showing more or less specific morphologic and even molecular characteristics. Our main goal is to merge the available morphologic and physiologic information, as well as to define the chief unanswered questions that should eventually be solved by future research.

BLOOD MICROVESSELS

Blood microvessel capillaries of the human and rodent parietal and visceral peritoneum have been classically reported to be the continuous type[14] (Fig. 1-1). However, the existence of fenestrated capillaries in the human parietal and rabbit diaphragmatic peritoneum,[15] as well as in the mesentery of mice,[16] has been reported (Fig. 1-2). The incidence of fenestrated capillaries in human parietal peritoneum appears to be low (1.7 percent of the total number of capillaries).[15] However, the presence of fenestrated capillaries in the mesentery, which contributes up to 49 percent of the total mesothelial dialyzing surface area in humans,[17] may be physiologically significant. Furthermore, it should be noted that the density distribution of submesothelial microvessels along the different portions of the peritoneum is heterogeneous. In rabbits, the mesentery appears as the most vascularized peritoneal segment, contributing 71.1 percent of the total number of observed capillaries. Reported diaphragmatic and parietal contributions to the total microvascular bed examined are 17.9 and 10.9 percent, respectively.[18]

The endothelial luminal surface-blood interface, which constitutes the first obstacle for solutes on the way to the peritoneal dialysate, is composed of the stagnant fluid film in the capillary lumen (the functional significance of which has been considered to be minor[8]) and the endothelial cell glycocalix. The latter, originally described by Luft[19] in other vascular beds, has also been observed on the surface of most cells[20] and at the luminal aspect of endothelial cells of peritoneal microvessels.[21-23]

The endothelial cell glycocalix is a regular, well-organized polymeric carpet, the major structural components of which are sialoconjugates, proteoglycans, and acidic polymers, which provide a fibrous network and impart an electronegative charge to the cell luminal membrane (Fig. 1-1, inset).[24-28] This polyanionic coat furnishes a nonthrombogenic surface[29] and contributes to the regulation of the transport of small and large molecules across the vascular wall, acting as a size, shape, and charge barrier.[27,28]

Therefore, the glycocalix can act as a physiologic barrier for anionic plasma proteins. In addition serum albumin, which has a net negative charge, can also bind anions as a result of the presence of cationic groups.[29,30] In this way, in the fiber matrix model of capillary permeability, the glycocalix is viewed as a meshwork of glycoprotein fibers which, by trapping circu-

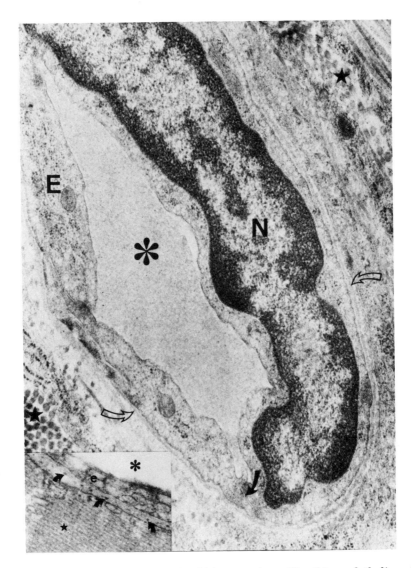

Fig. 1-1. Blood capillary of normal rabbit mesentery. The thin endothelium (E) is lying on a continuous and homogeneous basement membrane (open arrows). A tight junction (solid arrows) is apparently closing the intercellular cleft extended between the perivascular interstitial tissue and the capillary lumen (asterisk). Stars indicate bundles of collagen. N, nucleous of endothelial cell. (× 47,400.) (**Inset**) Partial view of a continuous capillary of rat parietal peritoneum. The animal was perfused with ruthenium-red. Periodic anionic sites (arrows) can be seen along the basement membrane lying under the endothelial cell (e). The asterisk shows the microvascular lumen. The star indicates bundles of collagen. (× 64,550.)

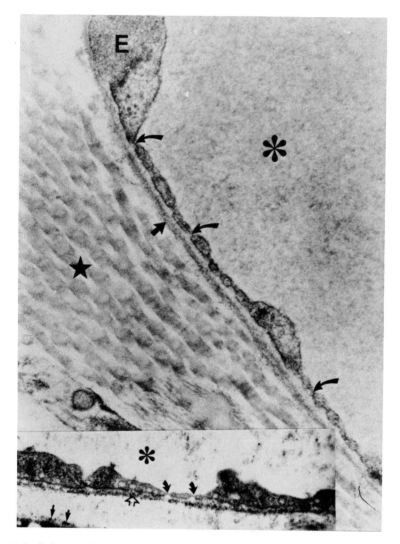

Fig. 1-2. Submesothelial fenestrated capillary of normal rabbit diaphragmatic peritoneum. The endothelial cell (E) shows fenestrations apparently closed by the diaphragms (curved arrows). A continuous basement membrane (short arrow) is interposed between the endothelial cell and the interstitial bundles of collagen (star). The asterisk indicates the microvascular lumen. ($\times$ 85,000.) (**Inset**) A mesenteric fenestrated capillary of a normal mouse. The specimen was obtained 4 hours after intraperitoneal injection of cationized ferritin. The endothelial cell (e) shows fenestrae with diaphragms (curved arrows). The large asterisk indicates the microvascular lumen. The small asterisk shows an uncoated plasmalemmal vesicle. Anionic fixed charges (open arrow) are regularly distributed along the subendothelial basement membrane. The straight black arrows show anionic fixed charges located on an interstitial fibroblast. ($\times$ 41,500.)

lating proteins, will eventually tighten itself, rendering the underlying endothelium less accessible to water and water-soluble molecules[29,30] and to anionic macromolecules.[31]

The plasmalemma of endothelial cells shows the trilaminar structure of the Robertson unit membrane,[32] which consists of a central lipid layer covered by two monolayers of protein. The overall thickness of the cell membrane is approximately 80 to 100 Å, each layer being approximately 30 Å thick.

It should be noted that, although glycolipids and sugar side chains of glycoproteins and many complex oligosaccharides are included in the outer surface of cell membranes, their presence in the opposite inner aspect of the membrane is minimal. This asymmetry of cell membranes mandates that a considerable amount of energy would eventually be required to move polar lipid molecules from one side of the membrane to the other.[33]

Furthermore, the different functional properties of cell membranes produced by different tissues indicate that the basic membrane unit can store a variety of enzymes and receptors, which can be exposed by using special cytochemical techniques.[34] Specialized areas of the cell membrane are involved in the complex process of pinocytosis, whereas others form the intercellular junctions.

Pinocytotic vesicles are conspicuously present in endothelial cells at both the basal and luminal aspects, as well as in the paranuclear cytoplasm (Fig. 1-3). They occupy approximately 7 percent of the cell volume, their mean diameter is approximately 700 Å, they have a round or oval shape, and are surrounded by a triple-layered membrane approximately 80 Å thick.[35,36]

The population density of pinocytotic vesicles varies considerably from one vascular segment to another, even within the same microvascular territory.[36] In the mouse diaphragm, arterioles show 200 vesicles/μm^2, 900 true capillaries/μm^2, 1,200 venular segments of capillaries/μm^2, and 600 postcapillary venules/μm^2.[36]

Most vesicles that open to the extracellular medium have necks with a diameter as small as 100 Å.[35] Transendothelial channels, formed by a chain of two or more vesicles opening simultaneously on both fronts of the endothelium, have been reported in the capillaries of mouse diaphragmatic muscle[36] as well as in the postcapillary venules of rabbit mesentery.[37]

The relative frequency of transendothelial channels has been found to be higher in true capillaries than in arterioles and venules, and highest in the venular segment of capillaries. Microvessels of frog mesentery showed a density distribution of three transendothelial channels for every 400 vascular profiles examined.[36,38] Palade's[39] prediction that endothelial pinocytotic vesicles are involved in transcellular transport is now generally accepted,[40–43] with few exceptions.[44] It has been proposed that vesicles can shuttle from one cell front to another or to the intercellular junction; taking up, transporting, and discharging their contents.[43] The energy source for vesicular movement remains unclear, although thermal energy is a possibility.[41] A 3- to 5-second median transit time for vesicles crossing capillary

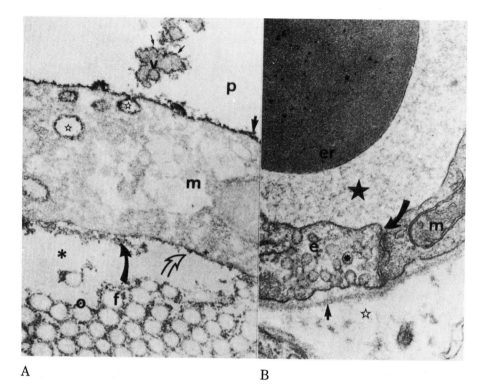

Fig. 1-3. (**A**) Mesenteric mesothelium of a rat perfused with ruthenium-red 24 hours after induction of septic (*Escherichia coli*) peritonitis. The microvilli (v) still show a glycocalix illuminated by ruthenium-red (small black arrows) as well as the luminal mesothelial cell plasmalemma (short black arrow). The mesothelial cell (m) shows the presence of coated vesicles (open stars). The submesothelial basement membrane (curved black arrow) is devoid of anionic fixed charges and, at times, disappears (open arrow). The interstitium is edematous (asterisk). Particles of ruthenium-red (open circle) are sporadically observed between the collagen fibers (f). (p, peritoneal space). (× 64,550.) (**B**) A continuous submesothelial diaphragmatic capillary obtained 24 hours after induction of septic (*E coli*) peritonitis from a rat perfused with ruthenium-red. The subendothelial basement membrane (short black arrow) is devoid of anionic fixed charges. The interstitial space (open star) is edematous. Coated pits and coated vesicles are not observed. er, Erythrocyte; black star, capillary lumen; curved black arrow, tight junction; e, endothelial cell; m, mitochondria. (× 34,600.)

endothelial and mesothelial cells of 0.3 to 0.5 μm thicknesses has been calculated, taking into account that approximately 40 percent of the released vesicles regain the plasmalemma on the opposite side of the cell.[42]

Since Lewis's[45] original description of pinocytosis in macrophages of the rat omentum, a full body of literature has been published. For many years, the process was thought to deal mainly with the cell's intake of fluid from the surrounding medium. However, later studies showed that, while metabolic inhibitors suppressed macromolecular uptake by pinocytosis,[46] fluid uptake remained unchanged, indicating that the underlying mechanisms of both processes are essentially different.[38] An important step forward was the demonstration of the preferential distribution of anionic sites at the luminal surface of capillary endothelium, coated pits, and coated vesicles, and their absence from plasmalemmal vesicles and transendothelial channels.[25,26] Further progress resulted in the demonstration of plasma membrane recycling[34] and receptor-mediated endocytosis.[47] It seems, therefore, that there are two different mechanisms and/or pathways for endocytosis. The first is a highly specific receptor-mediated pathway located in the coated pits (Fig. 1-4, inset) in which ligands first bind to receptors and are later internalized and delivered to the lysosomal compartment, while the receptor molecules are generally recycled back to the cell surface.[47-49] It should be noted that in a typical cultured cell, as many as 3,000 vesicles per minute can be formed[49] and that the same cell can internalize 50 percent of the plasma membrane in 1 hour.[47] Since cell volume and surface area remain unchanged during this process, it is evident that a simultaneous mechanism of exocytosis has to be functioning.[50] The second pinocytotic pathway is that of fluid-phase pinocytosis, which takes place through the system of uncoated plasmalemmal vesicles and transendothelial channels (the limiting membrane of which does not bind cationic tracers). This property would facilitate the reported transendothelial active transport of albumin.[51,52]

This population of plasmalemmal vesicles, which vastly outnumbers that of the coated pits and vesicles, seems to also internalize other substances not bound to receptors.[34,47,49] These observations support the hypothesis that the limiting membrane of uncoated plasmalemmal vesicles is chemically different from the plasma membrane, and that during their fusion, the two membranes do not mix.

In summary, macromolecules that permeate endothelia are selected according to charge in addition to size: cationic and anionic macromolecules follow different pathways across the endothelial layer of the capillary wall. Furthermore, histamine H_1 and H_2 receptors have been shown in the luminal plasma membrane of capillaries and, particularly, in the postcapillary venules of the mouse diaphragm.[53] The presence of these receptors in the peritoneum has also been documented in a study that showed increased permeability for proteins induced by histamine. This effect was blocked by histamine antagonists.[54,55]

Capillary endothelial cells are linked to each other by tight junctions or zonula occludens,[40,56-58] which apparently seal the intercellular cleft by close apposition or fusion of the external protein layers of the plasmalemma, completely obliterating the intercellular space (Fig. 1-1).

Postcapillary venules have loosely organized junctions with discontinuous ridges and grooves, of which 25 to 30 percent appear to be open, with a gap of 20 to 60 Å.[58] Occasionally, a gap or communicating junction can be observed between the endothelial cells of the mesenteric postcapillary venules.[37] It

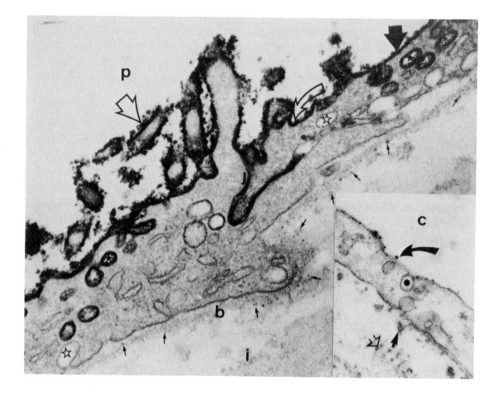

Fig. 1-4 Mesenteric mesothelium of a rat perfused with ruthenium-red. The cationic tracer illuminates the glycocalix of microvilli (short open arrow), as well as that of the luminal aspect of the mesothelial cell (short black arrow). Ruthenium-red can also be seen along a substantial part of the tight junction (j), the coated pits (curved open arrow), and the coated vesicles (black stars). Pinocytotic vesicles (open stars) are devoid of ruthenium-red staining. The submesothelial basement membrane (b) shows periodic anionic fixed charges (small arrows). p, Peritoneal space; i, interstitium. (× 50,720.) (**Inset**) A mesenteric continuous capillary of a mouse. The specimen was obtained 4 hours after intraperitoneal injection of cationized ferritin. Particles of this tracer can be observed on the luminal aspect of the plasmalemma of the endothelial cell (curved black arrow) and in the subendothelial basement membrane (short black arrow) and interstitial tissue (open arrow). c, Capillary lumen; asterisk, coated vesicle. (× 41,500.)

has been suggested that these junctions prevent the passage of molecules with a radius larger than that of peroxidase (MW, 1,900 d; radius, 20 Å).[58]

The actual tightness of the junctions has been one of the most debated topics in microvascular physiology since the formulation of the pore theory, which postulated the existence of small pores (40 to 50 Å radius), permeable to water and small lipid-insoluble solutes; and large pores (120 to 350 Å radius), permeable to molecules of higher molecular weight and size, including proteins.[59,60] The calculated frequency ratio of large to small pores is approximately 1 : 34,000. Based on physiologic studies, the role of the small pores has been attributed to the intercellular junctions. The passage of water and small ions would occur through a tortuous pathway resulting from discontinuities in the fusion line of the limiting endothelial cell plasmalemma.[61] In this context, the permeability of continuous capillaries would be regulated by the surface area available for passive diffusion of small solutes at the interfaces between adjacent endothelial cells.

The idea that open interendothelial cell junctions could be the pathway for transcapillary water and solutes exchange was morphologically substantiated by electron microscopic studies that showed open intercellular junctions in postcapillary venules of rat cremaster injected with histamine and serotonin.[62] In vivo studies showed that histamine induces albumin leakage at the level of postcapillary venules of cat mesentery. It was then suggested that large solutes migrate primarily across the venous end of capillaries and small venules.[63] It should be noted, however, that these studies reproduced an experimental situation of acute inflammation that can hardly be extrapolated to conditions of normal physiology.

Starling and Tubby,[5,6,64] maintained that both the direction and rate of fluid transfer through the capillary wall were proportional to the algebraic sum of the effective hydrostatic pressure in the capillaries and the osmotic pressure of plasma proteins. However, Starling[5,6] recognized that capillary walls were not completely impermeable to plasma proteins, and that the interstitial fluid contained plasma proteins at lower concentrations than plasma. Experimental studies later showed that all fractions of plasma proteins are represented in lymph, although not in the same proportions observed in plasma,[65] and that protein, which normally escapes from the circulating plasma into the intravascular fluid, returns to the blood stream via the lymphatics.[66-68] The fact that more than half of what is usually called plasma protein resides in the interstitial compartment caused a reevaluation of Starling's[5,6] hypothesis by Renkin,[69] which led to the conclusion that microvessels have two large pore systems.[70] The first is the static large pore system, which functions as the dominant macromolecular transport pathway under normal conditions. Its carrying capacity is fixed and, according to Renkin,[71] may be mediated by vesicles or chains of vesicles. The second is the variable large pore system, which is normally quiescent and under direct physiologic regulation and which may eventually be influenced by pharmacologic agents.

The static system can explain the solute fluxes across the normal, intact microvascular membrane under physiologic conditions. The second large pore system is defined by Grega et al.[70] as a mediator-stimulated, energy-dependent, and receptor-activated macromolecular transport pathway that is subject to direct regulation. The development of inflammatory edema is primarily due to the increase in protein efflux from blood microvessels, which virtually eliminates the transmural osmotic pressure gradients.[72] Rapid glucose absorption and reduction of ultrafiltration are observed in peritoneal dialysis patients during episodes of acute peritonitis.[73]

It has been shown that any inflammatory reaction, usually mediated by histamine and other vasoactive peptides, is characterized by a significant increase in capillary permeability to plasma proteins.[74,75] Peritonitis[73,76] and/or intraperitoneal injection of histamine[77] induce accumulation of plasma proteins and leukocytes in the peritoneal cavity. However, anti-inflammatory drugs can reduce the abnormal permeability to proteins without preventing the migration of leukocytes.[78] This fact indicates that exudation of plasma proteins and migration of leukocytes from blood microvessels are two different processes with quite different pathways.[79] We observed open interendothelial junctions in samples of peritoneum taken from patients during an episode of peritonitis.[80] Furthermore, peritoneal microvessels from rats with induced septic peritonitis showed a significant reduction of the endothelial cell glycocalix[81,82] (Fig. 1-3B). This decrease in cell-negative surface charge has been shown to be associated with cell contraction.[83] This could account for the eventual opening of interendothelial cell junctions (Fig. 1-3B), which do not appear open in normal microvessels fixed in their undisturbed state.[84]

The luminal endothelial cell glycocalix extends into the tight junctions,[20] whose wider parts contain a network of fibrous molecules that could modulate the passage of water-soluble substances according to their molecular weight, their net electric charge, and the chemical interactions between the solutes and the side chains of the fibrous network.[30]

Endothelial cells of fenestrated capillaries are pierced by fenestrae (20 to 120 nm in diameter) which on routine transmission electron microscopy, appear to be opened or closed by diaphragms (Fig. 1-2). Fenestrae are not static structures. It has been shown that they can increase during acute inflammation and under the influence of sexual hormones.[14] The use of electron-dense cationic tracers revealed the presence of high concentrations of negative fixed charges on the blood front of fenestral diaphragms in several microvascular beds,[25,26,45] which render fenestrated capillaries less permeable to anionic macromolecules than continuous macromolecules.[25,26,43,85] In this way, recent studies have shown the existence of anionic fixed charges on fenestral diaphragms of peritoneal fenestrated microvessels.[86] (Fig. 1-2, inset). The luminal aspect of the endothelial cells showed an irregular distribution of anionic sites, suggesting the existence of differentiated microdomains representing different transport-related organelles, as observed in other microvascular beds.[25,26] The basement membrane of true capillaries is normally a thin sheet at the interface between the abluminal aspect of the endothelial cell and the connective tissue (Fig. 1-1). In postcapillary venules, it is interposed between the endothelial and perithelial cells. Generally uniform for a given structure, the thickness of the basement membranes vary among the different parts of the body; in capillaries of normal rabbit mesentery, it is 234 ± 95 nm.[37]

The biochemical composition of basement membranes is only partially known. Several proteoglycans, which have been identified in different vascular beds,[24,87,88] furnish basement membranes with most of their strong electronegative charge. Labeling these substances with electron-dense cationic tracers showed their presence as anionic fixed charges regularly distributed along all three layers of basement membranes in several microvascular beds,[87–90] as well as in the microvessels of rat and mouse mesentery, and diaphragmatic and parietal peritoneum (Fig. 1-1, inset, and Fig. 1-5, inset),[21–23] and even along the basement membrane of mouse mesenteric fenestrated capillaries (Fig. 1-2, inset).

Therefore, it can be inferred that the microvascular basement membrane functions as a highly selective barrier for macromolecular anionic proteins. This approach is supported further by experimental studies that revealed a significant increase in the permeability of the glomerular basement membrane by anionic macromolecules after enzymatic degradation of glycosaminoglycans[87,89] and increased peritoneal permeability by protein after neutralization of anionic sites with protamine sulfate.[54,55] The density distribution of anionic fixed charges on the peritoneal microvascular basement membrane is significantly decreased during septic peritonitis (Fig. 1-3B),[91] a condition that, as previously stated, is known to induce enhanced protein losses in peritoneal dialysate effluent.

To summarize the role of blood microvessels in the peritoneal dialysis system, it seems evident that even though relatively simple models of passive diffusion show good accordance with experimental data, the transfer of solutes from the vascular compartment to the interstitial space in normal tissue is a perplexing process. The pore theory was essentially based on theoretical physiologic inferences that lacked a deeper knowledge of the nature of the microvascular membrane. The existence of charged polymers at the endothelial cell surface, in the interendothelial cell junctions, and on the subendothelial basement membrane is expected to induce decreased passage of ions with the same charge; binding to the polymer, and slower diffusion of ions of the opposite sign. Coated pits and coated vesicles, responsible for receptor-mediated endocytosis, represent a type of microdomain morphologically, biochemically, and physiologically different from plasmalemmal vesicles. The main function of the latter is the transfer of albumin and fluid phase pinocytosis. The transcapillary transfer of anionic macromolecules during acute inflammation is a consequence of the opening of specific pathways within the microvascular wall, unrelated to those pathways involved in the exchange of solutes in situations of normal physiology. Agents known to affect cellular metabolic and physiologic processes modify the effectiveness and selectivity of the capillary barrier. This loss of selectivity will eventually transform the microvascular living membrane into an unselective, highly porous membrane, similar to those currently used in clinical plasmapheresis. As stated by Curry,[92] "We are only at the beginning of our understanding of the relation between the metabolic functions of the endothelial cells and the transport processes."

THE INTERSTITIAL SPACE

The submesothelial connective tissue consists of fibroblasts, mast cell macrophages, occasional monocytes, mesothelial cell precursors, and a three-dimensional collagen fiber network embedded in a gel-like matrix. Fibroblasts have an electronegative surface coat that can be stained with the cationic tracer ruthenium-red.[22,23]

Compact bundles of collagen are generally interposed between the blood vessels and the mesothelial layer (Fig. 1-1 and Fig. 1-5, inset). One of the conspicuous components of the amorphous connective substance is hyaluronic acid, which is capable of binding substantial amounts of water. This property can be fully appreciated during peritonitis, when interstitial edema is prominent (Fig. 1-3).[91] Such a substantial increase in the volume of distribution of the interstitial compartment could eventually influence the passage of small uncharged solutes, like glucose. It may be speculated that the significantly accelerated elimination rate of glucose from the peritoneal dialysate that has been observed during peritonitis[73] could result, at least in part, from the challenge of a considerably higher volume of distribution offered by the interstitial compartment. It should also be noted that changes in the length and diameter of the microvessels depend on the interstitial pressure, which is negative in situations of normal physiology and becomes highly positive when edema develops.[93]

Hyaluronic acid and proteoglycans form a gel-like structure with the collagen fibers that is endowed with fixed anionic sites (Fig. 1-3A, and Fig. 1-5, inset).[22,23] This network of polymers acts as a filter and affects the transfer of both solvents and solutes.[94] The resistance to the passage of water through the interstitial tissue is regulated by the distribution and concentration of glycosaminoglycans. Transfer of anionic plasma proteins should be affected by the presence of anionic sites. Experimental data suggest that the interstitial matrix of the rat mesentery is extremely dense and offers a significant resistance to the diffusion of macromolecules.[95] Therefore, it may be speculated that the role of the interstitial matrix in solute transport is considerably more prominent than has been suggested by whole-organ studies.

LYMPHATICS

The first stage of lymph collection occurs through a system of interstitial, nonendothelial channels or low-resistance pathways known as pre-initial lymphatics,[96,97] which have also been found in the cat and rabbit mesentery.[98] This most peripheral part of the lymph vessel system is a completely open net of tissue channels which drain, at least in the cat mesentery, mainly along the paravascular area of the venous microvasculature into a network of 0.5-mm long, irregularly shaped endothelial tubes approximately 20 to 30 μ)m in width[99]; by the time these tubes are completely filled, they can reach a maximal diameter of up to 75 μm.[68] These endothelial tubes, defined as the

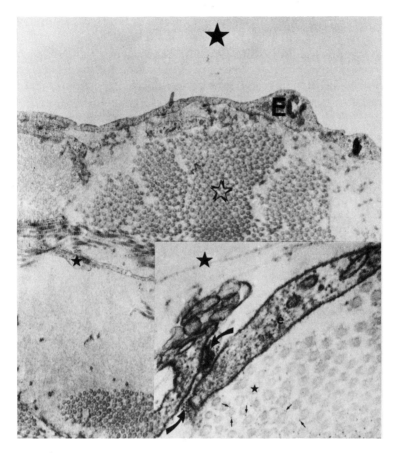

Fig. 1-5. Diaphragmatic lacuna of normal rabbit mesentery. An extremely thin endothelial cell (E) is facing the lacunar lumen (large black star). Notice the absence of subendothelial basement membrane. The interstitial space is occupied by bundles of collagen (open star). The small black star indicates a fibroblast. ($\times$ 22,750.) **(Inset)** A mesenteric lymphatic capillary of a normal mouse. The specimen was obtained 4 hours after intraperitoneal injection of cationized ferritin. The curved arrows show the cationic tracer traversing the open intercellular cleft which allows communication between the subendothelial interstitial space (small arrow) and the lymphatic capillary lumen (large star). The small arrows point out particles of cationized ferritin illuminating the external coating of collagen fibers. Notice the absence of subendothelial basement membrane (e, endothelial cells) and subendothelial anionic fixed charges. Cationized ferritin also decorates the endothelial cell plasmalemma. ($\times$ 87,000.)

initial lymphatics,[68,98] are formed by a single endothelial layer lying on the basement membrane that is only sporadically present.[68]

The total surface area of pre-initial and initial lymphatics seems to be smaller than the total exchange area of blood microvessels.[100] Other studies of the cat and rabbit mesentery showed the additional presence of flat, blind, saccular structures up to 40 μm wide, with a wall made up of a simple layer of thin endothelial cells devoid of basement membrane.[99,100]

Initial lymphatics drain into lympatic capillaries which, at least in the rabbit, occupy approximately 4 percent of the abluminal aspect of the mesenteric mesothelial surface.[37] Lymphatic capillaries are generally wider and more irregular than blood capillaries and show a diameter ranging from 15 to 40 μm.[101] Their luminal aspect is limited by a continuous layer of thin endothelial cells that have an average thickness of approximately 0.3 μm in nonnuclear areas.[35,102] The luminal aspect of lymphatic endothelium shows cationic as well as anionic fixed charges, with clear predominance of the latter[103] (Fig. 1-4, inset).

Nuclei are flattened and elongated, with an irregular outline and a thin peripheral rim of dense chromatin. Pinocytotic vesicles[35,101] and transendothelial channels, similar to those described for blood microvessels, are commonly observed. Coated pits and coated vesicles have also been observed[103] (Fig. 1-4, inset).

In addition, endothelial cells contain an abundant supply of fine actin-like filaments 40 to 60 Å in diameter, usually arranged in bundles parallel to the long axis of the cell. It has been suggested that these filaments represent the contractile element of the lymphatic capillary wall.[102,104]

Several types of interendothelial cell junctions have been described. Approximately 2 percent of the whole junctional system consists of open junctions showing gaps up to 100 nm in width[68] that can sometimes be as wide as 1,000 nm[104] (Fig. 1-4, inset). Ten percent of the junctions are zonula adherens, whereas the rest are tight junctions.[68] It should be mentioned that a small percentage of open junctions (from 1 to 6 percent) can account for a substantial lymphatic permeability.[68] Anionic fixed charges have been observed in junctional infundibuli[103] (Fig. 1-4, inset).

A subendothelial basement membrane may be present, but may show numerous interruptions. However, there are many places in which it vanishes.[68,101,102] Consequently, anionic fixed charges are rarely found along the abluminal aspect of lymphatic capillary endothelial cells[103] (Fig. 1-4, inset). On the other hand, areas devoid of basement membrane show anchoring filaments. These structures reside in the electron-dense layer of the abluminal aspect of the plasmalemma of the endothelial cell and extend into the connective tissue, binding the lymphatic capillary to the adjacent interstitium.[102,104]

The diaphragmatic lymphatic capillary net is organized as a plexus along the submesothelial surface,[105] which drains through an intercommunicating microvascular system into a plexus on the pleural side of the diaphragm.[66] The distribution of the whole diaphragmatic lymphatic network is irregular and varies in different species. In the rabbit, lymphatics are particularly abundant in the central tendinous area,[106] whereas they are essentially confined to the muscular portion in humans.[66] A prominent feature of diaphragmatic lymphatics is the presence of flattened, elongated cisternae approximately 0.3 to 0.6 cm in length, with a long axis that is parallel to the long axis of the muscle fibers[105,107] (Fig. 1-4).

The monolayer endothelial lining of the lymphatic lacunae is thin and shows no tight junctions. Adjacent cells usually overlap, leaving an open basal interface that can be as wide as 12 μm. The cytoplasm of endothelial cells, basement membrane, and anchoring filaments of lymphatic lacunae are similar to those structures described for lymphatic capillaries. While anionic sites have not been observed, the glycocalix of cisternal endothelium becomes heavily decorated by cationized ferritin, which also appears along open intercellular clefts.[108,109]

The century-old controversy concerning the existence of stomata (open intermesothelial communications between the abdominal cavity and the submesothelial diaphragmatic lymphatics, originally described by Von Recklinghausen in 1871[1]) was finally solved by electron microscopic studies that demonstrated both their presence[107,108] and the passage of particles from the abdominal cavity into the subdiaphragmatic lymphatics.[106] These studies also confirm the results of the experiments performed by Allen,[110] who showed the passage of frog erythrocytes through stomata of the mouse diaphragmatic peritoneum and their appearance within submesothelial lymphatics.

Stomata can be found only between mesothelial cells overlying lacunae. In these areas, mesothelial cells are more cuboidal,[107,111] and cover the luminal aspect of the stomata joining adjacent lymphatic endothelial cells. Together, both cell types line the channel that communicates with the abdominal cavity and the lacunar lumen.[107,109] At the sites of the stomata and their channels, mesothelial and endothelial cells contain actin-like filaments.[112] Cationized ferritin has been observed decorating the glycocalix of the mesothelial and lymphatic endothelial cells located along the stomata,[108] as well as the coated pits and coated vesicles of both types of cells.[109] Diaphragmatic lymphatic lacunae, regularly connected by transverse anastomosis[106] and capillaries from the whole peritoneal lymphatic network, including the rich lymphatic omental plexus,[113] drain into a system of precollector, small-caliber lymph vessels that have a poorly developed smooth muscle layer underlying the endothelium. These vessels, which have semilunar valves,[114] drain in turn into the larger collecting vessels, whose diameters range from 40 to 200 μm.[115] The luminal aspect of the endothelial layer shows a sequence of valvular segments approximately 0.5 to 2.0 mm in length, with a semilunar bicuspidal valve at the distal end of each.[66,115] The smooth muscle cell layer underlying the subendothelial basement membrane shows a spiral arrangement around the endothelial tube that becomes more pronounced toward the downstream end of the intervalvular segment.[116] This portion of the lymphatic collector between two consecutive values is called the lymphangion, and defines the anatomic and functional unit of the collecting lymphatic system.[116]

The innervation of lymph vessels was studied in the dog and cat mesentery by means of silver stains.[117] It was shown that large lymphatic collectors have myelinated fibers that remain on the adventitial surface and nonmyelinated nerve fibers that penetrate into the region of the valve attachment and are considered to be the motor supply to the smooth muscle. Bovine mesenteric collecting lymphatics show adrenergic nerve fibers in the media as well as in the adventitia. In human mesenteric lymph collectors, neurotransmitters are both adrenergic[118] and cholinergic, the former being prevalent. Lymphatic capillaries are devoid of innervation.[119]

Since Starling's reports,[5,6] it has been accepted that besides the removal of excess interstitial tissue fluid, the lymphatic system has the special function of absorbing protein. Normally, capillaries leak protein, which will not re-enter the blood vessels unless delivered by the lymphatic system.[120] It is generally accepted that the rate of lymph formation is equal to the net capillary efflux under normal physiologic conditions in order for interstitial fluid volume to remain constant.[121] However, the mechanism(s) involved in the formation of lymph at the level of the most peripheral part of the lymphatic system is still controversial. According to Allen,[122] who formulated the hydraulic theory, lymph formation is the result of hydraulic forces across the initial lymphatics. Assuming that interstitial pressure is negative,[93] any rise will also increase the initial lymphatic flow, and edema will eventually develop when the lymphatic drainage capacity is exceeded.[123] In this context, during formation of edema, the anchoring filaments are supposed to pull the vessels open, thus preventing them from collapsing under the increased interstitial tissue pressure.[104] This theory is also supported by experimental studies that have shown a close correlation between fluid absorption from the peritoneal cavity and intra-abdominal pressures[124] well within the range of values observed in clinical peritoneal dialysis.[125,126] However, part of the absorbed fluid seems to enter the tissue spaces limiting the peritoneal cavity; this fluid will later drain through the local lymphatic network.[127]

The osmotic theory of lymph formation[128] postulates the existence of a protein-concentrating mechanism at the level of the initial lymphatics, the main result of which would be that only 10 to 40 percent of the fluid initially within the lymphatic network would flow downstream, back to the blood compartment, and the remaining fluid would be filtered out from the lymphatic as a protein-free solution. This process would eventually cause protein concentration and osmotic gradients between the contents of the initial lymphatics and the surrounding interstitial fluid.[128] Other investigators have proposed a vesicular theory of lymph formation, which holds that pinocytotic vesicles provide the major route for transendothelial transport of protein, thereby creating the oncotic gradient needed for further fluid flow between adjacent cells or through transendothelial channels.[51,129] This hypothesis is supported by recent studies that have shown active transendothelial transport of albumin.[52,130] On the other hand, it has been suggested that the three mechanisms postulated are not necessarily exclusive, in the sense that some or all could function simultaneously. However, the relative influence of each could vary in different areas of the initial lymphatic network.[131] In this way, the formation of lymph in the diaphragmatic lymphatics is dependent on intra-abdominal pressure and on the presence of stomata.[131] The absorptive mechanism requires the integrity of the diaphragmatic peritoneum,[132] as well as the normal sequence of contraction and relaxation of the diaphragm occurring during the respiratory movements.[133,135] The scarcity of stomatal and lacunar subendothelial basement membrane and absence of subendothelial anionic sites[109] are expected to facilitate the passage of electronegative albumin from the interstitial space into the lacunar lumen. The condition of stomata can be influenced by drugs: carbachol has been shown to substantially decrease the number of patent stomata, whereas succinylcholine had the opposite effect.[136] The amount of fluid and protein absorbed by omental lymphatics is much smaller than that absorbed by the diaphragm.[66,133]

Lymph drained from the interstitium slowly moves downstream through lymphatic capillaries, which do not undergo contractions.[137] The observed velocity of particles (diameter up to 5 μm) in this portion of the system is 1 μm/min.[137] Capillary lymph drains into large (40 to 200 μm diameter) collecting channels and moves against a positive pressure gradient due to peristaltic, rhythmic contractions of consecutive lymphangions[99,115,116,137] with frequencies ranging from 4 to 12 contractions/min.[115,116] Within each lymphangion, hydrostatic pressure increases to a threshold of approximately 12 cm of water, after which the proximal valve is closed and the distal, downstream valve is opened. The cycle is then repeated in the following segment.[115] These contractions are generated by myogenic stimuli (hydrostatic pressure of 5 to 7 cm water),[67,115] and influenced by activation of α-adrenoreceptors,[118] increases in temperature (in the range of 33 to 40°C),[138] changes in calcium concentration,[139] and vasoactive peptides, such as bradykinin,[140,141] serotonin, PGF2a, norepinephrine, histamine, dopamine, acetylcholine, and leukotrienes B_4, C_4, and D_4.[119,140–143] Lymph flows from collectors to the thoracic duct and the right lymph duct and finally drains into the subclavian veins. The role of peritoneal lymphatics during peritoneal dialysis is analyzed in Chapter 2 and elsewhere.[144]

THE MESOTHELIUM

This monolayer of flat, elongated cells represents the fifth resistance encountered by water and solutes in their path between the intravascular compartment and the peritoneal dialysate fluid.[8] The average thickness of normal resting mesothelium ranges from 0.6 to 2 μm,[7,37] whereas the macroscopically measured mesothelial surface area in human adults ranges from 1.72 to 2.08 m².[17,145] These values can be substantially higher, as discussed below.

The mesothelial luminal surface/dialysate interface is formed by the stagnant fluid film of dialysate and the luminal aspect of mesothelial cells. The functional significance of this barrier can be extrapolated, at least in part, from studies in which peritoneal clearances for urea and creatinine were significantly increased by stirring the dialysate through external vibration applied to the abdominal wall.[146] When stained specifically, mesothelial cell plasmalemma shows the typical Robertson's membrane unit observed in all cell membranes.[32] Experimental studies of mice and rats[21,80–82,109] using the electron-dense cationic tracers ruthenium-red (MW, 551 d) and cationized ferritin (MW, 44,5000 d) revealed the existence of anionic fixed charges on the glycocalix of the plasmalemma of mesothelial cells (Fig. 1-5). This coating furnishes the mesothelial cell with an electronegative charge that most likely plays a significant role in the transfer of anionic macromolecules, such as plasma proteins, and charged small molecules; this role is similar to that described for microvascular endothelium. These charges disappear early in the course of experimental septic peritonitis[91] (Fig. 1-3).

The luminal aspect of the plasmalemma of the mesothelial cell has numerous microvilli (Fig. 1-5), the density distribution of which has been reported to be higher in visceral than in parietal peritoneum.[147] It has been speculated that the presence of mesothelial microvilli could increase the actual peritoneal surface area to 40 m^2.[80] The plasmalemma limiting the luminal aspect of microvilli also shows an electronegatively charged glycocalix, similar to that observed in the rest of the luminal cell membrane (Fig. 1-5).

Coated pits and coated vesicles have been observed on the luminal side of the mesothelial cells (Fig. 1-5).[80] Uncoated plasmalemmal vesicles appear at both the basal and the luminal border, as well as in the paranuclear cytoplasm,[2] and occasionally form transcellular channels[37] similar to those described in endothelial cells of blood capillaries.[36]

The physiologic role of vesicles described for endothelial cells of blood and lymphatic capillaries also applies to those observed in mesothelium. Metabolic inhibitors substantially reduce the transendothelial transport of macromolecules.[148,149]

Mesothelial cell boundaries are tortuous, with adjacent cells that often tend to overlap. Tight junctions close the luminal side of the intercellular boundaries (Fig. 1-5).[2,4,150] When studied in the horizontal plane using the freeze-fracture technique, these junctional contact areas were defined as cell extensions and serrated, finger-like processes that overlapped the adjacent cell structure.[151] Desmosomes have also been observed near the cellular luminal front, as have gap or communicating junctions.[152] Completely open intercellular interfaces have not been observed in normal, resting mesothelium.[2,37]

Studies performed on rats and mice perfused with ruthenium-red revealed that intermesothelial cell junctions were stained just at the level of their infundibulum, even though this electron-dense cationic tracer sometimes illuminated the junctional complex, staining approximately 50 percent of its length (Fig. 1-5). Septic peritonitis can induce a substantial decrease in ruthenium-red staining at the level of tight junctions, which have been observed wide open during the transmesothelial paracellular migration of leukocytes.[91] It is tempting to speculate that the protein-rich edema of submesothelial connective tissue could increase several times the interstitial volume of distribution, thereby restricting the free diffusion of small uncharged molecules. On the other hand, the large number of single K$^+$ channels in the mesothelial apical membrane of the frog mesentery and their high rate of conduction suggest an important role for these channels in the transmesothelial passage of K^+ ions.[153] Hence, even though we cannot solve the current controversy regarding transmesothelial and/or paramesothelial transfer, it appears that different solutes may also have different pathways.

The submesothelial basement membrane normally appears as a hyaline, homogeneous, and continuous layer at the abluminal aspect of visceral, parietal, and diaphragmatic mesothelial cells (Fig. 1-5). An exception to this, the functional significance of which is unknown, is the omental mesothelium of mice and humans, which lacks basement membrane.[154] The submesothelial basement membranes of the visceral, parietal, and diaphragmatic peritoneum of rats and mice perfused with ruthenium-red consistently showed anionic fixed charges periodically distributed along the lamina lucida and the lamina reticularis that, at times, formed double rows[80-82] (Fig. 1-5). Heparan sulfate proteoglycans from basement membranes seem to have a core protein different from that present in the glycocalix of the cells.[155] Acute inflammation similar to that which occurs during experimental murine septic peritonitis induces a substantial decrease of these anionic charges, up to absolute disappearance[91] (Fig. 1-3, left).

It has been shown that neutralization of peritoneal anionic sites by intraperitoneal injection of protamine sulfate results in a significant increase in protein concentration in the dialysate, without significant changes in concentration ratios of small uncharged solutes.[54,55] Therefore, the electric charge of solutes should play a role in their passage across the electronegative submesothelial basement membrane. This applies, at least, to macromolecular plasma proteins.

CONCLUSION

Ten years after its conception, the interpretation of the peritoneal dialysis system as described by Nolph[8] is still the only rational framework for analyzing the mechanisms involved in water and solute exchanges occurring during peritoneal dialysis.

Some basic, evolving concepts generate a better understanding and an increasing thirst for knowledge of the inner mechanisms acting at each of the different stages of the system. As previously stated, some areas of the peritoneal microvasculature have fenestrated capillaries furnished with anionic fixed charges that are also present in continuous capillaries, in the submesothelial connective tissue, in the submesothelial basement membrane, and on the luminal surface of the mesothelial cells. Consequently, neutralization of the peritoneal negative charges by cationic substances increases the transperitoneal passage of anionic plasma proteins. On the other hand, experimental studies have shown that endothelial cells can actively transport albumin. The existence of single K^+ channels in the apical membrane of peritoneal cells has been demonstrated. Peritoneal permeability is sensitive to changes in temperature, as well as to various drugs and metabolic inhibitors. Furthermore, the role of peritoneal lymphatics during peritoneal dialysis has only recently been described. All of this information is in marked contrast with the impressive stability of diffusional fluxes across artificial membranes. Hence, a different image, one of the peritoneum as a living dialyzing membrane,[64,156,157] is developing. The location, specificity, and functional characteristics of the multiple water and solutes transperitoneal pathways challenge and stimulate present and future research.

REFERENCES

1. Von Recklinghausen: Das lymph gefassystem. p. 214. Stricker IM (ed): Handbuch der lehre von den Geweben. Englemann, Leipzig, 1871
2. Odor L: Observations of the rat mesothelium with the electron and phase microscopes. Am J Anat 95: 433, 1954
3. Palade GE: Transport in quanta across the endothelium of blood capillaries. Anat Rec 136: 254, 1960 (abstr.)
4. Baradi AF, Hope J: Observations on ultrastructure of rabbit mesothelium. Exp Cell Res 34: 33, 1964
5. Starling, EH: On the absorption of fluid from the connective tissue spaces. J Physiol (London) 19: 312, 1896
6. Starling EH: Physiological factors involved in the causation of dropsy. Lancet 1: 1331, 1896
7. Gosselin RE, Berndt WD: Diffusional transport of solutes through mesentery and peritoneum. J Theor Biol 3: 487, 1962
8. Nolph KD: The peritoneal dialysis system. Contrib Nephrol 17: 44, 1979
9. Ganter G: Ueber die Beseitigung giftiger Stoffe aus dem Blute durch Dialyse. Münch Med Wochschr 70: 1478, 1923
10. Boen ST: Kinetics of peritoneal dialysis. A comparison with the artificial kidney. Medicine 40: 243, 1961
11. Tenckhoff H, Schechter H: A bacteriologically safe peritoneal access device for repeated peritoneal dialysis. Trans Am Soc Artif Internal Organs 14: 181, 1968
12. Popovich RP, Moncrief JW, Decherd JF, et al: Preliminary verification of the low dialysis clearance hypothesis via a novel equilibrium peritoneal dialysis technique. p. 646. In Abstracts of the American Society for Artificial Internal Organs. Vol 5. 1976
13. Oreopoulos DG, Robson M, Izatt S, et al: A simple and safe technique for continuous ambulatory peritoneal dialysis (CAPD). Trans Am Soc Artif Internal Organs 24: 484, 1978
14. Wolff JR: Ultrastructure of the terminal vascular bed as related to function. p. 95. In Kaley G, Altura BM (eds): Microcirculation. Vol. 1. University Park Press, Baltimore, 1977
15. Gotloib L, Shostak A, Bar-Sella P, Eiali V: Fenestrated capillaries in human parietal and rabbit diaphragmatic peritoneum. Nephron 41: 200, 1985
16. Gotloib L, Shostak A, Jaichenko J, Galdi P: Fenestrated capillaries in mice mesenteric peritoneum. Int J Artif Organs (in press)
17. Esperanca MJ, Collins DL: Peritoneal dialysis efficiency in relation to body weight. J Pediatr Surg 1: 162, 1966

18. Gotloib L, Shostak A, Bar-Sella P, Eiali V: Heterogeneous density and ultrastructure of rabbit's peritoneal microvasculature. Int J Artif Organs 7: 123, 1984

19. Luft JH: Fine structure of capillary and endocapillary layer as revealed by ruthenium-red. Fed Proc 25: 1173, 1966

20. Danon D: Blood vessel surface charge analysis by electron microscopy. p. 415. In Hanck G, Irwin JW (eds): Sixth European Conference on Microcirculation. S Karger AG, New York, 1970

21. Gotloib L: Anatomical basis of peritoneal permeabiity. p. 3. In La Greca G, Chiaramonte S, Fabris A, et al (eds): Peritoneal Dialysis. Wichtig, Milano, 1986

22. Gotloib L, Shostak A, Bar-Sella P, Cohen R: Continuous mesothelial injury and regeneration during long term peritoneal dialysis. Peritoneal Dialysis Bull 7: 148, 1987

23. Gotloib L, Bar-Sella P, Jaichenko J, Shostak A: Ruthenium-red stained polyanionic fixed charges in peritoneal microvessels. Nephron 47: 22, 1987

24. Ausprunk DB, Boudreau CL, Nelson DA: Proteoglycans in the microvasculature. II. Histochemical localization in proliferating capillaries of the rabbit cornea. Am J Pathol 103: 367, 1981

25. Simionescu N, Simionescu M, Palade GE: Differentiated microdomains on the luminal surface of capillary endothelium. I. Preferential distribution of anionic sites. J Cell Biol 90: 605, 1981

26. Simionescu M, Simionescu N, Silbert J, Palade G: Differentiated microdomains on the luminal surface of the capillary endothelium. II. Partial characterization of their anionic sites. J Cell Biol 90: 614, 1981

27. Schneeberger EE, Hamelin M: Interactions of serum proteins with lung endothelial glycocalyx: its effect on endothelial permeability. Am J Physiol 247: H206, 1984

28. Ryan US: The endothelial surface and responses to injury. Fed Proc 45: 101, 1986

29. Turner MR, Clough G, Michel CC: The effects of cationized ferritin and native ferritin upon the filtration coefficient of single frog capillaries. Evidence that proteins in the endothelial cell coat influence permeability. Microvasc Res 25: 205, 1983

30. Curry FE, Michel CC: A fiber matrix model of capillary permeability. Microvasc Res 20: 96, 1980

31. Simionescu M, Simionescu N, Santoro F, Palade GE: Differentiated microdomains of the luminal plasmalemma of murine muscle capillaries: segmental variations in young and old animals. J Cell Biol 100: 1396, 1985

32. Robertson JD: Molecular structure of biological membranes. p. 1404. In Lima de Faria A (ed): Handbook of Molecular Cytology. North Holland, Amsterdam, 1969

33. Goldberg DM, Riordan JR: Role of membranes in disease. Clin Physiol Biochem 4: 305, 1986

34. Steinman RM, Mellman IS, Muller WA, Cohn ZA: Endocytosis and the recycling of plasma membrane. J Cell Biol 96: 1, 1983

35. Casley-Smith, JR: The dimensions and numbers of small vesicles in cells, endothelial and mesothelial and the significance of these for endothelial permeability. J Microsc 90: 251, 1969

36. Simionescu M, Simionescu N, Palade GE: Structural basis of permeability in

sequential segments of the microvasculature. II. Pathways followed by micro-peroxidase across the endothelium. Microvasc Res 15: 17, 1978

37. Gotloib L, Digenis GE, Rabinovich S, et al: Ultrastructure of normal rabbit mesentery. Nephron 34: 248, 1983

38. Williams SK, Mathews MA, Wagner RC: Metabolic studies on the micropinocytotic process in endothelial cells. Microvasc Res 18: 175, 1979

39. Palade GE: Fine structure of blood capillaries. J Appl Physiol 24: 1424, 1953 (abstr.)

40. Majno G: Ultrastructure of the vascular membrane. p. 2293. In Handbook of Physiology. Section II. Circulation. American Physiology Society, Washington, 1965

41. Karnovsky MJ, Shea SM: Transcapillary transport by pinocytosis. Microvasc Res 2: 353, 1970

42. Casley-Smith JR, Chin JC: The passage of cytoplasmic vesicles across endothelial and mesothelial cells. J Microsc 93: 167, 1971.

43. Simionescu N: Cellular aspects of transcapillary exchange. Physiol Rev 63: 1536, 1983

44. Frokjaer-Jensen J: The plasmalemmal vesicular system in capillary endothelium. Prog Appl Microcirc 1: 17, 1983

45. Lewis WH: Pinocytosis. Bull John's Hopkins Hosp 49: 17, 1931

46. Yokomura E, Sogabe K, Nakatsuka A, Kubo T: The mechanism of phagocytosis. I. Effect of metabolic inhibitors on the phagocytosis of iron colloid particles by ascites macrophages. Acta Med Okayama 21: 93, 1967

47. Goldstein JL, Anderson RGW, Brown MS: Coated pits, coated vesicles and receptor mediated endocytosis. Nature 279: 679, 1979

48. Silverstein SC, Steinman RM, Cohen ZA: Endocytosis. Annu Rev Biochem 46: 669, 1977

49. Pastan I, Willingham MC: The pathway of endocytosis. p. 1. In Pastan I, Willingham MC (eds): Endocytosis. Plenum, New York, 1985

50. Helenius A, Mellman I, Wall D, Hubbard A: Endosomes. Trends Biochem Sci 8: 245, 1983

51. O'Morchoe ChCC, Jones WR III, Jarosz HM, et al: Temperature dependence of protein transport across lymphatic endothelium in vitro. J Cell Biol 98: 629, 1984

52. Shasby DM, Shasby SS: Active transendothelial transport of albumin from interstitium to lumen. Circ Res 57: 903, 1985

53. Antohe F, Heltianu C, Simionescu N: Further evidence for the distribution and nature of histamine receptors of microvascular endothelium. Microcirc Endothelium Lymphatics 3: 163, 1986

54. Shostak A, Hirszel P, Maher JF: Effects of histamine and its receptor antagonists on peritoneal permeability. Kidney Int 34: 786, 1988

55. Shostak A, Galdi P, Jaichenko J, Gotloib L: Protamine sulfate induces enhanced peritoneal permeability to proteins. Presented at the 21st Annual Meeting of the American Society of Nephrology, San Antonio, 1988

56. Farquhar MG, Palade GE: Junctional complexes in various epithelia. J Cell Biol 17: 375, 1963

57. Simionescu M, Simionescu N, Palade GE: Segmental differentiation of cell junctions in the vascular endothelium. The microvasculature. J Cell Biol 67: 863, 1975

58. Palade GE, Simionescu M, Simionescu N: Structural aspects of the permeability of the "microvascular endothelium." Acta Physiol Scand, suppl., 463: 11

59. Pappenheimer JR: Passage of molecules through capillary walls. Physiol Rev 33: 387, 1953

60. Grotte G: Passage of dextran molecules across the blood-lymph barrier. Acta Chir Scand, suppl, 211: 1, 1956

61. Pappenheimer JR, Renkin EM, Borrero LM: Filtration, diffusion and molecular sieving through peripheral capillary membranes. A contribution to the pore theory of capillary permeability. Am J Physiol 167: 13, 1951

62. Majno G, Palade GE, Schoeff GI: Studies on inflammation. II. The site of action of histamine and serotonin along the vascular tree. A topographic study J Biophys Biochem Cytol 11: 607, 1961

63. Nakamura Y, Wayland H: Macromolecular transport in the cat mesentery. Microvasc Res 9: 1, 1975

64. Starling EH, Tubby AH: On absorption from and secretion into the serous cavities. J Physiol (London), 16: 140, 1894

65. Perlman GE, Glenn WWK, Kaufman D: Changes in the electrophoretic pattern in lymph and serum in experimental burns. J Clin Invest 22: 627, 1943

66. Yoffey J, Courtice FC: Lymphatic, Lymph and Lymphoid Tissue. E. Arnold Limited, London, 1956

67. Ohhashi T, Azuma T, Sakaguchi M: Active and passive mechanical characteristics of bovine mesenteric lymphatics. Am J Physiol 239: H88, 1980

68. Casley-Smith JR: Lymph and lymphatics p. 423. In Kaley G, Altura BM (eds): Microcirculation. Vol. 4. University Park Press, Baltimore, 1981

69. Renkin EM: Some consequences of capillary permeability to macromolecules: Starling's hypothesis reconsidered. Am J Physiol 250: H706, 1986

70. Grega, GJ, Adamski SW, Dobbins DE: Physiological and pharmacological evidence for the regulation of permeability. Fed Proc 45: 86, 1986

71. Renkin EM: Multiple ways of capillary permeability. Cir Res 41: 735, 1977

72. Grega GJ, Svensjo E, Haddy FJ: Macromolecular permeability of the microvascular membrane. Physiological and pharmacological regulation. Microcirculation 1: 325, 1981

73. Rubin J, Ray R, Barnes T, Bower J: Peritoneal abnormalities during infectious episodes of continuous ambulatory peritoneal dialysis. Nephron 29: 124, 1981

74. Menkin V: Effects of cortisone on the mechanism of increased capillary permeability to trypan blue in inflammation. Am J Physiol 166: 509, 1951

75. Arfors KE, Rutili G, Svensjo E: Microvascular transport of macromolecules in normal and inflammatory conditions. Acta Physiol Scand, suppl., 463: 93, 1979

76. Berlyne GM, Jones HJ, Hewitt V, Nilwarangkur S: Protein loss in peritoneal dialysis. Lancet 1: 738, 1964

77. Northover BJ: The permeability to plasma proteins of the peritoneal blood vessels of the mouse, and the effect of substances that alter permeability. J Pathol Bacteriol 85: 361, 1963

78. Northover BJ: The effect of various anti-inflammatory drugs on the accumulation of leucocytes in the peritoneal cavity of mice. J Pathol Bacteriol 88: 332, 1964

79. Delaunay A, Pages J: L'inhibition de diapedese par les endotoxines bacteriennes et son mecanisme. Ann Inst Pasteur 71: 431–439, 1945

80. Gotloib L, Shostak A: Ultrastructural morphology of the peritoneum: new findings and speculations on transfer of solutes and water during peritoneal dialysis. Peritoneal Dialysis Bull 7: 119, 1987

81. Gotloib L, Shostak A, Jaichenko J, Galdi P: Decreased density distribution of

mesenteric and diaphragmatic microvascular anionic charges during murine abdominal sepsis. Resuscitation 16: 179, 1988

82. Gotloib L, Shostak A, Jaichenko J: Ruthenium-red stained anionic charges of rat and mice mesothelial cells and basal lamina: the peritoneum is a negatively charged dialyzing membrane. Nephron 1: 65, 1988

83. Majno G, Grilmore V, Leventhal M: On the mechanism of vascular leakage caused by histamine-type mediators. Circ Res 21: 833, 1967

84. Gabbiani G, Majno G: Fine structure of endothelium. p. 133. In Kaley G, Altura BM (eds): Microcirculation. Vol. 1. University Park Press, Baltimore, 1977

85. Charonis AS, Wissig SL: Anionic sites in basement membranes. Differences in their electrostatic properties in continuous and fenestrated capillaries. Microvasc Res 25: 265, 1983

86. Gotloib L, Shostak A, Jaichenko J, et al: Cationized ferritin decorates the anionic fixed charges of mice mesenteric fenestrated capillaries. (submitted for publication)

87. Kanwar YS, Linker A, Farquhar MG: Increased permeability of the glomerular basement membrane to ferritin after removal of glycosaminoglycans (heparan sulfate) by enzyme digestion. J Cell Biol 86: 688, 1980

88. Simionescu M, Simionescu N, Palade GE: Partial chemical characterization of the anionic sites in the basal lamina of fenestrated capillaries. Microvasc Res 28: 352, 1984

89. Chang RLS, Deen WM, Robertson ChR, Brenner BM: Permselectivity of the glomerular capillary wall. IV. Restricted transport of polyanions. Kidney Int 8: 212, 1975

90. Bankston PW, Milici AJ: A survey of the binding of polycationic ferritin in several fenestrated capillary beds: Indication of heterogeneity in the luminal glycocalyx of fenestral diaphragms. Microvasc Res 26: 36, 1983

91. Gotloib L, Shostak A, Jaichenko J: Loss of mesothelial and microvascular fixed anionic charges during murine experimentally induced septic peritonitis. Nephron 51: 77, 1989

92. Curry FE: Determinants of capillary permeability: a review of mechanisms based on single capillary studies in the frog. Circ Res 59: 367, 1986

93. Guyton AC: A concept of negative interstitial pressure based on pressures in implanted perforated capsules. Circ Res 12: 399, 1963.

94. Comper WD, Laurent TC: Physiological function of connective tissue polysaccharides. Physiol Rev 58: 255, 1978

95. Fox JR, Wayland H: Interstitial diffusion of macromolecules in rat mesentery. Microvasc Res 18: 255, 1979

96. Ottaviani G, Azzali G: Ultrastructure of lymphatic vessels in some functional conditions. p. 325. In Comel M, Laszt L (eds): Morphology and Histochemistry of the Vascular Wall. S Karger AG, Basel, 1966

97. Foldi M, Csanda E, Simon M, et al: Lymphagenic haemoangiopathy— prelymphatic pathways in the wall of cerebral and cervical blood vessels. Angiologica 5: 250, 1968

98. Hauck G: The connective tissue space in view of lymphology. Experientia 38: 1121, 1982

99. Crone C: Exchange of molecules between plasma, interstitial tissue and lymphatics. Pflugers Arch, suppl, 336: S65, 1972

100. Wayland H, Silberberg A: Meeting report. Blood to lymph transport. Microvasc Res 15: 367, 1978

101. Leak LV: Electron microscopic observations on lymphatic capillaries and the structural components of the connective tissue-lymph interface. Microvasc Res 2: 361, 1970
102. Leak LV, Burke JF: Fine structure of lymphatic capillaries and the adjoining connective tissue area. Am J Anat 118: 785, 1966
103. Jones WR, O'Morchoe CCC, Jarosz HM, O'Morchoe GJ: Distribution of charged sites on lymphatic endothelium. Lymphology 19: 5, 1986
104. Leak LV, Burke JF: Ultrastructural studies on the lymphatic anchoring filaments. J Cell Biol 36: 129, 1968
105. McCallum WG: On the mechanisms of absorption of granular materials from the peritoneum. Bull Johns Hopkins Hosp 14: 105, 1903
106. French JE, Florey HW, Morris B: The absorption of particles by the lymphatics of the diaphragm. Q J Exp Physiol 45: 88, 1959
107. Tsilibarry EC, Wissig SL: Absorption from the peritoneal cavity. SEM study of the mesothelium covering the peritoneal surface of the muscular portion of the diaphragm. Am J Anat 149: 127, 1977
108. Leak, LV: Polycationic ferritin binding to diaphragmatic mesothelial and lymphatic endothelial cells. J Cell Biol 95: 103, 1982
109. Leak LV: Distribution of cell surface charges on mesothelium and lymphatic endothelium. Microvasc Res 31: 18, 1986
110. Allen L: The peritoneal stomata. Anat Rec 67: 89, 1937
111. Leak LV, Rahil K: Permeability of the diaphragmatic mesothelium: the ultra-structural basis for "stomata." Am J Anat 151: 557, 1978
112. Leak LV: Permeability of peritoneal mesothelium: a TEM and SEM study. J Cell Biol 70: 423, 1976 (abstr.)
113. Simer PH: Omental lymphatics in man. Anat Res 63: 253, 1935
114. Robinson B: The Peritoneum. p. 13. WT Keener, Chicago, 1897
115. Hargens AR, Zweifach BW: Contractile stimuli in collecting lymph vessels. Am J Physiol 233: H57, 1977
116. Horstmann E: Anatomie und physiologie des lymphgefa B systems im bauchraum. p. 1. In Bartelheimer H, Heisig N (eds): Actuelle Gastroentero-logie, Verh. Thieme, Suttgart, 1968
117. Vajda J: Innervation of lymph vessels. Acta Morphol Acad Sci Hung 14: 197, 1966
118. Ohhashi T, Kobayashi S, Tsukahara S, Azuma T: Innervation of bovine mesenteric lymphatics: from the histochemical point of view. Microvasc Res 24: 377, 1982
119. Fruschelli C, Gerli R, Alessandrini C, Sacchi G: Il Controllo Neurohumorale della Contralita dei Vasi Linfatici. p. 2. In Firenze (ed): Atti della Societa Italiana di Anatomica 39 Convegno Nazionale, 19–21 Settembre, 1983. I Sedicicesimo
120. Drinker CK, Field ME: The protein of mammalian lymph and the relation of lymph to tissue fluid. Am J Physiol 97: 32, 1931
121. Hogan RD, Unthank JL: The initial lymphatics as sensors of interstitial volume. Microvasc Res 31: 317, 1986
122. Allen L: Volume and pressure changes in terminal lymphatics. Am J Physiol 123: 1938
123. Guyton AC: Interstitial fluid pressure. Physiol Rev 51: 527, 1971
124. Zink J, Greenway CV: Control of ascites absorption in anesthetized cats: effects of intraperitoneal pressure, protein and furosemide diuresis. Gastroenterology 73: 1119, 1977

125. Gotloib L, Mines M, Garmizo AL, Varka I: Hemodynamic effects of increasing intra-abdominal pressure in peritoneal dialysis. Peritoneal Dialysis Bull 1: 41, 1981
126. Gotloib L, Garmizo AL, Varka I, Mines M: Reduction of vital capacity due to increased intra-abdominal pressure during peritoneal dialysis. Peritoneal Dialysis Bull 1: 63, 1981
127. Flessner MP, Parker RJ, Sieber SM: Peritoneal lymphatic uptake of fibrinogen and erythrocytes in the rat. Am J Physiol 244: H89, 1983
128. Casley-Smith JR: A fine structural study of variations in protein concentration in lacteals during compression and relaxation. Lymphology 12: 59, 1978
129. Dobbins WO, Rollins EL: Intestinal mucosa lymphatic permeability: An electron microscopic study of endothelial vesicles and cell junctions. J Ultrastruct Res 33: 29, 1970
130. Shasby DM, Peterson MW: Effects of albumin concentration on endothelial albumin transport in vitro. Am J Physiol 253: H654, 1987
131. Albertine KH, O'Morchoe CC: Renal lymphatic ultrastructure and translymphatic transport. Microvasc Res 19: 338, 1980
132. Lill SR, Parsons RH, Buhac I: Permeability of the diaphragm and fluid resorption from the peritoneal cavity in the rat. Gastroenterology 76: 997, 1979
133. Higgins GM, Beaver MG, Lemon WS: Phrenic neurectomy and peritoneal absorption. Am J Anat 45: 137, 1930
134. Allen L, Vogt E: A mechanism of lymphatic absorption from serous cavities. Am J Physiol 119: 776, 1937
135. Allen L: On the penetrability of the lymphatics of the diaphragm. Anat Rec 124: 639, 1956
136. Tsilibarry EC, Wissig SL: Lymphatic absorption from the peritoneal cavity: regulation of patency of mesothelial stomata. Microvasc Res 25: 22, 1983
137. Rhodin JA, Lim Sue S: Combined intravital microscopy and electron microscopy of the blind beginnings of the mesentery lymphatic capillaries of the rat mesentery. Acta Physiol Scand suppl., 463: 51, 1979
138. Yasuda A, Ohshima N: In situ observations of spontaneous contractions of the peripheral lymphatic vessels in the rat mesentery: effects of temperature. Experientia 40: 342, 1984
139. McHale NG, Allen JM: The effect of external Ca2+ concentration on the contractility of bovine mesenteric lymphatics. Microvasc Res 26: 182, 1983
140. Johnston MG, Fever C: Supression of lymphatic vessel contractility with inhibitors of arachidonic acid metabolism. J Pharmacol Exp Ther 266: 603, 1983
141. Unthank JL, Hogan RD: The effect of vasoactive agents on the contractions of the initial lymphatics of the bat's wing. Blood Vessels 24: 31, 1987
142. Ohhashi T, Kawai Y, Azuma T: The responses of lymphatic smooth muscles to vasoactive substances. Pflugers Arch 375: 183, 1978
143. Ohhashi T, Azuma T: Variegated effects of prostaglandins on spontaneous activity in bovine mesenteric lymphatics. Microvasc Res 27: 71, 1984
144. Nolph KD, Mactier R, Khanna R, et al: The kinetics of ultrafiltration during peritoneal dialysis: the role of lymphatics. Kidney Int 32: 219, 1987
145. Putiloff PV: Materials for the study of the laws of growth of the human body in relation to the surface areas of different systems: the trial on Russian subjects of planigraphic anatomy as a means of exact anthropometry. Presented at the Siberian branch of the Russian Geographic Society, October 29, 1884. Omsk, 1886

146. Rudoy J, Kohan R, Ben-Ari, J: Externally applied abdominal vibration as a method for improving efficiency in peritoneal dialysis. Nephron 46: 364, 1987
147. Baradi AF, Rao SN: A scanning electron microscope study of mouse peritoneal mesothelium. Tissue Cell, 8: 159, 1976
148. Fedorko ME, Hirsch JG, Fried B: Studies on transport of macromolecules and small particles across mesothelial cells of mouse omentum. II. Kinetic features and metabolic requirements. Exp Cell Res 69: 313, 1971
149. Rasio EA: Metabolic control of permeability in isolated mesentery. Am J Physiol 226: 962, 1974
150. Fukata H: Electron microscopic study on normal rat peritoneal mesothelium and its changes in absorption of particulate iron dextran complex. Acta Pathol Jpn 13: 309, 1963
151. Simionescu M, Simionescu N: Organization of cell junctions in the peritoneal mesothelium. J Cell Biol 74: 98, 1977
152. Whitaker D, Papadimitriou JM, Walters MNI: The mesothelium and its reactions: a review. CRC Crit Rev Toxicol 10: 81, 1982
153. Grygorczyk R, Simon M: Single K^+ channels in the apical membrane of amphibian peritoneum. Biochim Biophys Acta 861: 385, 1986
154. Felix DM, Dalton AJ: A comparison of mesothelial cells and macrophages in mice after the intraperitoneal inoculation of melamine granules. J Biophys Biochem Cytol 2: suppl. 2, 109, 1956
155. Couchman JR: Heterogeneous distribution of a basement membrane heparan sulphate proteoglycan in rat tissues. J Cell Biol 105: 1901, 1987
156. Putnam TJ: The living peritoneum as a dialysing membrane. Am J Physiol 63: 548, 1923
157. Gotloib L, Oreopoulos DG: Transfer across the peritoneum: passive or active? Nephron 29: 201, 1981

2

Kinetics of Ultrafiltration With Glucose and Alternative Osmotic Agents

Robert A. Mactier

INTRODUCTION

Replacement of renal function with peritoneal dialysis serves as an excellent example of applied physiology. Fluid and solute transport during peritoneal dialysis has been assumed to be almost exclusively between the capillaries located within the peritoneal interstitium and the initially hypertonic dialysis solution infused into the peritoneal cavity. Transcapillary transport should therefore favor net removal of water and unwanted solutes in the drained dialysate at the end of each exchange. However, the efficiency of the technique is limited by peritoneal blood flow rates, resistance sites to trans-peritoneal transport (endothelial layer, interstitium, mesothelium, and fluid films), and dialysate flow rates. For these reasons, Nolph et al[1] have com-pared peritoneal dialysis to a relatively low efficiency hemodialysis system. Adequate control of end-stage renal failure is achieved by treating patients for longer periods of time each week (intermittent peritoneal dialysis [IPD]) or continuously (continuous ambulatory peritoneal dialysis [CAPD]).

The substantive increase in the number of patients treated with CAPD during the past decade has promoted renewed interest in the physiology of peritoneal dialysis, especially after long-dwell exchanges. Ultrafiltration in peritoneal dialysis is induced by transperitoneal osmotic pressure, and all of the currently available commercial dialysis solutions are rendered hyper-tonic to plasma by the addition of varying concentrations of glucose. However, glucose has proved to be a less than ideal osmotic agent for CAPD, so other potential substitutes have been evaluated. This chapter aims to review recent developments in the kinetics of ultrafiltration with glucose-based dialysis solutions and to summarize the search for effective and safe alternative osmotic agents.

ULTRAFILTRATION KINETICS WITH GLUCOSE-BASED DIALYSIS SOLUTIONS

Transcapillary Ultrafiltration

During peritoneal dialysis, water flux into the peritoneal cavity is induced by the transmembrane osmotic pressure gradient generated by the infused hypertonic dextrose dialysis solution. Nolph[2] reviewed the indirect evidence indicating that the source of ultrafiltrate is primarily the peritoneal capillar-ies. However, it has not been established whether the glucose concentration gradient is transcapillary, transmesothelial, or both. The transcapillary os-motic gradient is likely to be the most important since the mesothelium is not an effective barrier to glucose absorption from the dialysate and peritoneal ultrafiltration capacity is reduced by hyperglycemia.

The transcapillary ultrafiltration rate (Jw) during the dwell time reflects the prevailing transmembrane osmotic gradient and is equal to the product of peritoneal hydraulic permeability (Lp), effective membrane area (A), and the sum of hydrostatic (ΔP) and osmotic pressure ($\Delta \pi$) gradients, as follows:

(1) $$Jw = Lp.A (\Delta P + \Delta \pi)$$

Consequently, transcapillary ultrafiltration is maximum at time zero and decreases exponentially as the dialysate glucose concentration is dissipated by a combination of dilution by the ultrafiltrate and transperitoneal glucose absorption (Fig. 2-1). As osmotic equilibrium is approached, transcapillary ultrafiltration ceases and peak intraperitoneal volume is observed. The dwell time required for the dialysis solution to reach osmotic equilibrium depends on the osmotic agent load and its absorbance rate.[3] For any given patient, increasing the osmolality and/or volume of the dialysis solution prolongs the dwell time until peak intraperitoneal volume occurs (Fig. 2-1), since more time is required to absorb the higher glucose load (Fig. 2-2). Increasing the osmolality of the dialysis solution also results in higher initial transcapillary ultrafiltration rates and higher maximum intraperitoneal volumes (Fig. 2-1). Accordingly the ultrafiltration volume for any given patient after standardized exchanges correlates linearly with the osmolality of the dialysis solution.[4] After peak ultrafiltration, the rate of net fluid absorption is similar irrespective of the initial osmolality or volume of the dialysis solution. From analysis of each patient's drain volumes after a series of exchanges of different dwell times, Twardowski et al.[5] and Rubin et al.[6]

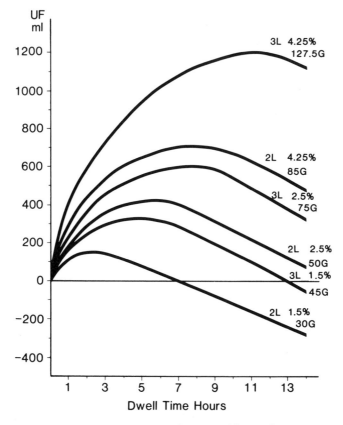

Fig. 2-1. Ultrafiltration profiles during exchanges with varying concentrations and volumes of glucose dialysis solutions. (From Twardowski et al,[3] with permission.)

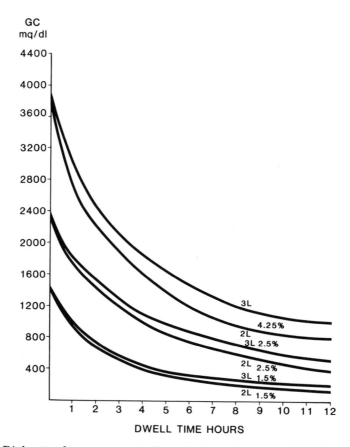

Fig. 2-2. Dialysate glucose concentrations during exchanges with different volumes and initial concentrations of glucose dialysis solutions.

observed that fluid absorption after peak intraperitoneal volume proceeded at an almost linear rate, averaging 40 ml/hr. Thus, long-dwell CAPD exchanges with 1.36 percent (anhydrous) dextrose dialysis solutions frequently result in drain volumes that are lower than infusion volumes.[6] An osmotic agent that has lower absorbance rates and produces more sustained transcapillary ultrafiltration than glucose would be more suited for long-dwell exchanges.

Lymphatic Absorption

Uptake of fluid and solutes from the peritoneal cavity may occur by two mechanisms: (1) absorption by the peritoneal capillaries (transcapillary absorption) or (2) absorption by the peritoneal cavity lymphatics (translymphatic absorption).

Whereas transcapillary fluid movement is determined by the balance of hydrostatic and osmotic transperitoneal pressure gradients, the peritoneal lymphatics continuously absorb intraperitoneal fluid by convective flow, regardless of the tonicity of the dialysis solution.[7] Consequently, fluid absorption via the peritoneal lymphatics is cumulative from the beginning of the dwell time. Lymphatic drainage from the peritoneal cavity is mainly via specialized end lymphatics (stomata) located on the undersurface of the diaphragmatic peritoneum.[8] These stomata were observed by von Recklinghausen as early as 1863. More recently, investigators have delineated the ultrastructure of the stomata and confirmed that intraperitoneal fluid, solutes, particles, and cells enter the underlying lymphatic lacunae by extracellular pathways[9,10] (Fig. 2-3). Absorption into the subdiaphragmatic lymphatics is promoted by the excursions of the diaphragm during respiration.[11] The pathways of lymphatic drainage from the peritoneal cavity to the great veins have been recently summarized.[12] Thus, the physiologic role of the peritoneal lymphatics is to act as a one-way pathway, returning excess intraperitoneal fluid and proteins to the systemic circulation. Under normal conditions, the rate of lymphatic drainage of serous fluid equals its rate of formation, and only a small volume of isosmotic fluid is maintained within the peritoneal cavity. The lymphatic absorption rate is increased, however, if there is an increase in intraperitoneal fluid volume, intraperitoneal hydrostatic pressure, or rate and depth of respiration.[8] These factors should also influence lymphatic flow rates in peritoneal dialysis[12] and in all forms of ascites in which there is no reduction in patency of the subdiaphragmatic lymphatics.[13]

Transperitoneal movement of solutes exhibits transport asymmetry (Fig. 2-4). All solutes are transported from the peritoneal capillaries into the peritoneal cavity at rates related to their molecular weight, charge, and configuration. In contrast, large intraperitoneal solutes with molecular weights greater than 20,000 demonstrate minimal direct uptake into the peritoneal capillaries and are absorbed from the peritoneal cavity almost exclusively by the peritoneal lymphatics.[14] Smaller intraperitoneal solutes may be absorbed into either the peritoneal capillaries or the lymphatics (Fig. 2-3). Moreover, intraperitoneal fluid is drained by the lymphatics without change in the prevailing concentration of index macromolecules.[15] Therefore, rates of lymphatic drainage from the peritoneal cavity have been estimated by assuming that the sole pathway for absorption of intraperitoneal macromolecules is via convective flow into the lymphatics.[16,17]

The absorption rates observed following intraperitoneal infusion of isosmotic plasma or blood in normal animals and humans suggest that the peritoneal cavity lymphatics have considerable drainage capacity.[18–21] Indeed, intraperitoneal blood transfusions have been used to effectively correct anemia in neonates and fetuses.[22,23] Transcapillary fluid fluxes, however, preclude direct estimation of lymphatic flow rates during hypertonic peritoneal dialysis exchanges. Lymphatic absorption in CAPD has been estimated indirectly from the mass transfer rate of index macromolecules from the peritoneal cavity[7,12,24] or from the rate of mass transfer of intraperitoneal

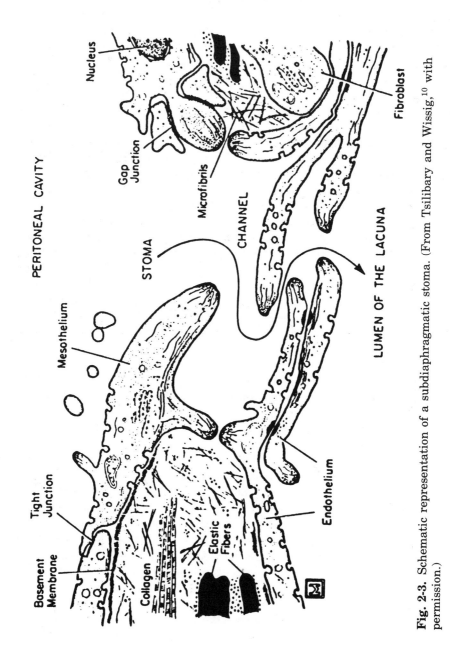

Fig. 2-3. Schematic representation of a subdiaphragmatic stoma. (From Tsilibary and Wissig,[10] with permission.)

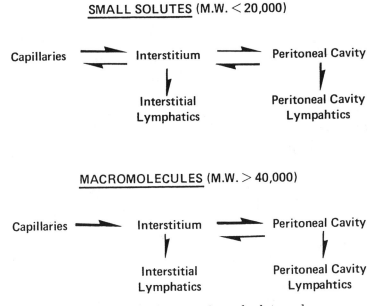

Fig. 2-4. Pathways of transperitoneal solute exchange.

radiolabeled colloids to the blood.[25] Since the intraperitoneal concentration of an index macromolecule is unaltered by the lymphatic absorption of intraperitoneal fluid,[14,15] any decrease in the dialysate colloid concentration during the exchange is the result of net influx of fluid from the peritoneal microcirculation. Consequently, cumulative net transcapillary ultrafiltration during CAPD exchanges may be calculated concurrently from the dilution of the initial dialysate marker macromolecule concentration.[26] Using this approach, Nolph et al.[7] demonstrated that lymphatic drainage during hypertonic peritoneal dialysis exchanges proceeds at an almost constant rate during the dwell time, whereas transcapillary ultrafiltration decreases at an exponential rate from time zero (Fig. 2-5). Peak intraperitoneal volume occurs when the transcapillary ultrafiltration rate has decreased to equal the lymphatic absorption rate (Fig. 2-6). Therefore, maximum ultrafiltration volume is observed before osmolar equilibrium is reached and before transcapillary ultrafiltration ceases (Fig. 2-6). Thereafter, the lymphatic absorption rate exceeds the transcapillary ultrafiltration rate and net fluid absorption begins. Due to solute sieving with transcapillary ultrafiltration,[27] a transperitoneal glucose concentration gradient persists after osmolar equilibrium is first observed and glucose equilibrium does not occur until much later in the dwell time (Fig. 2-6).

Measured Net Ultrafiltration

Assuming that the residual intraperitoneal fluid volume remains constant, the measured net ultrafiltration volume (ΔV) at the end of each exchange equals the dialysate drain volume minus the infusion volume, but

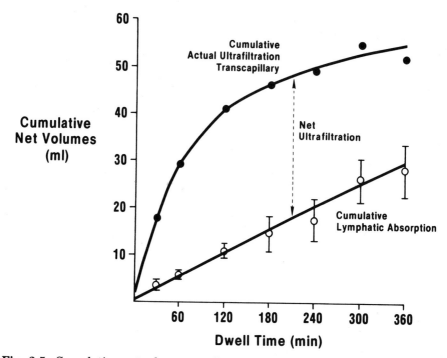

Fig. 2-5. Cumulative actual transcapillary ultrafiltration, lymphatic absorption, and net ultrafiltration during hypertonic dextrose peritoneal dialysis exchanges in rats.

physiologically represents the difference between cumulative net transcapillary ultrafiltration *into* the peritoneal cavity (Jw) and total lymphatic drainage *out of* the peritoneal cavity over the dwell time (J_L) (Fig. 2-7). Thus, incorporating equation 1,

$$(2) \qquad \delta V = Lp.A\ (\Delta P + \Delta\pi) - J_L$$

The terminology net transcapillary ultrafiltration refers to the total net influx of fluid from the peritoneal capillaries into the peritoneal cavity in response to the osmotic pressure of the dialysis solution. This definition recognizes that there may be bidirectional water flux during the exchange, yet indicates that inflow into the peritoneal cavity dominates and that only the *net* fluid transport can be estimated.[26] The resultant net influx of fluid would equal measured net ultrafiltration if it was not for the constant drainage via the peritoneal lymphatics (Fig. 2-7).

Using the aforementioned methods, lymphatic absorption during 4-hour exchanges using 2 L of 2.5 percent dextrose dialysis solution with 30 g of human albumin as marker solute averaged 358 ± 47 ml and reduced cumulative net transcapillary ultrafiltration at the end of the exchanges by 58 ± 7 percent.[26] When extrapolated to four exchanges per day, lymphatic drainage reduced the potential daily net ultrafiltration volume by 83 percent, the

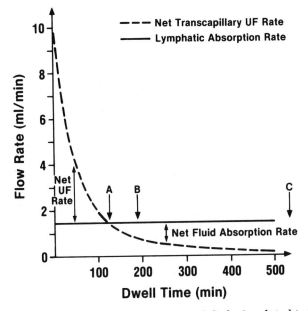

Fig. 2-6. Kinetics of ultrafiltration during peritoneal dialysis related to key events. Arrow A indicates time of peak ultrafiltration; arrow B represents osmolar equilibrium; and arrow C delineates hypothetical glucose equilibrium.

daily drain volume by 19 percent, the daily urea clearance by 17 percent, and the daily creatinine clearance by 16 percent. These estimates of lymphatic drainage may be greater than in active CAPD patients since all of the patients were supine throughout the study exchanges which may have enhanced fluid contact with the subdiaphragmatic lymphatics.[16] Alternatively, due to the increase in intraperitoneal hydrostatic pressure when patients are in the upright position, lymphatic absorption may be expected to increase when patients are ambulatory. Nevertheless, the above findings indicate that cumulative lymphatic absorption significantly reduces net ultrafiltration volumes and solute clearances in CAPD patients. In short-dwell exchanges, net transcapillary ultrafiltration greatly exceeds lymphatic absorption, so the reduction in the dialysate drain volume due to lymphatic drainage is relatively minor. However, by neglecting the translymphatic absorption of water and solutes during the dwell time, the efficiency of the peritoneum as a dialyzing membrane is likely to have been underestimated. The lymphatic absorption of intraperitoneal fluid and solutes also has other potential adverse sequelae on peritoneal dialysis (Table 2-1).

Interpatient Variation in Ultrafiltration Capacity

Peritoneal ultrafiltration capacity in CAPD patients has been assessed by measuring the net ultrafiltration volume (drain volume minus infusion volume) after timed exchanges using 4.25 percent or 2.5 percent dextrose dialysis solution.[28–30] For interpatient and intrapatient comparisons to be valid,

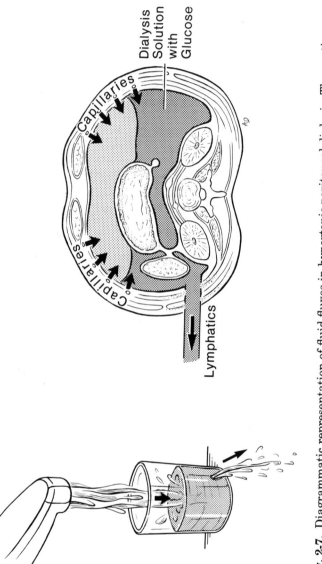

Fig. 2-7. Diagrammatic representation of fluid fluxes in hypertonic peritoneal dialysis. The continuous leakage of fluid from the beaker simulates the role of lymphatic drainage in peritoneal dialysis.

Table 2-1. Adverse Effects of
Lymphatic Absorption in
Peritoneal Dialysis

Loss of ultrafiltration
Reduction in solute clearances
Absorption of all osmotic agents
Absorption of particulate contaminants
  and bacteria
Absorption of index macromolecules
  used in indicator dilution estimates
  of dialysate volume

study exchanges must be standardized. Under such conditions, Nikolakakis et al[28] observed that the coefficient of variation for measured net ultrafiltration volumes after sequential identical exchanges in a patient was less than 5 percent, even without corrections for dialysate residual volumes. However, in similar study exchanges in CAPD populations, measured ultrafiltration volumes showed wide interindividual variation.[29,30] As already discussed, the net ultrafiltration volume at the end of each exchange reflects the balance of net transcapillary ultrafiltration into and lymphatic drainage out of the peritoneal cavity during the dwell time (equation 2). Therefore, either or both of these factors may contribute to the differences in peritoneal ultrafiltration capacity observed among CAPD patients.

From equation 1, it is evident that transcapillary ultrafiltration during exchanges using the same dialysis solution is dependent on differences in peritoneal permeability × area (Lp.A). The transmembrane osmotic pressure ($\Delta\pi$) at each time point during an exchange is equal to the sum of the product of the prevailing osmolar concentration gradient (ΔC) and the peritoneal reflection coefficient (σ) of each solute. That is

$$(3) \qquad \Delta\pi = (\sigma_1 \cdot C_1 + \sigma_2 C_2 + \sigma n \cdot Cn)$$

Consequently, transcapillary ultrafiltration will be reduced in patients with high peritoneal permeability × area because of two interrelated mechanisms: the high diffusive permeability of the peritoneum dissipates the transperitoneal glucose concentration gradient more quickly during the dwell time; and at any given osmolar gradient, the lower peritoneal reflection coefficient for glucose generates less osmotic pressure and, thus, lower water flux.

The relative contributions of transcapillary ultrafiltration and lymphatic absorption to variability in ultrafiltration capacity were assessed in patients with average (mean $\pm$ 1 SD) and high (greater than 1 SD above the mean) transperitoneal glucose transport rates (Fig. 2-8).[26] Measured ultrafiltration volumes and cumulative transcapillary ultrafiltration were significantly lower in the patients with rapid dialysate glucose absorption, whereas lymphatic drainage over the dwell time was similar in both groups (Fig. 2-9). Thus, reduced transcapillary ultrafiltration is the major factor leading to

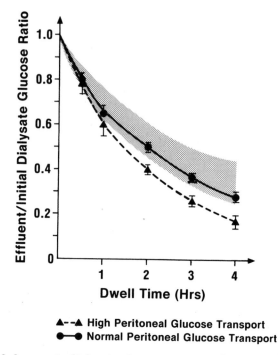

Fig. 2-8. Serial changes in dialysate glucose concentration ratios during exchanges with 2 L of 2.5 percent dextrose dialysis solution in CAPD patients with average and high solute peritoneal transport rates. (From Mactier et al,[26] with permission.)

poor ultrafiltration capacity in patients with high peritoneal permeability × area. After any given dwell time in these patients, lymphatic drainage negates a relatively greater proportion of the transcapillary ultrafiltrate, so peak ultrafiltration is observed earlier in the dwell time (Fig. 2-9). Shorter exchanges, such as daily ambulatory peritoneal dialysis (DAPD) with the peritoneal cavity empty overnight, should therefore be used in patients with rapid dialysate glucose absorption in order to capture maximum ultrafiltration. Otherwise, ultrafiltration failure may supervene if the patient loses residual urine volume or is unable to restrict daily fluid intake.

Intrapatient Variation in Ultrafiltration Capacity

Loss of ultrafiltration capacity over time in CAPD patients has been observed frequently, especially in Europe.[31–33] The reduction in drain volumes usually results from a persistent increase in peritoneal permeability × area and increased dialysate glucose absorption rates (type 1 membrane failure). Even if glucose absorption from the dialysate progressively increases with the duration of peritoneal dialysis, this may not be clinically evident since patients may compensate by using extra hypertonic exchanges.[32]

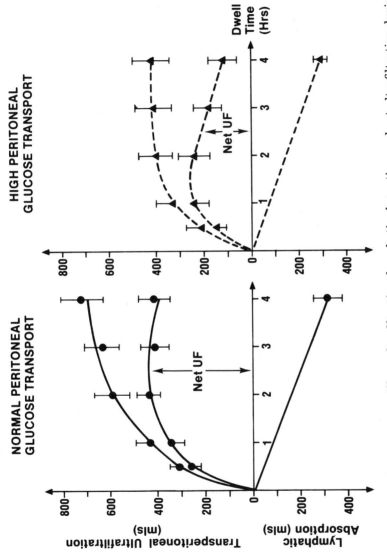

Fig. 2-9. Cumulative transcapillary ultrafiltration, lymphatic absorption, and net ultrafiltration during exchanges using 2 L of 2.5 percent dextrose dialysis solution in CAPD patients with average and high peritoneal solute transport rates.

The pathogenesis of a persistent increase in peritoneal solute transport rates is uncertain. Similar but transient increases in peritoneal permeability × area occur during episodes of peritonitis.[34,35] However, long-term peritoneal ultrafiltration capacity is unrelated to the number of prior episodes of peritonitis.[28,31] Increased peritoneal permeability × area has been associated with loss of the structural integrity of the meosthelial layer[36] and has been attributed to the chronic use of dialysis solutions containing acetate.[31,33] Consequently, commercially available dialysis solutions now only contain lactate as buffer base. The almost continuous exposure of the peritoneum to nonphysiologic, hypertonic dialysis solutions has also been suspected of leading to permanent increases in peritoneal transport rates[37] and has prompted the search for effective, almost isosmolar, osmotic agents.

Poor ultrafiltration capacity may less commonly be associated with low peritoneal solute transport rates (type II membrane failure).[36] The combination of inadequate solute clearances and ultrafiltration may herald the development of sclerosing encapsulating peritonitis or massive intraperitoneal adhesions and usually necessitates discontinuation of CAPD.[38] The encroachment of fibrosis within the peritoneum presumably lowers peritoneal permeability × area and thereby impairs transcapillary ultrafiltration despite the presence of an effective transperitoneal osmotic gradient.

Disadvantages of Glucose as an Osmotic Agent

The requirements for an ideal osmotic agent for peritoneal dialysis are well-established (Table 2-2). To a certain extent, glucose (molecular weight, 180) fulfills all of the first seven criteria. However, as a low molecular weight osmotic agent, glucose exhibits high peritoneal diffusive permeability, is relatively quickly absorbed from the dialysis solution, and is therefore unable to achieve sustained transcapillary ultrafiltration. This factor did not

Table 2-2. Properties of an Ideal
Osmotic Agent

Effective osmotic agent at low concentrations
Easily metabolized
Nonimmunogenic
Inexpensive
Nutritional value if absorbed
Nontoxic (systemically or to the peritoneum)
Ease of manufacture and sterilization
Slowly absorbed
Does not cause metabolic or biochemical derangement
Does not inhibit local host defenses

pose difficulties with short-dwell exchange techniques, such as IPD, but has become important with the routine use of long-dwell exchanges in CAPD. Glucose-based dialysis solutions may also predispose CAPD patients to obesity, hypertriglyceridemia, hyperinsulinemia, and glucose intolerance.[39-41] These unwanted sequelae are related to the absorption of 150 to 300 g of glucose from the dialysate each day, which has been calculated to represent up to one third of the total daily caloric intake of CAPD patients.[40] The ill effects mentioned above are more likely to develop the more frequently hypertonic exchanges are used each day. The high osmolality and low pH of fresh glucose-based dialysis solutions have been shown to compromise phagocytic and bactericidal activity in vitro.[42] However, the impairment of the above local host defense mechanisms is not evident later in the dwell time once the dialysate has reached physiologic pH and its osmolality has decreased. For these reasons, it has been proposed that rapid lavage exchanges should not be performed when CAPD-associated peritonitis occurs. The low initial pH of glucose dialysis solutions is also presumed to be a cause of inflow pain, which is observed in a small proportion of CAPD patients.

The glucose in dialysis solutions is not entirely stable and undergoes spontaneous degradation with aging or heating to intermediate products, which include 5-hydroxymethylfurfural, formic, and levulinic acids.[43] The accumulation of these glucose degradation products with the regular use of almost time-expired, hypertonic, lactate-buffered glucose dialysis solutions has been associated with abdominal pain on infusion and reversible loss of ultrafiltration capacity.[43] These observations emphasize the importance of assessing the long-term, often insidious, effects of dialysis solutions on the integrity of the peritoneum as a dialyzing membrane. Prospective studies are needed to determine whether ultrafiltration capacity decreases with the long-term use of hypertonic glucose dialysis solutions, as is suspected.[37] These disadvantages of glucose-based solutions (Table 2-3) have prompted the search for alternative osmotic agents for CAPD.

Table 2-3. Disadvantages of Glucose as an Osmotic Agent

Short ultrafiltration profile
Glucose intolerance and increased
  insulin requirements
Hyperlipidemia
Obesity
Inflow pain
Impaired phagocytosis
Accumulation of glucose degradation
  products with aging of dialysis
  solution
Disruption of integrity of peritoneum
  as a dialyzing membrane?

KINETICS OF ULTRAFILTRATION WITH ALTERNATIVE OSMOTIC AGENTS

The agents that have been investigated may be divided conveniently into two groups, the alternative low molecular weight osmotic agents and the large molecular weight osmotic agents.

Alternative Low Molecular Weight Osmotic Agents

The alternative low molecular weight osmotic agents have been evaluated because of their potential metabolic advantages rather than their improved ultrafiltration profiles. At any given concentration of a solute (g/L), the number of osmotically active molecules (mOsm/kg) is inversely related to the solute's molecular weight (Fig. 2-10). Thus, when added in the same

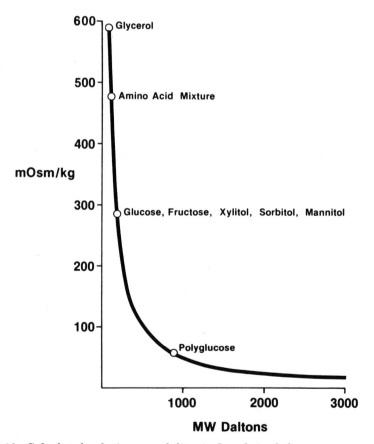

Fig. 2-10. Calculated solution osmolality (mOsm/kg) of the same concentration (5 percent) of solutes of different molecular weight. (From Twardowski et al,[3] with permission.)

concentrations, lower molecular weight solutes have higher osmolality and produce higher initial transcapillary ultrafiltration rates. However, the peritoneal diffusive permeability of an osmotic agent is also determined by its molecular weight. Lower molecular weight osmotic agents are therefore more rapidly absorbed from the dialysate, the transperitoneal osmolar gradient is dissipated more quickly, and the peak ultrafiltration volume is observed earlier in the dwell time. Representative ultrafiltration patterns induced by the same concentration of osmotic agents of different molecular weight are depicted in Figure 2-11.

Fructose and sugar alcohols (such as xylitol and sorbitol) have similar molecular weights to glucose, so generate comparable ultrafiltration kinetics. These agents were considered to be possible substitutes for glucose since they are metabolized in the liver independently of insulin. However, their absorption rate from the dialysis solution exceeded their metabolic rate, resulting in the development of hyperosmolar syndromes,[44-47] and their use as osmotic agents has been abandoned.

Glycerol (molecular weight, 90)-based solutions have also been assessed since they have higher osmolality per unit mass (Fig. 2-10) and higher pH than glucose solutions. Because it did not require insulin for metabolism, it had also been anticipated that glycerol would help achieve good control of glycemia in diabetic CAPD patients.[48] However, because of its lower molecu-

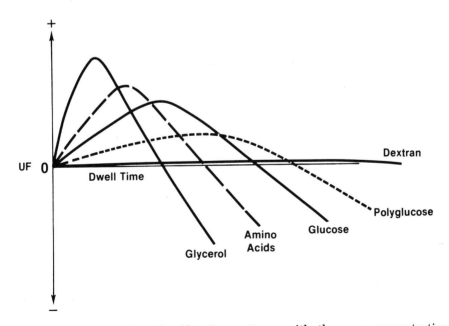

Fig. 2-11. Representative ultrafiltration patterns with the same concentration (5 percent) of osmotic agents of different molecular weight. (From Twardowski et al,[3] with permission.)

lar weight, glycerol is absorbed more rapidly from the dialysate and generates net ultrafiltration of shorter duration (Fig. 2-11).[49-51] During exchanges comparing 0.85 percent glycerol and 1.36 percent glucose, 1.40 percent glycerol and 2.27 percent glucose, and 2.50 percent glycerol and 3.86 percent glucose solutions, net calculated ultrafiltration volumes were similar within the first 2 hours of dwell time but were thereafter higher with the glucose-based solutions.[50] Glycerol solutions also generate lower net ultrafiltration per unit caloric load than glucose-based solutions.[49,51] Despite its shorter duration of effective ultrafiltration, glycerol solutions may be of value in diabetic CAPD patients.[52] Even though glycerol was well-tolerated by diabetic patients and achieved good biochemical control, adequate ultrafiltration, and smooth control of glycemia while requiring less insulin, these potential benefits were offset by the development of high serum glycerol levels, an increase in serum triglycerides, and an increased risk of developing a hyperosmolar syndrome. Glycerol appears to offer no significant advantages as an osmotic agent for most CAPD patients.

Amino acid-containing dialysis solutions were introduced as osmotic agents to try to avoid the obligatory protein and amino acid losses observed with glucose solutions.[53] This rationale was first applied in 1968 by Gjessing,[54] who added amino acids to the dialysis solution to improve the protein intake of peritoneal dialysis patients. Recently, amino acid mixtures (molecular weight ranging from 75 to 214) have been shown to be osmotic agents as effective as glucose; 2 percent and 1 percent amino acid solutions produced similar ultrafiltration volumes to 4.25 percent and 2.5 percent glucose dialysis solutions, respectively.[55,56] Moreover, at the end of 6-hour exchanges, more than 90 percent of the infused amino acids were absorbed from the peritoneal cavity.[55] The use of alternating 1 percent amino acid and glucose solutions over a period of 4 weeks was well-tolerated by patients, produced adequate ultrafiltration, and led to improved nutritional status as indicated by an increase in total body nitrogen and serum transferrin levels.[56] However, the chronic use of amino acid solutions was associated with increasing serum urea levels and worsening acidosis, and current high manufacturing costs may limit the more widespread use of amino acids in CAPD solutions.

High Molecular Weight Osmotic Agents

The high peritoneal diffusive permeability and relatively low reflection coefficient of small solutes restricts their effectiveness as osmotic agents to short-dwell exchanges (Fig. 2-11). This limitation has been countered to a certain extent by the clinical use of CAPD dialysis solutions with high initial glucose concentrations. However, these hypertonic solutions may have several long-term disadvantages (Table 2-3). Sustained transcapillary ultrafiltration during long-dwell exchanges may be better achieved with large molecular weight solutes as osmotic agents. Even though such solutes have the low diffusive permeability and high reflection coefficient required of osmotic agents suitable for long-dwell times, several problems still arise, such as the following:

1. High concentrations are necessary to produce an osmolar gradient with large molecular weight solutes (Fig. 2-10), which may result in high solution viscosity and poor dialysate inflow and outflow rates. The poor ultrafiltration characteristics previously accorded to dextran dialysis solutions[57] may almost certainly be attributed to the insufficient molar concentrations of dextran used in the study solution (1 mmol/L) as well as the short duration of the exchanges.

2. The lower osmolar gradient provided by a dialysis solution containing an uncharged, high molecular weight solute as an osmotic agent will generate relatively poor initial transcapillary ultrafiltration rates and provide inadequate ultrafiltration volumes after short-dwell exchanges. Increased osmotic effectiveness per unit mass of solute has been achieved using synthetic charged polymers, but all of these macromolecules have proved to be toxic and are unsuitable for clinical use.[58] However, despite the lack of a significant initial osmolar gradient, solutions containing large molecular weight solutes can induce slow and sustained fluid flux from the peritoneal capillaries by a mechanism similar to colloid osmosis. For example, a 5 percent glucose polymer solution (average molecular weight, 16,800; osmolality, 302 mOsm/kg) produced higher net ultrafiltration volumes than 1.36 percent glucose solution (initial osmolality, 332 mOsm/kg) after both 6- and 12-hour dwell times.[59] The use of this soluble polymeric form of glucose, isolated from the fractionation of hydrolyzed corn starch, attained a better ultrafiltration profile than glucose in long duration exchanges without exposing the peritoneum to the potential adverse effects of unphysiologic, high osmolality solutions.[37] In addition, at the end of the 6- and 12-hour exchanges, 14 percent and 28 percent of glucose polymer had been absorbed compared with 62 percent and 83 percent of glucose, indicating that glucose polymer provides a much lower obligatory caloric load per unit ultrafiltrate drained after long exchanges.[59]

3. Nevertheless, the observed absorption rates of all macromolecules from the peritoneal cavity are much higher than the rates of diffusive transport predicted from their molecular weight.[60] Indeed, the percentage absorption of intraperitoneal large solutes of different molecular weight is similar (Table 2-4), mainly due to convective flow into the peritoneal lymphatics. The fractional absorption rates of intraperitoneal gelatins of varying sizes were also almost identical[62] and provide further evidence that bulk flow into the lymphatics is virtually the sole pathway for absorption of intraperitoneal solutes with molecular weights greater than 20,000.[17] Thus, drainage via the lymphatics will lead to the systemic accumulation and potential toxicity of all large solute osmotic agents, regardless of their molecular weight. Moreover, increasing the molecular weight of an osmotic agent beyond 20,000 would not reduce its rate of peritoneal absorption significantly, but

Table 2-4. Absorption of Solutes During 6-Hour Peritoneal Dialysis Exchanges

Dialysis Solution	Solute	Molecular Weight	Percentage of Absorption	Source
0.85% Glycerol	Glycerol	90	93 ± 3	Lindholm et al[50]
2% Amino acids	Amino acid	75–214	90	Williams et al[54]
1.36% Glucose	Glucose	180	74 ± 4	Lindholm et al[50]
3.86% Glucose	Glucose	180	70 ± 12	Lindholm et al[50]
5% Glucose polymer	Polyglucose	16,800	14 ± 3	Mistry et al[58]
3.86% Glucose	Hemoglobin	34,000	19 ± 3	De Paepe et al[60]
3.86% Glucose	^{131}I-Albumin	68,000	18 ± 1	De Paepe et al[60]

would greatly increase the solute mass required to generate the same ultra-filtration profile. This consideration may be important when choosing the optimum size of an osmotic agent for long exchanges.

The specific disadvantages of alternative osmotic agents to glucose are summarized in Table 2-5.

Future Osmotic Agents

It is apparent that no single osmotic agent is ideal for both short- and long-duration exchanges. Glucose in varying concentrations continues to be the only osmotic agent used in commercial peritoneal dialysis solutions. Of the alternative low and large molecular weight agents evaluated so far, amino acid and polyglucose solutions appear to have the greatest potential. The initial promise offered by the use of polyglucose during long exchanges may, however, be limited by the accumulation of its poorly metabolized disaccharides in the blood. Albumin would be a good osmotic agent for long duration exchanges since it is relatively slowly absorbed, it generates greater osmotic pressure than predicted from its osmolality because of its negative charges at physiologic pH, and it may decrease or avoid negative nitrogen balance. At present, its use is prohibited by cost and limited availability, but its manufacture by recombinant DNA technology may be possible in the future.

Another approach for the future is to use mixtures of osmotic agents in

Table 2-5. Disadvantages of Alternative Osmotic Agents

Solute	Disadvantages
Glycerol	Short duration of ultrafiltration, hyperosmolality, increased serum glycerol levels
Fructose, sorbitol	Hyperosmolar syndrome
Xylitol	Lactic acidosis, hyperosmolality
Amino acids	Elevated serum urea, acidosis, cost
Polyglucose	Increased serum maltose
Cross-linked gelatins	Immunogenicity, high nitrogen load
Synthetic polymers	Toxicity
Albumin	Expense, limited availability

dialysis solutions to obtain the additional benefits of their metabolic effects and different ultrafiltration profiles. Potential mixtures of osmotic agents that merit evaluation include amino acids combined with either glucose polymer or glycerol. However, none of the present alternatives offer definite advantages over glucose, and the search for safe and effective osmotic agents for long-term CAPD continues.

REFERENCES

1. Nolph KD, Miller F, Rubin J, Popovich R: New directions in peritoneal dialysis concepts and applications. Kidney Int, suppl. 18, pp. S111, 1980
2. Nolph KD: Peritoneal Dialysis. p. 277. In Drukker W, Parsons FM, Maher JF (eds): Replacement of Renal Function by Dialysis. Martinus Nijhoff Publishing, The Hague, 1978
3. Twardowski ZJ, Khanna R, Nolph KD: Osmotic agents and ultrafiltration in peritoneal dialysis. Nephron 42: 93, 1986
4. Krediet RT, Boeschoten EW, Zuyderhoudt FMJ, Arisz L: The relationship between peritoneal glucose absorption and body fluid loss by ultrafiltration during continuous ambulatory peritoneal dialysis. Clin Nephrol 27: 51, 1987
5. Twardowski Z, Ksiazek A, Majdan M, et al: Kinetics of continuous ambulatory peritoneal dialysis (CAPD) with four exchanges per day. Clin Nephrol 15: 119, 1981
6. Rubin J, Nolph KD, Popovich RP, et al: Drainage volumes during continuous ambulatory peritoneal dialysis. J Am Soc Artif Internal Organs 2: 54, 1979
7. Nolph KD, Mactier RA, Khanna R, et al: The kinetics of ultrafiltration in peritoneal dialysis: the role of lymphatics. Kidney Int 32: 219, 1987
8. Courtice FC, Simmonds WJ: Physiological significance of lymph drainage of the serous cavities and lungs. Physiol Rev 31: 419, 1954
9. Casley-Smith JR: Endothelial permeability—the passage of particles into and out of diaphragmatic lymphatics. Q J Exp Physiol 49: 365, 1964
10. Tsilibary EC, Wissig SL: Light and electron microscope observations of the lymphatic drainage units of the peritoneal cavity of rodents. Am J Anat 180: 195, 1987
11. Bettendorf U: Lymph flow mechanism of the subperitoneal diaphragmatic lymphatics. Lymphology 11: 111, 1978
12. Mactier RA, Khanna R, Twardowski ZJ, Nolph KD: Role of peritoneal cavity lymphatic absorption in peritoneal dialysis. Kidney Int 32: 165, 1987
13. Coates G, Bush RS, Aspin N: A study of ascites using lymphoscintigraphy with ^{99}m Tc sulfur colloid. Radiology 107: 577, 1973
14. Flessner MF, Dedrick RL, Schultz RS: Exchange of macromolecules between peritoneal cavity and plasma. Am J Physiol 248: H15, 1985
15. Henriksen JH, Lassen NA, Parving H, Winkler K: Filtration as the main transport mechanism of protein exchange between plasma and the peritoneal cavity in hepatic cirrhosis. Scand J Clin Lab Invest 40: 503, 1980
16. Courtice FC, Steinbeck AW: The effects of lymphatic obstruction and of posture on the absorption of proteins from the peritoneal cavity. Aust J Exp Biol Med Sci 29: 451, 1951
17. Flessner MF, Parker RJ, Sieber SM: Peritoneal lymphatic uptake of fibrinogen and erythrocytes in the rat. Am J Physiol 244: H89, 1983

18. Hedenstedt S: Elliptocyte transfusions as a method in studies on blood destruction, blood volume and peritoneal resorption. Acta Chir Scand 95: suppl 128, 105, 1947
19. Courtice FC, Steinbeck AW: The lymphatic drainage of plasma from the peritoneal cavity of the cat. Aust J Exp Biol Med Sci 28: 161, 1950
20. Courtice FC, Harding J, Steinbeck AW: The removal of free red blood cells from the peritoneal cavity of animals. Aust J Exp Biol Med Sci 31: 215, 1953
21. Raybuck HE, Allen L, Harms WS: Absorption of serum from the peritoneal cavity. Am J Physiol 199: 1021, 1960
22. Scopes JW: Intraperitoneal transfusion of blood in newborn babies. Lancet 1: 1027, 1963
23. Liley AW: Intrauterine transfusion of the fetus in haemolytic disease. Br Med J 2: 1107, 1963
24. Krediet RT, Struijk DG, Boeschoten EW, et al: Autologous haemoglobin for the measurement of intraperitoneal volume and lymphatic absorption in CAPD. Peritoneal Dialysis International. 8: 83, 1988
25. Rippe B, Stelin G, Ahlmen J: Lymph flow from the peritoneal cavity in CAPD patients. p. 24. In Maher JF, Winchester JF (eds): Frontiers in Peritoneal Dialysis. New York, Field, Rich & Associates, 1986
26. Mactier RA, Khanna R, Twardowski ZJ, et al: Contribution of lymphatic absorption to loss of ultrafiltration and solute clearances in continuous ambulatory peritoneal dialysis. J Clin Invest 80: 1311, 1987
27. Nolph KD, Hano JE, Teschan PE: Peritoneal sodium transport during hypertonic peritoneal dialysis: Physiologic mechanisms and clinical implications. Ann Intern Med 70: 931, 1969
28. Nikolakakis N, Rodger RSC, Goodship THJ, et al: The assessment of peritoneal function using a single hypertonic exchange. Peritoneal Dialysis Bull 5: 186, 1985
29. International Co-operative Study: A survey of ultrafiltration in continuous ambulatory peritoneal dialysis. Peritoneal Dialysis Bull 4: 137, 1984
30. Twardowski ZJ, Nolph KD, Khanna R, et al: Peritoneal equilibration test. Peritoneal Dialysis Bull 7: 138, 1987
31. Slingeneyer A, Canaud B, Mion C: Permanent loss of ultrafiltration capacity of the peritoneum in long-term peritoneal dialysis: an epidemiological study. Nephron 33: 133, 1983
32. Wideroe TE, Smeby LC, Mjaaland S, et al: Long-term changes in transperitoneal water transport during continuous ambulatory peritoneal dialysis. Nephron 38: 238, 1984
33. Faller B, Marichal JF: Loss of ultrafiltration in continuous ambulatory peritoneal dialysis: A role for acetate. Peritoneal Dialysis Bull 4: 10, 1984
34. Krediet RT, Zuyderhoudt FMJ, Boeschoten EW, Arisz L: Alterations in peritoneal transport of water and solutes during peritonitis in continuous ambulatory peritoneal dialysis. Eur J Clin Invest 17: 43, 1987
35. Raja RM, Kramer MS, Barber K: Solute transport and ultrafiltration during peritonitis in CAPD patients. J Am Soc Artif Internal Organs 7: 8, 1984
36. Verger C, Larpent L, Dumontet M: Prognostic value of peritoneal equilibration curves in CAPD patients. p. 83. In Maher JF, Winchester JF (eds): Frontiers in Peritoneal Dialysis. Field, Rich & Associates, New York, 1986
37. Ota K, Mineshima M, Watanabe N, Naganuma S: Functional deterioration of the peritoneum: does it occur in the absence of peritonitis? Nephrol Dial Transplant 2: 30, 1987

38. Slingeneyer A, Mion C, Mourad G, et al: Progressive sclerosing peritonitis: a late and severe complication of maintenance peritoneal dialysis. Trans Am Soc Artif Internal Organs 29: 633, 1983

39. Nolph KD, Rosenfeld PS, Powell JT, Danforth E: Peritoneal glucose transport and hyperglycaemia during peritoneal dialysis. Am J Med Sci 259: 272, 1970

40. Grodstein GP, Blumenkrantz MJ, Kopple JD, et al: Glucose absorption during continuous ambulatory peritoneal dialysis. Kidney Int 19: 564, 1981

41. Cattran D: The significance of lipid abnormalities in patients receiving dialysis therapy. Peritoneal Dialysis Bull 3: 29, 1983

42. Duwe AK, Vas SI, Weatherhead JW: Effects of the composition of peritoneal dialysis fluid on chemiluminescence, phagocytosis and bactericidal activity in vitro. Infect Immun 33: 130, 1981

43. Henderson IS, Couper IA, Lumsden A: Potentially irritant glucose metabolites in unused CAPD fluid. p. 261. In Maher JF, Winchester JF (eds): Frontiers in Peritoneal Dialysis. Field, Rich and Associates, New York, 1986

44. Raja RM, Moros JG, Kramer MS, Rosenbaum JL: Hyperosmolal coma complicating peritoneal dialysis with sorbital dialysate. Ann Intern Med 73: 993, 1970

45. Raja RM, Kramer MS, Manchanda R, et al: Peritoneal dialysis with fructose dialysate—prevention of hyperglycaemia and hyperosmolality. Ann Intern Med 79: 511, 1973

46. Vidt DG: Recommendations on choice of peritoneal dialysis solutions. Ann Intern Med 78: 144, 1973

47. Bazzato G, Coli U, Landinis S, et al: Xylitol and low dosage of insulin: new perspectives for diabetic uraemic patients on CAPD. Peritoneal Dialysis Bull 2: 161, 1982

48. Heaton A, Ward MK, Johnston DG, et al: Short term studies on the use of glycerol as an osmotic agent in continuous ambulatory peritoneal dialysis. Clin Sci 67: 121, 1984

49. Daniels FH, Leonard EF, Cortell S: Glucose and glycerol compared as osmotic agents for peritoneal dialysis. Kidney Int 25: 20, 1984

50. Heaton A, Ward MK, Johnston DG, et al: Evaluation of glycerol as an osmotic agent for continuous ambulatory peritoneal dialysis in end-stage renal failure. Clin Sci 70: 23, 1986

51. Lindholm B, Werynski A, Bergstrom J: Kinetics of peritoneal dialysis with glycerol and glucose as osmotic agents. Trans Am Soc Artif Internal Organs 33: 19, 1987

52. Matthys E, Dolkart R, Lameire N: Extended use of a glycerol containing dialysate in the treatment of diabetic CAPD patients. Peritoneal Dialysis Bull 7: 10, 1987

53. Blumenkrantz MJ: Protein and nitrogen metabolism during CAPD: comparison with hemodialysis. p. 192. In: Atkins R, Thomson N, Farrell PC (eds): Peritoneal Dialysis. Edinburgh, Churchill Livingstone, 1981

54. Gjessing J: Addition of amino acids to peritoneal dialysis fluid. Lancet 2: 82, 1968

55. Williams PF, Marliss EB, Anderson GH, et al: Amino acid absorption following intraperitoneal administration in CAPD patients. Peritoneal Dialysis Bull 2: 124, 1982

56. Oren A, Wu G, Anderson GH, et al: Effective use of amino acid dialysate over 4 weeks in CAPD patients. Peritoneal Dialysis Bull 3: 66, 1983

57. Gjessing J: Use of dextran as a dialysing fluid in peritoneal dialysis. Acta Med Scand 185: 237, 1969

58. Twardowski ZJ, Moore HL, McGary TJ, et al: Polymers as osmotic agents for peritoneal dialysis. Peritoneal Dialysis Bull 4: S125, 1984
59. Mistry CD, Gokal R, Mallick NP: Ultrafiltration with an isosmotic solution during long peritoneal dialysis exchanges. Lancet 2: 178, 1987
60. Babb AL, Johansen PJ, Stand MJ, et al: Bidirectional permeability of the human peritoneum to middle molecules. Proc Eur Dialysis Transplant Assoc 10: 247, 1973
61. De Paepe M, Kips J, Belpaire F, Lameire N: Comparison of different volume markers in peritoneal dialysis. p. 279. In Maher JF, Winchester JF (eds): Frontiers in Peritoneal Dialysis. Field, Rich and Associates, New York, 1986
62. Cheek TR, Twardowski ZJ, Moore HL, Nolph KD: Absorption of inulin and high molecular weight gelatin isocyanate solution from the peritoneal cavity of rats. Proceedings of the IVth International Symposium on Peritoneal Dialysis. Plenum, New York (in press)

Pharmacologic Manipulations of Peritoneal Transport

Sunder M. Lal
Karl D. Nolph

INTRODUCTION

Peritoneal dialysis has become an accepted modality of treatment for end stage renal disease.[1,2] The mass transport rates and clearances of solutes depend on various factors, including peritoneal membrane area and permeability, which are determined by effective total pore area and mean pore size, by the blood flow rate, and especially by the dialysate flow rate.[3-6] Due to inherent limitations, such as the peritoneal dialysis solution flow rate and fluid film resistances, small molecular weight solute clearances are lower during peritoneal dialysis than during hemodialysis. Peritoneal solute clearances have been found to be reduced in the presence of significant vascular disease, such as diabetes mellitus and scleroderma.[7]

Previous investigators have attempted to enhance the peritoneal solute transport by increasing the infused dialysate volume, cycle frequency, solution temperature, pH, and/or osmolality or with pharmacologic agents administered orally or systemically.[8–11] Modest increases in creatinine clearance and blood urea nitrogen clearance were observed with an externally applied abdominal vibratory device, presumably by enhanced mixing and decreased fluid film resistance.[12]

The peritoneum is considered to be a composite biologic membrane (endothelium, interstitium, and mesothelium), unlike the synthetic membranes used during hemodialysis. The anatomic details and the proposed physiologic transport mechanisms involved in peritoneal dialysis have been described elsewhere.[13]

MECHANISMS OF SOLUTE (DIFFUSIVE AND CONVECTIVE) TRANSPORT: MASS TRANSFER RATES

The net solute removal of substances not present in the instilled dialysis solution is calculated as the product of drainage volume and the concentration of the solute in the dialysate. The clearance of a solute is calculated as (dialysate ÷ serum concentration) × (drainage volume ÷ cycle time). In continuous ambulatory peritoneal dialysis (CAPD) with longer dwell times (ranging from 4 to 10 hours), the dialysate to plasma solute ratio approaches 1.0 for small molecular weight solutes like urea and creatinine. Hence, the major limiting factor for the smaller solute clearances in CAPD is the dialysate flow rate and not the peritoneal membrane permeability or the surface area. In a given peritoneal dialysis cycle, the instantaneous net mass transfer rates, the osmotic pressure gradient, and the ultrafiltration rates are maximum near the end of instillation. These factors result in peak solute transport due to diffusion and convective processes for a given exchange.[3,4,14] The theoretic instantaneous diffusive clearances near the time the exchange begins are used to study the peritoneal membrane area and permeability characteristics and are termed the mass transfer area coefficients (ml/min). Based on the changing ratios of dialysate to plasma concentrations over time, mathmatic models have been proposed to calculate mass transfer area coefficients.[15–18]

Glucose is used as an osmotic agent in peritoneal dialysis. Increases in the dialysate glucose concentrations, osmolality, and infused volume result in enhanced ultrafiltration rates. These increases in drainage volume are associated with increases in solute clearance due to convection.[19,20] A hypothetical model explaining the mechanism of ultrafiltration in peritoneal dialysis was described by Nolph et al in 1981.[21]

PHARMACOLOGIC MANIPULATION OF PERITONEAL TRANSPORT

Various vasoactive and osmotic agents have been used either orally, intraperitoneally, or intravenously in an attempt to enhance peritoneal solute clearances and to maintain adequate ultrafiltration rates with minimal metabolic abnormalities or side effects. These agents and the role of prostaglandins have been well summarized in detail elsewhere.[13,22]

In this chapter, we summarize the data from recent studies concerning pharmacologic manipulation of peritoneal ultrafiltration rates and solute transport characteristics.

Calcium channel blockers (verapamil, diltiazem), angiotensin-converting enzyme inhibitors (captopril), and dipyridamole modulate capillary blood flow by affecting either vascular tone or platelet adhesion. The effects of these agents and those of cytochalasin D, a phenylalanine-derived fungal metabolite, on peritoneal solute transport in recently published animal experiments are reviewed in this chapter.

Calcium Channel Blockers

Peritoneal dialysis with 1.5 percent Dianeal solution containing calcium channel blockers performed on Sprague-Dawley rats showed increases in urea dialysate to plasma ratios and urea clearances.[23,24] The dialysate protein concentrations either decreased or remained unchanged.

Verapamil in different doses (3, 6, and 12 mg/kg) showed a delayed increase in urea dialysate to plasma ratios (16 to 44 percent) while the dialysate protein concentrations decreased (38 to 56 percent).

With diltiazem (15 and 50 mg/kg)-containing exchanges, the urea dialysate to plasma ratios increased by 25 percent. Increases in urea dialysate to plasma ratios of 52 to 71 percent were noted during the post-diltiazem control exchanges. The dialysate protein concentration did not increase significantly. Calcium channel blockers had no effect on the peritoneal ultrafiltration rates. All these changes, which are summarized in Figures 3-1 and 3-2, were observed in the presence of systemic hypotension and were thought to be secondary to increases in capillary blood flow without alterations in the peritoneal membrane permeability and/or surface area.

Converting Enzyme Inhibitors

The effects of intraperitoneally administered captopril, an angiotensin-converting enzyme inhibitor, on peritoneal solute transport in a rat model were reported by Lal et al.[25] Rats treated with high doses of captopril

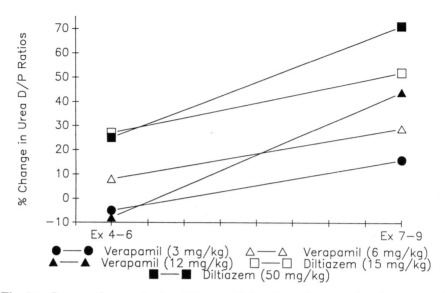

Fig. 3-1. Percent changes (ex 1 − 3) in urea dialysate to plasma ratios of rats treated with different doses of verapamil and diltiazem. (Data from Lal et al.[23,24])

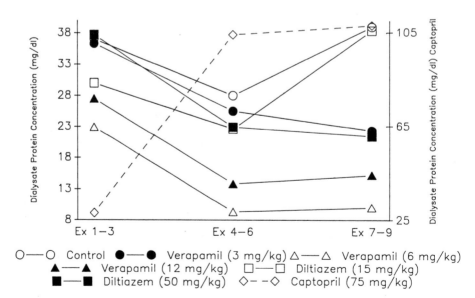

Fig. 3-2. Effect of verapamil, diltiazem, and captopril on the dialysate protein concentration in rat study groups. (Data from Lal et al.[23-25])

(75 mg/exchange; range, 259 to 268 mg/kg) showed a delayed significant increase (30 percent) in urea dialysate to plasma ratios and dialysate protein losses both during and following the drug-containing exchanges (Fig. 3-2). These changes were accompanied by enhanced glucose absorption. The animals were hypotensive. The observed changes in the peritoneal solute transport in association with systemic hypotension were considered to be suggestive of increases in blood flow, capillary permeability, and/or surface area, secondary to modulation of the effect of angiotensin II on the peritoneal vasculature.

Dipyridamole

Using two groups of patients, Reams et al.[26] reported the effects of oral dipyridamole on the peritoneal clearances of urea, creatinine, and inulin and on the ultrafiltration rates. Seven patients received a single oral dose of dipyridamole (75 mg), while 17 patients in a multiple-dose study were randomized to receive either a placebo or 75 mg of dipyridamole three times a day. Neither of the study groups showed an effect of dipyridamole on the peritoneal solute transfer or clearance rates. In contrast, Maher et al.[27] noted increases in peritoneal transport rates in patients with vascular disease; this effect was attributed to the anti-platelet aggregating effect of dipyridamole.

Cytochalasin D

The effects of intraperitoneally administered cytochalasin D on the peritoneal transport of solutes and water fluxes was studied in rabbits.[28] Cytochalasin D is a phenylalanine-derived secondary metabolite of fungi and is known to destabilize the cell junctions at concentrations above 5 μg/ml.[29,30] In a rabbit model, increases in the dosage of cytochalasin D (325 to 475 to 920 μg/kg) were associated with significant increases in both the urea (49 percent) and creatinine (67 percent) clearances (Fig. 3-3) and with a reduction in the ultrafiltration rates. The greater increases in creatinine clearance than in urea clearance were interpreted as an effect on permeability. The decrease in ultrafiltration rate was thought to be a result of enhanced influx of glucose and the dissipation of osmotic gradient. The dialysate protein and glucose concentrations, however, were not reported.

PHARMACOLOGIC MANIPULATION OF ULTRAFILTRATION RATES

Glucose is commonly used as an osmotic agent during peritoneal dialysis. Glucose has some disadvantages, such as the mandatory lower pH during sterilization, which may impair leukocytic/phagocytic responses. After ab-

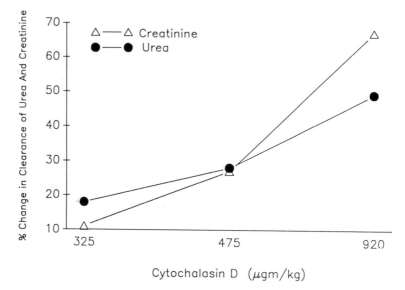

Fig. 3-3. Percent changes in urea and creatinine clearance of rabbits treated with cytochalasin D. (Data from Hirszel et al.[28])

sorption, metabolic abnormalities such as hyperglycemia, hyperinsulinemia, hypertriglyceridemia, and obesity can result.

The effects of various charged and uncharged molecular osmotic agents, including amino acids, albumin, dextran sulfate, polyacrylate, polyethylenimine, gelatin, cross-linked gelatins, glucose, fructose, polyglucose, and neutral dextrans, on the ultrafiltration rates in humans and animals were recently reviewed by Twardowski et al.[31] They concluded that despite its drawbacks, glucose still seems to be the best osmotic agent available for peritoneal dialysis.

Various agents in the human and animal experiments have been found to increase ultrafiltration rates. These agents are hypothesized to influence ultrafiltration rates by osmotic effects (glycerol), by decreasing lymphatic absorption rates (phosphatidylcholine, neostigmine), by decreasing fluid film resistances and surface tension (chlorpromazine, amphotericin-B, phosphatidylcholine), or by modulating the response of peritoneal lymphocytes and macrophages and their secretions with calcium antagonists (verapamil). Recent results with these agents are discussed below.

Osmotic Agents Other Than Glucose

In a rat model, McGary et al.[32] reported the effects of intraperitoneally administered polycation (polyethylenimine) compared with the standard dextrose-containing dialysis solution. Rats treated with the high molecular weight polycation showed significant increases in the phosphate clearance and sustained ultrafiltration rates. However, all rats given polycation died before the completion of the experiments and swollen mesothelial cells with intercellular gaps were seen histologically.

Thirteen diabetic CAPD patients were treated with 1.4 g/dl or 2.5 g/dl glycerol solutions for 2.5 to 42.5 months.[33,34] The increases in hematocrit observed 6 months after treatment were sustained at the 24-month follow-up. Biochemical parameters, including urea, creatinine, liver function tests, and serum cholesterol, were stable and the corrected triglyceride levels were not significantly different in the long-term follow-up. Glycerol-containing dialysate maintained ultrafiltration rates and the protein losses were insignificant. Blood sugar control was satisfactory; these patients required approximately 67 U of intraperitoneal insulin, compared with the 99 U of insulin required while using dextrose as an osmotic agent reported by Grefberg et al.[35] There are disadvantages of using glycerol as an osmotic agent. The plasma osmolalites in patients using 2.5 percent glycerol were higher compared with those using 1.4 percent glycerol and those using conventional dextrose-containing dialysate (324, 312, and 308 mOsm/kg, respectively). Matthys et al.[33,34] described a CAPD patient using 2.5 percent glycerol solution for 42 months who developed a hyperosmolar state and sustained an acute myocardial infarction. This patient also developed hyperglycemia, moderately severe lactic acidosis, and elevated levels of glycerol. For reasons that are not clear, the use of glycerol-containing dialysate solution was associated with an unusually high rate (44 percent) of culture-negative peritonitis.

Calcium Antagonists and Enhancement of Ultrafiltration Rates

The effects of the calcium channel blocker verapamil on peritoneal lymphocyte and macrophage calcium concentrations and their respective secretory products, interferon-Y and interleukin-l, were determined serially in 10 CAPD patients with poor ultrafiltration rates ($\leq$ 300 ml) and in patients with normal ultrafiltration characteristics.[36] Similar in vitro studies were also performed. Patients on CAPD with low ultrafiltration rates were treated with 1.5 mg of verapamil added to 2 L of 2.27 percent dextrose dialysis solution for 6 months. Progressive decreases in the intracellular calcium concentrations were seen within peritoneal lymphocytes and macrophages (Fig. 3-4). Similarly, the levels of their secretory products, interferon-Y and interleukin-l, progressively decreased (Fig. 3-5). Comparable results were observed in in vitro studies. Significant increases in the drainage volume in CAPD patients with low ultrafiltration rates were seen only after a few months of verapamil therapy (Fig. 3-6). The investigators postulate that increases in lymphokine concentrations probably stimulate fibroblastic proliferation, resulting in peritoneal structural and functional alterations with loss of ultrafiltration characteristics. Perhaps verapamil increases ultrafiltration by interfering with these pathophysiologic mechanisms.

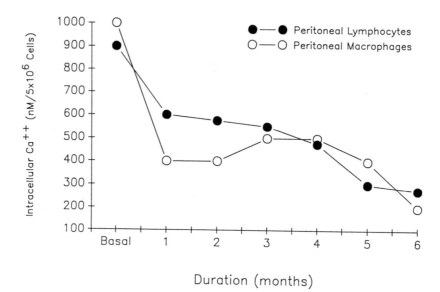

Fig. 3-4. Peritoneal lymphocyte and macrophage intracellular calcium concentrations before and during verapamil therapy in CAPD patients. (Data from Lamperi et al.[36])

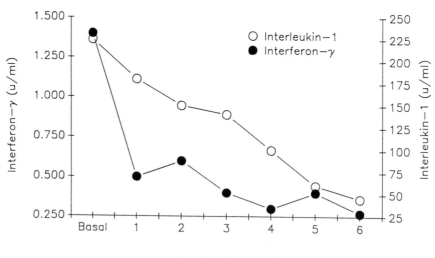

Fig. 3-5. Interferon-Y and interleukin-l levels in the peritoneal effluent before and during verapamil therapy in CAPD patients with low ultrafiltration rates. (Data from Lamperi et al.[36])

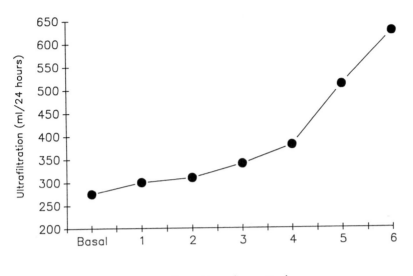

Fig. 3-6. Ultrafiltration rates before and during verapamil therapy in CAPD patients with low ultrafiltration rates. (Data from Lamperi et al.[36])

Drugs Increasing Ultrafiltration Rates by Decreasing the Surface Tension, Increasing Hydraulic Permeability, and/or Decreasing Lymphatic Absorption Rates

In 12 CAPD patients, intraperitoneal chlorpromazine (2 mg/L exchanges) was reported by Indraprasit and Sooksriwongse[37] to significantly increase (more than 50 percent) the ultrafiltration rates (85 ± 23 ml to 138 ± 16 ml/exchange) and the clearances of urea and inulin. The effects on dialysate to plasma ratios of urea, creatinine, or phosphorous were not reported. These increments were not accompanied by any changes in the dialysate osmolality or protein concentration and were postulated to result from changes in the fluid film resistances. These investigators also noticed lowered dialysate surface tension in vitro and hypothesized that the agent diminishes the thickness of the stagnant fluid layers and enhances water transport across the peritoneum.

Maher et al[38] showed that intraperitoneal amphotericin B in rabbits caused modest but insignificant increases in potassium clearances. There were no changes in the urea and phosphate clearances. The osmolality of the intraperitoneal fluid remained unchanged, but ultrafiltration rates increased more than 70 percent. Increases in the amphotericin B dosage did not cause parallel increases in the ultrafiltration rates and solute clearances. These investigators proposed that increases in the ultrafiltration rates, in the absence of increases in the osmotic gradient across the peritoneal membrane, were a result of increases in the ultrafiltration coefficient. These changes were not observed following intravenous administration of amphotericin B,[39] suggesting that the drug acts on the serosal side of the mesothelium or vasculature.

The peritoneal effluent in CAPD patients was reported to contain a phospholipid surface active material, identified on thin layer chromatography as positively charged phosphatidylcholine.[40] Lower levels of phosphatidylcholine were found in the peritoneal effluent of patients who underwent CAPD for a long time or who had lower ultrafiltration rates and/or high peritonitis rates.[41] Intraperitoneal administration of phosphatidylcholine (50 mg/L of dialysis solution) in CAPD patients with low ultrafiltration rates resulted in increases in the ultrafiltration rates (298 versus 937 ml) with concomitant increases in the urea and creatinine clearances (convective transport). Similar increases and sustained ultrafiltration rates were observed following intravenous and prolonged oral therapy with phosphatidylcholine. These changes were observed in the absence of alterations in the dialysate osmolality. The increases in urea and creatinine clearance and enhanced ultrafiltration rates were not seen in CAPD patients with normal ultrafiltration rates. DiPaola et al.[42] postulated that the positively charged choline binds to the negative charges on the mesothelial surface, thereby decreasing the surface tension and thickness of the stagnant fluid films over the mesothelium. These changes result in enhanced water fluxes. Comparable changes were observed in rabbit experiments.[43] In vitro studies performed on isolated rabbit mesentery revealed increased transmembrane fluxes of water, urea, and glucose after the addition of phosphatidylcholine only on the mesothelial side. These responses were blunted by adding a cationic dye (Alcian blue) before the addition of phosphatidylcholine.

In groups of Sprague-Dawley rats, Mactier et al.[44] studied the effects of intraperitoneally administered neostigmine, phosphatidylcholine, aminophylline, hydralazine, indomethacin, furosemide, and vasopressin on the lymphatic flow and net ultrafiltration rates. The addition of intraperitoneal neostigmine to the dialysis solution led to decreases in the lymphatic flow rate (Fig. 3-7), increasing the measured net ultrafiltration rates. The dialysate to plasma ratios for urea, creatinine, and phosphate showed no increases. The authors postulate that acetylcholine or drugs increasing diaphragmatic acetylcholine tissue concentrations decrease the lymphatic flow rates either directly, by decreasing the subdiaphragmatic stomal diameters (the entry ports to diaphragmatic lymphatics), or secondarily, by increasing diaphragmatic tone. No significant changes in the lymphatic flow rates were observed with furosemide, aminophylline, hydralazine, indomethacin, and vasopressin. Mactier et al.[45] performed studies in a rat model to evaluate lymphatic flow rates, net ultrafiltration rates, and the solute transport across the peritoneal membrane during 4-hour peritoneal dialysis exchanges with and without phosphatidylcholine. The net transcapillary ultrafiltration rates (lymphatic absorption and net measured ultrafiltration rates) were reported to be comparable in various groups, but due to a reduction in lymphatic absorption rates, the net measured ultrafiltration rates were in-

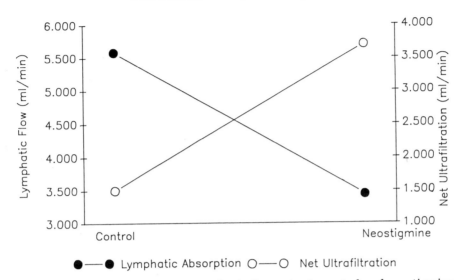

Fig. 3-7. Net ultrafiltration and lymphatic flow rates in control and neostigmine-treated rats. (Data from Mactier et al.[44])

creased only in groups of rats treated with phosphatidylcholine (Fig. 3-8). In rats treated with phosphatidylcholine, India ink particles placed in dialysis solution were seen in neither the diaphragmatic and retrosternal lymphatics nor in the mediastinal and mesenteric lymph nodes. In contrast, groups of rats not treated with phosphatidylcholine showed increased accumulation of

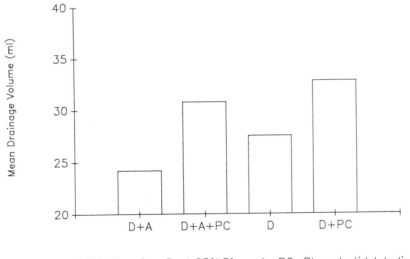

Fig. 3-8. Mean drainage volume in rats treated with hypertonic dextrose solution alone or with albumin and/or phosphatidylcholine. (Data from Mactier et al.[45])

India ink in the lymphatics and the draining mediastinal and mesenteric lymph nodes. These results were interpreted to be suggestive of reduction in lymphatic absorption with phosphatidylcholine and increases in the net measured ultrafiltration rates. These observations are in contrast to DiPalo et al.[42] who noted no increases in the net ultrafiltration rates with oral, intravenous, or intraperitoneally administered phosphatidylcholine in CAPD patients with normal ultrafiltration rates.

ACKNOWLEDGMENT

We wish to thank Joyce Schlemper for outstanding secretarial assistance.

REFERENCES

1. Nolph KD: Continuous ambulatory peritoneal dialysis. Am J Nephrol 1: 1, 1981
2. Oreopoulos DG: Chronic peritoneal dialysis. Clin Nephrol 9: 165, 1978
3. Henderson LW: Peritoneal ultrafiltration dialysis. Enhanced urea transfer using hypertonic dialysis fluid. J Clin Invest 45: 950, 1966
4. Henderson L: Ultrafiltration with peritoneal dialysis. p. 124. In Nolph KD: (ed): Peritoneal Dialysis. Martinus Nijhoff Publishing, The Hague, 1981
5. Popovich RP, Moncrief JW: Kinetic modeling of peritoneal transport. Contrib Nephrol 17: 59, 1977
6. Randerson DH, Farrell PC: Mass transfer properties of the human peritoneum. Am Soc Artif Internal Organs J 3: 140, 1980
7. Nolph KD, Miller L, Husted FC, Hirszel P: Peritoneal clearances in scleroderma and diabetes mellitus: effects of intraperitoneal isoproterenol. Int Urol Nephrol 8: 161, 1976
8. DeSanto NG, Capodicasa G, Capasso G, Giordano C: Development of means to augment peritoneal urea clearances: the synergistic effects of combining high dialysate temperature and high dialysate flow rates with dextrose and nitroprusside. Artif Organs 5: 409, 1981
9. Nolph KD, Ghods AJ, Brown PA, Twardowski ZJ: Effects of intraperitoneal nitroprusside on peritoneal clearances in man with variations of dose, frequency of administration and dwell times. Nephron 24: 114, 1979
10. Robson M, Oreopoulos DG, Izatt S, et al: Influence of exchange volume and dialysate flow rate on solute clearance in peritoneal dialysis. Kidney Int 14: 486, 1978
11. Twardowski ZJ, Nolph KD, Prowant BF, Moore HL: Efficiency of high volume low frequency continuous ambulatory peritoneal dialysis (CAPD). Trans Am Soc Artif Internal Organs 29: 53, 1983
12. Rudoy J, Kohan RE, Ben-Ari J: Externally applied abdominal vibration as a method for improving efficiency in peritoneal dialysis. Nephron 46: 364, 1987
13. Nolph KD: Peritoneal dialysis. p. 1847. In Brenner BM, Rector FC, Jr. (eds): The Kidney. Vol. 2. WB Saunders, Philadelphia, 1986
14. Zelman A, Giser D, Whittam PJ, et al: Augmentation of peritoneal dialysis efficiency with programmed hyper/hypoosmotic dialysate. Trans Am Soc Artif Internal Organs 23: 203, 1977

15. Felt J, Richard C, McCaffrey C, Levy M: Peritoneal clearance of creatinine and insulin during dialysis in dogs: effect of splanchnic vasodilators. Kidney Int 16: 459, 1979

16. Lanciault G, Jacobson ED: The gastrointestinal circulation. Gastroenterology 71: 851, 1976

17. Messina EJ, Weiner R, Kaley G: Prostaglandins and local circulatory control. Fed Proc 35: 2367, 1976

18. Steinhauer HB, Gunter B, Schollmeyer P: Enhanced peritoneal generation of vasoactive prostaglandins during peritonitis in patients undergoing CAPD. p. 604. In Maher JF, Winchester JF (eds): Frontiers in Peritoneal Dialysis. Field, Rich & Associates, New York, 1986

19. Daugirdas JT, Ing TS, Gandhi VC, et al: Kinetics of peritoneal fluid absorption in patients with chronic renal failure. J Lab Clin Med 95: 351, 1980

20. Rubin J, Nolph KD, Popovich RP, et al: Drainage volumes during CAPD. Am Soc Artif Int Organs J 2: 54, 1979

21. Nolph KD, Miller FN, Pyle WK, et al: An hypothesis to explain the ultrafiltration characteristics of peritoneal dialysis. Editorial review. Kidney Int 20: 543, 1981

22. Maher JF, Hirszel P: Pharmacologic manipulation of Peritoneal Transport. p. 267. In Nolph KD (ed): Peritoneal Dialysis. Martinus Nijhoff Publishing, Boston, 1985

23. Lal SM, Nolph KD, Moore HL, Khanna R: Effects of calcium channel blockers (Verapamil, Diltiazem) on peritoneal transport. Trans Am Soc Artif Internal Organs 32: 564, 1986

24. Lal SM, Nolph KD, Moore HS, Khanna R: Calcium channel blockers enhance urea transport without increasing protein loss. Clin Res 34: 40A, 1986

25. Lal SM, Moore HL, Nolph KD: Effects of intraperitoneal captopril on peritoneal transport in rats. Peritoneal Dialysis Bull 7: 80, 1987

26. Reams GP, Young M, Sorkin M, et al: Effects of dipyridamole on peritoneal clearances. Uremia Invest 9: 27, 1985–86

27. Maher JF, Hirszel P, Galen MA: Enhanced transport with dipyridamole. Trans Am Soc Artif Internal Organs 23: 219, 1977

28. Hirszel P, Dodge K, Maher JF: Acceleration of peritoneal solute transport by cytochalasin D. Uremia Invest 8(2): 85, 1984–85

29. Miyaki Y, Kim J, Okada Y: Effect of cytochalasin D on fusion of cells by HVJ (Sendai virus). Exp Cell Res 116: 167, 1978

30. Schliwa M: Action of cytochalasin D on cytoskeletal networks. J Cell Biol 92: 79, 1982

31. Twardowski ZJ, Khanna R, Nolph KD: Osmotic agents and ultrafiltration in peritoneal dialysis. Nephron 42: 93, 1986

32. McGary TJ, Nolph KD, Moore HL, Kartinos NJ: Polycation as an alternative osmotic agent and phosphate binder in peritoneal dialysis. Uremia Invest 8: 79, 1984–85

33. Matthys E, Dolkart R, Lameire N: Extended use of a glycerol containing dialysate in diabetic CAPD patients. Peritoneal Dialysis Bull 7: 10, 1987

34. Matthys E, Dolkart R, Lameire N: Potential hazards of glycerol dialysate in diabetic CAPD patients. Peritoneal Dialysis Bull 7: 16, 1987

35. Grefberg N, Danielson BG, Nilsson P: Continuous ambulatory peritoneal dialysis in the treatment of end stage diabetic nephropathy. Acta Med Scand 215: 427, 1984

36. Lamperi S, Carozzi S, Nasini MG: Calcium antagonists improve ultrafiltration in patients on continuous ambulatory peritoneal dialysis. Trans Am Soc Artif Internal Organs 33: 657, 1987
37. Indraprasit S, Sooksriwonge C: Effect of chlorpromazine on peritoneal clearances. Nephron 40: 341, 1985
38. Maher JF, Hirszel P, Bennett RR, Chakrabarti E: Amphotericin B selectively increases peritoneal ultrafiltration. Am J Kidney Dis 4: 285, 1984
39. Maher JF, Hirszel P, Bennett RR, Chakrabarti E: Augmentation of peritoneal hydraulic permeability by amphotericin B: locus of action. Peritoneal Dialysis Bull 4: 229, 1984
40. Grahame GR, Torchia MG, Dankevich KA, Ferguson IA: Surface active material in peritoneal effluent of CAPD patients. Peritoneal Dialysis Bull 5: 109, 1985
41. DiPaolo N, Buoncristiani U, Gaggiotti E, et al: Improvement of impaired ultrafiltration after addition of phosphatidylcholine in patients on CAPD. Peritoneal Dialysis Bull 6: 45, 1986
42. DiPaolo N, Buoncristiani U, Capotondo L, et al: Phosphatidylcholine and peritoneal transport during peritoneal dialysis. Nephron 44: 365, 1986
43. Breborowicz A, Sombolos K, Rodela H, et al: Mechanism of phosphatidylcholine action during peritoneal dialysis. Peritoneal Dialysis Bull 7: 6, 1987
44. Mactier RA, Khanna R, Moore H, et al: Reduction of lymphatic absorption from the peritoneal cavity with intraperitoneal neostigmine, phosphatidylcholine and other drugs. p. 41. In La Greca G, Chiaramonte S, Fabris A, et al (eds): Peritoneal Dialysis. Wichtig Editorie, Milan, 1988
45. Mactier RA, Khanna R, Twardowski ZJ, et al: Influence of phosphatidylcholine on lymphatic absorption during peritoneal dialysis in the rat. Peritoneal Dialysis Int 8: 179, 1988

4

Dialysis Adequacy and New Cycler Techniques

Zbylut J. Twardowski

(Continues)

EARLY PERITONEAL DIALYSIS
Techniques

In the 1920s and 1930s, two techniques of peritoneal dialysis were developed: continuous flow and intermittent flow. In *continuous flow* peritoneal dialysis, dialysis solution is infused through a trocar or tubing into the upper abdomen and drained simultaneously through another trocar or tubing introduced into the lower abdomen. Some amount of fluid, retained in the peritoneal cavity during dialysis (sump volume), is drained at the end of the session.[1-4] In *intermittent flow* peritoneal dialysis, only a single trocar or rubber catheter is used. Fluid is infused into the peritoneal cavity, equilibrated for a short time, and drained as completely as possible through the same trocar or catheter.[5-7] Both techniques were constantly developing, and 101 cases were reported in the literature from 1923 to 1948.[8] Seventy-three patients were treated with the continuous technique and 22 were treated with the intermittent technique. Thirty-two of 63 patients with reversible renal diseases recovered; the results in chronic renal failure were uniformly unfavorable. The continuous flow technique was frequently used up to the late 1950s,[9,10] but became gradually less popular due to technical difficulties. Catheter holes were frequently occluded by the bowel and/or omentum due to the suction, patients suffered pain with rapid inflows, and fluid channeling between the catheters frequently decreased efficiency. During the same period, the intermittent technique was markedly improved.[11,12] In the 1960s, the continuous flow technique was mostly abandoned, and the intermittent flow technique was commonly used for treatment of acute renal failure.[13,14]

Regimens

The intermittent peritoneal dialysis (IPD) regimen for chronic renal failure was introduced in the early 1960s[15] and gained popularity after two crucial improvements made by Tenckhoff and colleagues: a safe and permanent chronic peritoneal access[16] and an automated sterilization and delivery system of dialysis solution that allowed therapy at home.[17] The method, however, could not compete successfully with hemodialysis because of low efficiency, resulting in inadequate dialysis and a shorter technique survival than other forms of renal replacement therapy. All efforts to increase the efficiency of dialysis to shorten the time of dialysis proved unsuccessful, and peritoneal dialysis for chronic renal failure began to decline in the early 1970s.

A revival of peritoneal dialysis resulted from the concept of portable/wearable equilibrium peritoneal dialysis, using several long-dwell exchanges each day.[18] Initial clinical studies confirmed that adequate steady-state control of azotemia, hyperkalemia, acidosis, and sodium and water balance could be achieved in patients with end-stage renal failure using five 2-L volume exchanges per day, and the technique was renamed continuous ambulatory peritoneal dialysis (CAPD).[19,20] The concept and practice of CAPD are contrary to the objectives of IPD over the years: delivery of large amounts of fluid intraperitoneally to increase efficiency, and sophisticated automation. CAPD uses a manual method of fluid delivery and drainage and overcomes the inefficiency of IPD by a continuous dialysis regimen in the sense that the dialysis is performed around the clock every day whether the patient is ambulatory or asleep. Instead of the patient being confined to bed three to four times weekly with large amounts of fluid delivered into and drained from the peritoneal cavity, the CAPD patient infuses dialysis solution into the peritoneal cavity and returns to daily activities for several hours until the fluid becomes equilibrated with plasma; the fluid is then drained and replaced by fresh solution. During the past decade, CAPD has become the most common form of home dialysis.

TERMINOLOGY

Confusing peritoneal dialysis terminology developed throughout the years, particularly in relation to the terms continuous and intermittent which have been used to describe regimens and techniques.[21] The term regimen refers to the overall systematic plan of dialysis. The term technique refers to the peritoneal dialysis procedure by which a regimen is accomplished, particularly to the method of dialysis solution flow during a single dialysis session.

In intermittent flow peritoneal dialysis, three distinctive periods occur during a fluid exchange: inflow, dwell, and outflow. After the outflow, before the next inflow and during the dwell, the flow of fluid is interrupted, hence the term "intermittent." In the early 1960s, when Boen et al[15] introduced peritoneal dialysis for the treatment of chronic renal failure, the dialysis sessions were performed periodically (several times per week); consequently, the term "periodic peritoneal dialysis" was applied to this regimen. Single dialysis sessions were performed with the intermittent flow technique and the term "intermittent" gradually became synonymous with "periodic" and the latter term was abandoned.

In continuous flow peritoneal dialysis, dialysis solution flows continuously between two single lumen peritoneal catheters or between two lumens of the double lumen catheter during a single dialysis session, hence the term "continuous." In the late 1970s, after the introduction of CAPD, the term continuous was applied to the regimen and meant that the dialysis was performed around the clock with only brief, insignificant interruptions for infrequent exchanges. In fact, CAPD is performed with the intermittent flow technique.

In this chapter, when describing regimens performed periodically, the term intermittent peritoneal dialysis will be used. However, when describing techniques, the term intermittent flow peritoneal dialysis will be used in its original meaning.

ADEQUACY OF DIALYSIS

The ultimate goal of peritoneal dialysis is to achieve adequate dialysis. But what does it mean to provide adequate dialysis? A vast literature on the adequacy of hemodialysis is a peculiar combination of clinical opinions and scientific objectivity. The term is frequently used as two meanings: a dialysis prescription providing the best possible patient condition, and the condition of a patient achieved with a particular prescription. This latter meaning may be called a criterion of dialysis adequacy.

Criteria of Dialysis Adequacy

Hemodialysis

During the early years of chronic hemodialysis, a definition of adequate dialysis was based on clinical grounds, particularly on the absence of symptoms and signs of uremia.[22] In the early 1970s the definition was based on a mixture of clinical symptoms and laboratory data.[23,24] The National Institutes of Health-sponsored National Cooperative Dialysis Study (NCDS) used the overall morbidity and mortality rates as decisive objective criteria for the relative values of different dialysis prescriptions.[25]

Peritoneal Dialysis

The criteria of peritoneal dialysis adequacy are based mainly on clinical grounds (Table 4-1). The adequately dialyzed patient feels well, maintains a hematocrit level above 25 percent (without anabolic steroids or erythropoietin), has stable or increasing nerve conduction velocity (if not diabetic), and exhibits a well-controlled blood pressure. Manifestations of inadequate dialysis may be subtle and often develop insidiously. Most commonly, inadequate dialysis results in such symptoms as insomnia, weakness, dysgeusia, nausea, and anorexia leading to poor nutrition with wasting and loss of lean body weight. Blood urea nitrogen (BUN) may be low because of poor protein

Table 4-1. Basic Criteria of Dialysis Adequacy

Clinical
    The patient feels well and has well-controlled blood pressure and stable lean body mass.
    Absence of even subtle uremic symptoms: anorexia, astheny, nausea, emesis, dysgeusia, insomnia.

Laboratory
    Hematocrit > 25% (without erythropoietin and/or anabolic steroids).
    Stable nerve conduction velocity.

Chemistries
    Normal electrolytes.
    Serum creatinine < 20 mg/dl (in muscular persons).
    Serum creatinine < 15 mg/dl (in nonmuscular persons).

intake, but the creatinine level is usually high. There is no particular creatinine level at which all patients develop symptoms of underdialysis. According to my personal experience, serum creatinine levels above 20 mg/dl are associated with subtle underdialysis symptoms in the majority of peritoneal dialysis patients; however, serum creatinine levels above 15 mg/dl may be associated with inadequate dialysis, especially in nonmuscular persons.[26]

Prescription Providing Adequate Treatment

The degree of residual renal function, metabolic rate, and dialysis efficiency are the three major determinants of the dialysis prescription for adequate dialysis. The metabolite generation rate varies with dietary protein intake, body weight, and catabolic rate, while residual renal functions decrease with the duration of dialysis. In most dialyzed patients, residual renal function gradually deteriorates with time. Renal function decline rates vary among patients, but after 2 to 5 years of dialysis the urine output becomes negligible in almost every patient.[27-30] In hemodialysis, the efficiency of dialysis depends on blood and dialysis solution flow rates as well as the kind of dialyzer, and may be relatively easily manipulated. Peritoneal transport kinetics depend mainly on peritoneal membrane resistance, vary widely among patients, and are difficult to manipulate.[31-37] In some patients a dialysate to plasma equilibrium, even for urea, is not attained during long-dwell exchanges.[38]

Hemodialysis

The first quantitative approach to dialysis prescription for an adequate dose of hemodialysis was the dialysis index based on square meter-hour hypothesis. Assuming that middle molecules are the most important uremic toxins, Babb et al.[39] proposed that the combined clearances (dialysis and renal) of these molecules should exceed 3.0 ml/min (4.32 L/d or 30.24 L/wk) as a minimum adequate clearance. Urea kinetic modeling gradually came to the fore and replaced the dialysis index for providing a basic reference parameter to measure the individualized dose of dialysis.[40] In an analysis of the NCDS data, Gotch and Sargent[41] came to the conclusion that net normalized urea clearance, termed Kt/V, of more than 1.0 per dialysis (3.0 per week) provides adequate dialysis. Others postulated that a urea fractional index of 2,000 to 2,900 ml/wk/L body water provided sufficient dialysis.[42,43]

Peritoneal Dialysis

Popovich et al.[18] based the concept of CAPD on urea equilibration. Assuming that the urea equilibrates between plasma and dialysate at the end of the long-dwell exchange and that the urea nitrogen generation rate equals 8.2 g/d, simple calculations indicated that five 2-L exchanges plus 1.8 L of ultrafiltration would yield 11.8 L of urea clearance per day, which would

keep BUN below 70 mg/dl. Initial clinical studies confirmed these calculations[19]; however, five exchanges per day appeared to be cumbersome for the
majority of patients and four 2-L exchanges were recommended.[20] The
adequacy of this dialysis prescription has never been tested in a well-
controlled prospective study. Unfortunately, peritoneal dialysis was not included in the NCDS. Urea kinetic modeling has only recently been applied to
assess an adequate dose of peritoneal dialysis, and preliminary studies suggest that this may be a valuable method.[44]

For adequate IPD, Boen et al.[45] postulated a combined creatinine
clearance of 5.5 ml/min (7.92 l/d, or 55.44 L/wk) in a standard patient with a
body surface area of 1.73 m^2. Our clinical personal experience[26] indicates
that patients fulfilling criteria of adequate dialysis have at least a combined
creatinine clearance of 4.0 to 5.0 ml/min/1.73 m^2 (5.8 − 7.2 L/d; 40 to
50 L/wk).

In a continuous peritoneal dialysis regimen, a daily creatinine clearance
(K_{dd}) may be measured from an average dialysate creatinine concentration
(D_{av}) in total dialysate volume (V_t) drained per day:

$$K_{dd} = V_t \times \frac{D_{av}}{P}$$

An anuric CAPD patient with a daily drainage volume of 9.5 L may
achieve adequate dialysis (K_{dd} of 5.8 − 7.2 L/d) if the D_{av} to P ratio exceeds
0.61 to 0.76.

In an intermittent (periodic) peritoneal dialysis (IPD) regimen

$$K_{dw} = \frac{K_{di} \times T_d}{168}$$

in which, K_{dw} = the average weekly dialysis creatinine clearance, K_{di} = the
IPD clearance (ml/min), T_d = the IPD time (hs/wk), and 168 = the total
hours in 1 week.

An anuric patient with a K_{di} of 12.0 to 15.0 ml/min/1.73 m^2 may have
adequate dialysis with 56 hours of IPD per week.

MASS TRANSFER AREA COEFFICIENT

Dialysate to plasma ratios of solute concentrations change at different
rates in different patients on peritoneal dialysis, and peritoneal clearances
measured during standard intermittent peritoneal dialysis vary from patient to patient.[8,11,13,46-49]

The mass transfer area coefficient (MTAC) was introduced to separate
influences of dialysate flow rate and convective transport on solute
transfer.[50-54] This coefficient, based on kinetic models of the solute mass

transfer process, is the inverse of peritoneal diffusion resistance and represents the clearance rate that would be realized in the absence of both ultrafiltration and solute accumulation in the dialysate.

The MTAC measurement is seldom used in routine clinical practice as a guide in the selection of the optimal dialysis regimen because of the complexity of its calculations. Hiatt et al[55] published a nomogram to calculate MTAC from a single measurement of solute dialysate to plasma ratio at 4-, 5-, or 6-hour dwell times; however, such a recalculation does not have any advantage over a presentation of the result as a simple dialysate to plasma ratio.

ULTRAFILTRATION

In peritoneal dialysis, ultrafiltration is osmotically induced and the predominant transperitoneal osmotic pressure gradient is produced by the glucose concentration of the dialysis solution. Consequently, the net transcapillary ultrafiltration rate is maximal at the beginning of the exchange and decreases exponentially as the glucose concentration gradient is dissipated by a combination of transperitoneal glucose absorption and dilution by the ultrafiltrate.[54,56] The intraperitoneal volume increases until a maximum is reached when the net transcapillary ultrafiltration rate equals the peritoneal cavity lymphatic absorption rate.[57] Transcapillary ultrafiltration during exchanges using the same dialysis solution is primarily dependent on differences in peritoneal MTAC. Transperitoneal osmotic pressure is equal to the sum of the products of the osmotic gradient and peritoneal reflection coefficient of each solute. Because glucose creates most of the osmotic driving force, high peritoneal MTAC reduces cumulative transcapillary ultrafiltration by two related mechanisms: at any given osmotic gradient, the lower peritoneal reflection coefficient for glucose generates reduced osmotic driving force and diminished ultrafiltration; and rapid absorption of glucose from the dialysate dissipates the transperitoneal osmotic gradient more quickly during the dwell time.

Transcapillary ultrafiltration into the peritoneal cavity is negated by a variable rate of lymphatic drainage from the peritoneal cavity, but lymphatic absorption is independent of transcapillary MTAC for glucose.[58] Consequently, in patients with high peritoneal MTAC, peak ultrafiltration occurs earlier during dwell time and net positive ultrafiltration is shorter compared to patients with low MTAC (Fig. 4-1.)

PERITONEAL EQUILIBRATION TEST

Since 1983, we have been systematically measuring peritoneal transfer rates of urea, creatinine, glucose, protein, potassium, and sodium, as well as drain and residual volumes. For this purpose, the peritoneal equilibration

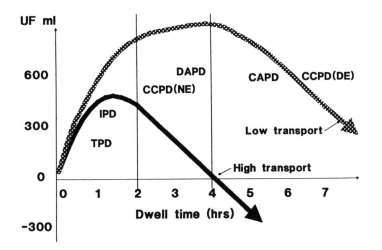

Fig. 4-1. Representative ultrafiltration curves during long-dwell exchanges in patients with high (high transport) and low (low transport) transperitoneal glucose absorption from the dialysate. In patients with high transperitoneal transport, peak ultrafiltration occurs early during dwell time and net positive ultrafiltration is of shorter duration compared with patients with low transport. In these patients, short-dwell exchange techniques such as IPD or tidal peritoneal dialysis (TPD) may be needed for adequate ultrafiltration. In patients with low transport rates, adequate ultrafiltration may be achieved with CAPD. Daytime (diurnal) ambulatory peritoneal dialysis (DAPD) and nocturnal exchanges (NE) of continuous cyclic peritoneal dialysis (CCPD) usually operate within an intermediate range of dwell times (2 to 4 hours) and are also acceptable to patients with high transport rates. From an ultrafiltration perspective, diurnal exchanges (DE) of CCPD are suitable only for patients with low transport rates.

test has been performed over a 4-hour dwell exchange with 2 L of 2.5 percent Dianeal solution. Excellent reproducibility was seen after tests were standardized for length of preceding exchange, inflow volume, inflow position, inflow rate, dwell time, dwell position, drain time, drain position, methods of obtaining and processing samples, and laboratory assays. Wide variations were found in the study population. Drain volume after a 4-hour dwell, the dialysate to plasma ratio of creatinine at 2 and 4 hours of dwell time, and the ratio of dialysate glucose at 2 and 4 hours of dwell time to dialysate glucose at 0 dwell time proved to be most valuable for prognostic and diagnostic purposes.[59,60] Recently, a simplified test assessing only these parameters was routinely performed in our institution. Details of our technique have already been published.[61,62] The baseline test is performed at the beginning of peritoneal dialysis treatment and the test is repeated in patients who have inadequate dialysis, inadequate ultrafiltration, or unexpected changes in serum chemistries.

Equilibration Test Results

Based on the results of 103 peritoneal equilibration tests, the transport rate is categorized as low, low average, high average, and high (Fig. 4-2). Dialysate to plasma ratios of creatinine at the 2- and 4-hour dwell times and the ratios of dialysate glucose at 2 and 4 hours of dwell to dialysate glucose at 0 dwell time are calculated and superimposed on standard curves.

Drain volumes are categorized using the same principle as for dialysate to plasma ratios (Fig. 4-3). Drain volumes correlate positively with the dialysate glucose at 0 dwell time and negatively with dialysate to plasma ratios of creatinine.

Ultrafiltration and Clearance Patterns in Relation to Solute Transport

Figures 4-1 and 4-4 portray the ultrafiltration and small molecular weight solute clearances versus dwell time in patients with extreme low and high transport rates using dialysis solution with 2.5 percent glucose concentrations. In patients with low transport rates, peak ultrafiltration occurs late during dwell time and net ultrafiltration is still obtained after a long dwell time (Fig. 4-1). Also, the dialysate to plasma ratios increase almost linearly

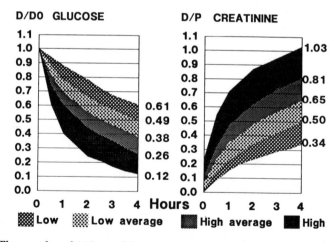

Fig. 4-2. The results of 103 equilibration tests. Areas shaded in different patterns portray results representing high, high-average, low-average, and low peritoneal transport rates. Creatinine concentration in dialysate and plasma is corrected for glucose interference. For creatinine, the higher the dialysate to plasma ratio (D/P), the higher the transfer rate. Because glucose transport direction is opposite to that of creatinine, the higher the concentration ratio of dialysate glucose at a particular dwell time to dialysate glucose at 0 dwell time, (D/D0), the lower the transfer rate. The numbers separate the four categories. (Data from Twardowski et al.[59,60])

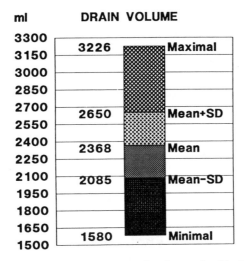

Fig. 4-3. Drain volumes after standardized 4-hour dwell time test exchanges (n = 94). Patients with high solute transport rates usually have low drain volumes, and vice versa. The stack bar areas are shaded in the patterns corresponding to categories portrayed in Fig. 4-2. (Data from Twardowski et al.[59,60])

during the dwell (Fig. 4-2); consequently, clearances per exchanges also increase almost linearly throughout the long dwell exchange (Fig. 4-4). In these patients, the time of dialysis is crucial for adequate clearances and they benefit from continuous regimens such as CAPD or continuous cyclic peritoneal dialysis (CCPD) with diurnal exchanges. Because of a well-maintained dialysate to plasma concentration gradient for an extended period during dwell, clearances per unit time are augmented relatively little by rapid exchange techniques such as IPD or tidal peritoneal dialysis (TPD). Consequently, intermittent techniques require long treatment times for adequate clearances. On the contrary, the patients with high peritoneal transport rates have poor ultrafiltration on standard CAPD with dwell times exceeding 4 hours. In these patients, peak ultrafiltration occurs early during the dwell time and is followed by dialysate absorption. If dialysate is drained after a 4-hour dwell, there is minimal or no net ultrafiltration (Fig. 4-1). Also, the mass transfer of small molecular weight solutes in long-dwell exchanges decreases proportionately with the reduction in drain volume (Fig. 4-4). After several hours of dwell, the clearance per exchange may be less than in patients with low peritoneal transport rates. Reducing the dwell time in patients with high transport rates captures maximum ultrafiltration while maintaining near complete equilibration of small molecular weight solutes and so increases net solute removal. These patients benefit from techniques using rapid exchanges and may achieve adequate clearances with IPD regimens. Patients with solute transport rates between these two extremes have intermediate patterns.

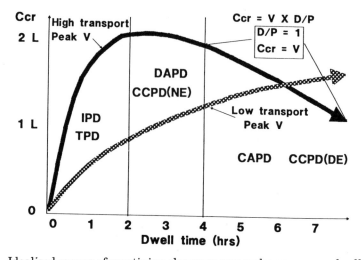

Fig. 4-4. Idealized curves of creatinine clearance per exchange versus dwell time in patients with extremely low and high peritoneal transport characteristics. In patients with low transport rates, clearances per exchange increase almost linearly throughout the long-dwell exchange, even after peak ultrafiltration is achieved. A well-maintained dialysate to plasma concentration gradient for an extended period during dwell restricts enhancement of clearances per unit time by rapid exchange techniques, such as IPD or TPD. These patients benefit from continuous regimens such as CAPD or continuous cyclic peritoneal dialysis (CCPD) with diurnal exchanges (DE) because the time of dialysis is crucial for adequate clearances. In patients with high transport, the clearance increases rapidly during the dwell and is nearly maximal at the peak ultrafiltration. The clearance changes little at the beginning of the dialysate absorption phase because the dialysate to plasma ratio still increases. After equilibrium (dialysate to plasma ratio = 1.0) is achieved, the clearance declines because it is identical with the dialysate volume, which is decreasing. Because of this phenomenon, creatinine clearance per exchange is lower with long-dwell times in patients with high peritoneal transport than that in patients with low peritoneal transport. Short-dwell exchange techniques such as IPD or TPD are beneficial in patients with high peritoneal transport not only for ultrafiltration but for solute removal. Long-dwell exchanges are unsuitable for these patients. Daytime (diurnal) ambulatory peritoneal dialysis (DAPD) and nocturnal exchanges (NE) of CCPD usually operate within an intermediate range of dwell times (2 to 4 hours) and also yield excellent clearances in patients with high transport rates.

Prognostic Value of Baseline Equilibration Test

Table 4-2 summarizes the prognostic usefulness of the baseline peritoneal equilibration test. The patients with high peritoneal transport rates have poor ultrafiltration and clearances on continuous regimens. They are ideal candidates for rapid exchange intermittent techniques (nightime intermittent peritoneal dialysis [NIPD], nocturnal tidal peritoneal dialysis [NTPD], diurnal ambulatory peritoneal dialysis [DAPD]).

The best candidates for standard-dose continuous peritoneal dialysis regimens are patients with high average peritoneal transport rates. They can

Table 4-2. Prognostic Value of the Baseline Peritoneal Equilibration Test Results in Patients with Well-Functioning Catheter After Break-in

Peritoneal Solute Transport	Drain Volume	Predicted Long-Term Response to Standard-Dose CAPD or CCPD After Loss of Residual Renal Functions		Preferred Dialysis Prescription After Loss of Residual Renal Functions
		Ultrafiltration	Dialysis	
High	Low	Poor	Adequate	NIPD, DAPD, NTPD[a]
High-average	Low-average	Adequate	Adequate	Standard-dose CAPD, CCPD, or NIPD[b]
Low-average	High-average	Good	Adequate or inadequate[c]	Standard-dose CAPD, CCPD, or NIPD[b] High-dose CAPD, CCPD, or NIPD[d]
Low	High	Excellent	Inadequate	High-dose CAPD, CCPD, or NIPD[d] or hemo-dialysis[e]

[a] NIPD (nightly intermittent peritoneal dialysis): intermittent peritoneal dialysis performed every night for 8 to 12 hours using 10 to 20 L of dialysis solution. The higher the peritoneal transport rate, the shorter the time of dialysis required for adequate clearances. In patients with high transport, a treatment time of 8 hours every night is usually sufficient. DAPD (daytime [diurnal] ambulatory peritoneal dialysis): ambulatory peritoneal dialysis performed only during daytime using three to four exchanges. NTPD (nightly [nocturnal] tidal peritoneal dialysis): nightly dialysis performed with the tidal technique.

[b] Standard-dose CAPD = CAPD with 7.5 to 9.0 L of dialysis solution used per 24 hours; standard-dose CCPD = CCPD with 6 to 8 L of dialysis solution used overnight and 2 L during the daytime; and standard-dose NIPD = 15 L of NIPD used for 10 hours every night.

[c] Inadequate dialysis likely in patients with body surface area >2.00 m².

[d] High-dose CAPD = CAPD with >9.0 L of dialysis solution used per 24 hours; high-dose CCPD = CCPD with >8 L of dialysis solution used overnight and/or >2 L during the daytime; and high-dose NIPD = 20 L NIPD used for 10 to 12 hours every night.

[e] Hemodialysis may be needed in patients with body surface area >2.00 m².

achieve adequate dialysis even after losing residual renal function and can obtain adequate ultrafiltration with moderate dialysis solution glucose concentrations. Adequate clearances may also be obtained with intermittent techniques using moderate weekly treatment time.

Most patients with low average peritoneal transport can be maintained on the standard-dose peritoneal dialysis; however, many may require a modified prescription (high-dose CAPD or high-dose CCPD) when residual renal function becomes negligible, particularly if they have high body surface area. These patients have excellent ultrafiltration with moderate dialysis solution glucose concentrations.

Finally, patients with low peritoneal transport rates usually have excellent ultrafiltration with low dialysis solution glucose concentration and are likely to develop symptoms of inadequate dialysis on standard CAPD when their residual renal function becomes negligible.[30,59,60]

Diagnostic Value of Repeated Equilibration Test

Table 4-3 portrays the diagnostic value of repeated tests in patients presenting with inadequate dialysis. An unchanged and high or high average peritoneal solute transport indicates noncompliance to a prescribed dialysis regimen. Inadequate dialysis in patients with low average or low peritoneal solute transport frequently occurs after a loss of residual renal function. To improve symptoms of underdialysis, a high-dose peritoneal dialysis prescription should be implemented.

A decreased transport test leading to inadequate dialysis may be either transient or permanent. Patients with a mild, transient decrease in peritoneal transport have high or high average drain volumes on repeated equilibration tests and normal fluid distribution on peritoneography. A permanent decrease in peritoneal transport, secondary to massive adhesions or sclerosing peritonitis, is associated with decreased ultrafiltration (see below).

The diagnostic value of the peritoneal equilibration test in the differential diagnosis of ultrafiltration loss is presented in Table 4-4. Insufficient ultrafiltration in a patient with stable, high peritoneal solute transport and stable, low drain volume without a change in residual volume indicates a loss of residual renal function and a necessity of change to NIPD or DAPD. The diagnosis should be confirmed by a 24-hour urine collection. A reported

Table 4-3. Diagnostic Value of Repeated Peritoneal Equilibration Test Compared with Baseline in Patients Presenting with Inadequate Dialysis

Peritoneal Solute Transport		Drain Volume	Most Likely Diagnosis	Other Diagnostic Test	Recommended Therapy
Baseline	Repeated				
High or high-average	High or high-average	Low or low-average	Dialysis noncompliance		Counseling
Low or low-average	Low or low-average	High or high-average	Loss of residual renal function	24° Urine collection	High-dose CAPD, CCPD, or NIPD[a]
High or high-average	Low or low-average	High or high-average	Unknown reason of decreased transport[b]	Peritoneography	High-dose CAPD, CCPD, or NIPD[a]
High or high-average	Low or low-average	Low or low-average	Massive adhesions[c] or sclerosing peritonitis	Laparotomy[d]	Permanent hemodialysis

[a] See notes to Table 4-1.

[b] Normal fluid distribution seen on peritoneography. The incidence of this change in peritoneal transport is low. Among over 300 peritoneal dialysis patients, I have seen only four such patients; two after transplant rejection had decreased transport lasting several months, two after severe peritonitis had permanent decrease in transport.

[c] Two patients could not be maintained on peritoneal dialysis after severe peritonitis. Peritoneography revealed multiple adhesion with fluid maldistribution.

[d] Peritoneography or gastrointestinal x-ray series may be sufficient for diagnosis.

Table 4-4. Diagnostic Value of Repeated Peritoneal Equilibration Test Compared with Baseline in Patients Presenting with Apparent or Actual Loss of Ultrafiltration

Loss of Ultra-filtration	Peritoneal Solute Transport	Drain Volume	Most Likely Diagnosis	Other Diagnostic Test	Recommended Therapy
Apparent	Stable, high	Stable, low	Loss of residual renal function	24° Urine collection	NIPD, DAPD,[c] NTPD[d]
Apparent	Stable <high[a]	Stable, >low[b]	High fluid intake	Dietary history	Counseling
Gradual	Stable	Lower	Excessive lymphatic absorption	Intraperitoneal albumin removal	NIPD, DAPD,[c] permanent hemodialysis
Gradual	Increased	Lower	Mesothelial alterations[e]	Peritoneography	Temporary hemodialysis; NIPD, DAPD[c]
Gradual	Decreased	Lower	Massive adhesions sclerosing peritonitis[f]	X-ray, laparotomy	Permanent hemodialysis
Sudden	Stable	Lower	Dialysate leak	Peritoneography	Temporary hemodialysis or supine peritoneal dialysis[g]
Sudden	Stable	Lower	Catheter malposition	Plain abdominal x-ray	Catheter repositioning

[a] <high, High-average, low-average, or low.
[b] >low, Low-average, high-average, or high.
[c] DAPD may be inadequate in patients with <high peritoneal transport rates.
[d] See explanations to Table 4-1.
[e] Type I ultrafiltration failure.
[f] Type II ultrafiltration failure.
[g] Peritoneal dialysis regimen in which the patient is supine during dialysis.

insufficient ultrafiltration in a patient with stable but less than high peritoneal solute transport and more than low drain volume indicates dietary indiscretions. Dietary counseling rather than change in dialysis prescription is needed.

A gradual decrease in ultrafiltration (Table 4-4) may result from three principal causes: excessive lymphatic absorption,[63] type I ultrafiltration failure (mesothelial alterations),[64] type II ultrafiltration failure (massive peritoneal adhesions or sclerosing peritonitis).[64] A combination of slow glucose absorption, slow urea equilibration, and a sodium concentration in dialysate equal to that in infused dialysis solution has been reported by Verger et al.[35] in sclerosing peritonitis.

A sudden decrease in ultrafiltration with a corresponding decrease in drain volume but without a change in peritoneal solute transport indicates either a dialysate leak or catheter malfunction. Localized abdominal edema indicates dialysate leak, which may be confirmed on computed tomography (CT) with intraperitoneal contrast[65]; however, small or intermittent leaks may not show on CT scan.[66] Catheter malfunction is usually easy to diagnose. Slow inflow and/or slow drainage are the most common signs of catheter malfunction. A plain x-ray film of the abdomen usually shows catheter tip malposition.

EMERGENCE OF NEWER TECHNIQUES

Intermittent peritoneal dialysis, the only form of peritoneal dialysis in the early 1970s, could not compete with hemodialysis because of short patient survival. A further decline in the number of IPD patients has been observed during the 1980s. Standard CAPD with four 2-L exchanges is the most widely used form of peritoneal dialysis at present; however, after 2 years of therapy, almost 34 percent of patients are transferred from CAPD.[67] Frequent peritonitis is the main reason for dropout, but over 70 percent of patients are transferred because of other medical and sociopsychologic problems.[67] Common medical complications leading to transfers are related to high intra-abdominal pressure, inadequate ultrafiltration, and inadequate dialysis. Newer modifications of peritoneal dialysis, such as CCPD, nightly (nocturnal) peritoneal dialysis (NPD), DAPD, and high volume peritoneal dialysis, allow continuation of peritoneal dialysis therapy in patients who experience inadequate dialysis or inadequate ultrafiltration on standard CAPD.[60-62] Patients with complications related to increased intra-abdominal pressure such as hernias, hemorrhoids, and abdominal leaks benefit from peritoneal dialysis performed in the supine position. For regimens decreasing dialysis time, an increased dialysis efficiency is of essential importance; thus, new techniques are being explored. Table 4-5 illustrates recent trends in the application of various peritoneal dialysis prescriptions in the United States. Whereas the number of IPD patients is rapidly decreasing and the number of CAPD patients is increasing slightly, there is a rapid growth of the CCPD patient population. Newer techniques are not yet reported separately and are probably included in the CCPD population. All

Table 4-5. Peritoneal Dialysis in the United States From 1980 to 1987 (Based on Data From the Health Care Financing Administration)

Patients as of	Total	IPD Home and Training (%)	IPD In Unit (%)	CAPD Home and Training (%)	CCPD Home and Training (%)
12/31/80	4,008	911 (22.7)	657 (16.4)	2,440 (60.9)	—
12/31/81	6,080	944 (15.5)	672 (11.1)	4,464 (73.4)	—
12/31/82	8,404	885 (10.5)	835 (9.9)	6,684 (79.5)	—
12/31/83	10,265	745 (7.3)	823 (8.0)	8,688 (84.7)	—
12/31/84	11,896	590 (5.0)	272 (2.3)	10,158 (85.4)	876 (7.4)
12/31/85	13,255	584 (4.4)	235 (1.8)	11,462 (86.5)	974 (7.3)
12/31/86	14,187	510 (3.6)	199 (1.4)	12,141 (85.6)	1,337 (9.4)
12/31/87	15,332	441 (2.9)	168 (1.1)	12,995 (84.8)	1,728 (11.3)

these modifications evolved from the older techniques, IPD and CAPD, incorporating their advantages and eliminating some of their disadvantages.

REASONS FOR INTERMITTENT PERITONEAL DIALYSIS FAILURE

As mentioned previously, IPD therapy for end-stage renal disease was associated with relatively short patient survival. Although survival rates were comparable to patients on hemodialysis during the initial 1 year of therapy, there was a sudden increase in mortality after the first or second year.[27–29,68] There were two main reasons for IPD failure, especially in patients who lost residual renal function: inadequate dialysis clearances and inadequate sodium balance resulting in thirst and poor blood pressure control.

Ahmad et al.[69] postulated that 51 hours per week is the minimum required dialysis time for anuric patients; in reality, however, a total dialysis time did not exceed 40 hs/wk in their patients. In patients with renal creatinine clearance exceeding 2 ml/min, a dialysis time of 30 hs/wk was sufficient for adequate dialysis. Failure to prolong dialysis time was probably the main reason for IPD failure after 2 years of treatment when residual renal functions diminished to negligible values.[69]

Inadequate sodium balance in IPD is due to the low sodium concentration in ultrafiltrate resulting from solute sieving. Convective net removal of sodium per liter of ultrafiltrate is usually well below extracellular fluid concentration. Thus, dialysate sodium concentration is initially reduced due to solute sieving with ultrafiltration and tends to increase later in the dwell time due to diffusion and diminished ultrafiltration rate.[59,70–72]

Dialysate sodium concentration decreases more in patients with low peritoneal transport characteristics.[59] Although the sieving effect creates a concentration gradient for some diffusion, during short dwell exchanges net electrolyte removal per liter of ultrafiltrate remains far below the extracellular fluid concentration and severe hypernatremia may develop.[73–74] Also, in patients who have chronically low serum sodium concentration, probably because of a reset osmostat, the sodium concentration gradient between dialysate and serum is so low that the sodium diffusion cannot compensate even for moderate sieving. Blood pressure control is difficult in both types of patients.

FEATURES OF CAPD COMPARED WITH HOME IPD

A summary comparison of CAPD and home IPD is shown in Table 4-6.

Table 4-6. Advantages and Disadvantages of CAPD Compared with Home IPD

Advantages	Disadvantages
Medical	
Adequate weekly clearances	More frequent peritonitis episodes
Sufficient sodium removal (absent thirst, usually well-controlled blood pressure)	Higher glucose absorption/ultrafiltration (obesity, lipid disturbances, relative malnutrition)
Steady blood chemistries	High intra-abdominal pressure with fluid (hernias, dialysate leaks, hemorrhoids)
	Aggravated low back pain
Psychosocial	
Simple equipment	Distorted body image
Easy travel	Inconvenient exchange schedule in employed and school-attending patients
No bed confinement for treatment	

Advantages of CAPD

Clearances

The main advantage of CAPD over IPD is higher dialysis clearances for solutes in all molecular rate ranges. A mean creatinine clearance is approximately 6.3 L/d (4.4 ml/min),[75] a value that provides adequate dialysis.

Sodium Balance, Thirst, and Blood Pressure Control

Sodium sieving occurs early during the dwell time when the ultrafiltration rate is high; however, the ultrafiltration rate diminishes rapidly with glucose absorption and a dissipation of the osmotic gradient. Simultaneously, due to a high sodium concentration gradient between plasma and dialysate, sodium diffusion rate increases. After several hours of dwell time, the ultrafiltration ceases and the continuing diffusion increases the dialysate sodium concentration. Usually, water and sodium losses are nearly proportional to water and sodium intakes, serum sodium does not increases, no thirst is present, and sodium removal is sufficient to control blood pressure.[61]

Psychosocial

Continuous ambulatory peritoneal dialysis is a simple procedure. It does not require machines and a suitable environment can be relatively easily created to perform dialysis exchanges; thus, there are essentially no restrictions for travel. The interruption of daily activities to perform exchanges is short. Intermittent peritoneal dialysis requires a bed confinement for prolonged periods, although most dialysis may be performed during the night. Machines for IPD require running water and/or electricity; thus, travel is difficult.

Disadvantages of Continuous Ambulatory Peritoneal Dialysis

Although the continuous presence of dialysis fluid in the peritoneal cavity is favorable for the dialysis clearances, sodium balance, and steady-state chemistries in CAPD patients, it is disadvantageous in several aspects.

Peritonitis

Peritonitis rates are higher in CAPD patients than in IPD patients. Vas[76] presented an attractive hypothesis to explain this phenomenon. Peritoneal defense mechanisms against infections are compromised with the presence of a nonphysiologic fluid in the peritoneal cavity. Immunoglobulin concentrations in the high-volume dialysate are lower than in the few milliliters of fluid that are normally present in the peritoneal cavity; bacterial opsonization is thus decreased. The phagocytes are also diluted in the fluid and their contact with bacteria, essential for effective phagocytosis, is hampered. Moreover, the efficiency of phagocytic cells decrease at the low pH and high osmolality of the dialysis solution. Intermittent peritoneal dialysis patients have long periods when the peritoneum is without solutions, and normal defense mechanisms may contain and eradicate a small bacterial inoculum.

Relative Malnutrition

Glucose absorption per milliliter of net ultrafiltration is higher in CAPD patients than in IPD patients and may reach 300 g/d.[77] This constant and high glucose absorption probably contributes to obesity and lipid disturbances and, coupled with abdominal distension, decreases appetite, leading to the documented trend of CAPD patients to store fat and develop relative malnutrition.[78]

Fluid Leaks, Hernias, and Hemorrhoids

Abdominal hernias are relatively common complications of CAPD. Several investigators have reported a 9 to 28 percent incidence of hernias in CAPD patients,[79–81] whereas only 2 to 3 percent of IPD patients develop hernias.[81] Also, hemorrhoids and abdominal and pericatheter leaks are frequent in CAPD patients.[82] Undoubtedly, it is related to the constant presence of fluid in the peritoneal cavity coupled with high intra-abdominal pressures in the vertical position during natural activities.[83] Intra-abdominal pressure in the supine position is negligible in relaxed patients.

Chronic Back Pain

Back pain is a frequent complication of CAPD, probably related to the change in body posture with the presence of fluid in the peritoneal cavity.[81]

Psychosocial Disadvantages

A protruding abdomen due to the chronic artificial ascites distorts the body image in many CAPD patients. Frequent CAPD exchanges during the daytime are tedious and inconvenient, especially for patients who work or attend school. Dialysis exchanges require a creation of a proper environment and are not easily performed outside the home or dialysis facility. If exchanges are performed under inappropriate conditions, the risk of peritoneal system contamination is increased.

CONTINUOUS CYCLIC PERITONEAL DIALYSIS

The possibility of combining positive features of CAPD and IPD with a reduction of the negative aspects was predicted by Scribner in 1979.[84] Soon thereafter, Diaz-Buxo et al.[85,86] introduced CCPD. Unlike CAPD, in which short dwell exchanges are performed during the daytime and one long dwell exchange occurs overnight, CCPD short dwell exchanges take place at night with an automatic cycling machine and one long dwell exchange is performed during the day. Originally, CCPD provided three overnight 2-L exchanges with one prolonged diurnal 2-L exchange. The number of nightly exchanges can be increased to five to augment clearances.[81]

Cyclers

Most current machines are designed after the model of Lasker et al.[87] using gravity for infusion and drainage of dialysate, and consist primarily of a fluid heater and timing mechanisms to actuate valves that control the gravity flow of fluid to and from the peritoneal cavity. Commercially available cyclers are intended to be used with premixed dialysis solutions supplied in plastic containers. Additional features include electronic scales, drain alarms, and ultrafiltration monitors. Figure 4-5 depicts a diagram of a commonly used PAC-X-2 cycler. The detailed description of cyclers can be found in a recently published article by the Emergency Care Research Institute.[88]

Indications to Continuous Cyclic Peritoneal Dialysis

According to Diaz-Buxo,[81] the advantages of CCPD include uninterrupted daytime activities; simplicity of adjusting a dialysis prescription contingent on the required efficiency by modifying the number of nightly exchanges; a reduction in the number of connection/disconnection procedures to two per day; and a decreased burden on the partner, if one is required, because all technical assistance takes place early in the morning and late in the evening.

Indications to CCPD are based on these advantages. Nissenson[89] and

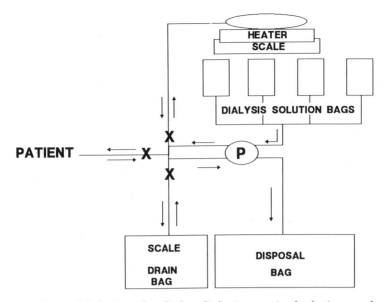

Fig. 4-5. Peritoneal dialysis cycler. Before dialysis, premixed solutions are hung and connected with the peritoneal dialysis catheter through a system of tubings with occlusors (X). The solution is pumped from solution bags into a heater bag on a scale and warmed to body temperature. A specified volume (determined gravimetrically) of warmed solution is delivered by gravity into the peritoneal cavity. After a predetermined time, the dialysate is drained by gravity into a drain bag and the volume is measured gravimetrically. Dialysate from the drain bag is pumped into a disposal bag.

Diaz-Buxo[81] recommend CCPD instead of CAPD for inadequate control of chemistries and/or fluid balance, recurrent abdominal hernias and leaks, frequent peritonitis on CAPD, and chronic low back pain. CCPD seems to be particularly useful in patients with low peritoneal solute transport rates requiring increased doses of dialysis. High-dose CCPD (Table 4-2) provides adequate dialysis in these patients.[56,60,90]

Psychosocial circumstances constitute an important incentive to opt for CCPD instead of CAPD. School children and employed patients are frequently unable or unwilling to perform exchanges during the day. When a partner is necessary, the convenience of CCPD becomes particularly attractive. Parents dialyzing children, relatives dialyzing the elderly, and debilitated patients usually prefer CCPD over CAPD. The compliance with a prescribed dialysis schedule seems to be improved on CCPD.

Disadvantages of Continuous Cyclic Peritoneal Dialysis

The main disadvantage of CCPD is the higher cost compared with CAPD. Travel is difficult with CCPD; however, if CCPD is chosen because of psychosocial reasons, CAPD may be performed during travel and vacation. For most patients, CAPD is still more attractive because it does not require machines and there are no sleep interruptions caused by machine alarms. Also, complications related to high intra-abdominal pressure with fluid are common if a regular diurnal exchange is used.

NIGHTLY PERITONEAL DIALYSIS

Nightly peritoneal dialysis (NPD) may be considered CCPD without long-dwell daytime exchanges. Nightly peritoneal dialysis performed with an intermittent flow technique is called nightly intermittent peritoneal dialysis (NIPD).

Incentives to and Disadvantages of Nightime Intermittent Peritoneal Dialysis

Since 1982, we have used NIPD in patients with complications related to high intra-abdominal pressure and poor ultrafiltration on CAPD due to high peritoneal transport rates. Table 4-7 portrays incentives to NIPD instead of CAPD or CCPD. The main disadvantage of NIPD is bed confinement during treatment and the need for a cycler. In patients with low peritoneal transport rates, the duration of the dialysis session may be excessively long. In such patients, the cost of dialysis is markedly higher than that of CAPD.

Currently Used Technique

All NIPD treatments are performed overnight on a peritoneal dialysis cycler with 1.5- to 2-L fill volumes of commercial peritoneal dialysis solutions. Total dialysis time ranges from 8 to 12 hours per night (56 to 84 hrs/wk). A total volume of used dialysis solution per dialysis ranges from 8 to 20 L (56 to 140 L/wk). The time of dialysis and dialysate dose are adjusted according to the patient's peritoneal membrane permeability area. The higher the

Table 4-7. Incentives to Use NIPD Instead of CAPD and CCPD

Medical
   Complications related to high intra-abdominal pressure (hernias, abdominal
      dialysate leaks, peritoneopleural leak, hemorrhoids, bladder prolapse)
   High peritoneal solute transport resulting in high glucose absorption with poor
      ultrafiltration
   Low back pain

Psychosocial
   Distorted body image due to protruding abdomen on continuous dialysis
   Convenient treatment time in employed and school-attending patients
      (compared with CAPD)
   Convenient dialysis schedule for helpers (compared with CAPD)

permeability, the shorter the session times and the lower the volume of dialysis solution used per treatment. An attempt is made to achieve creatinine clearance of 5.8 to 7.2 L/d per 1.73 m^2 body surface area (40 to 50 L/wk/1.73 m^2). Drain time is restricted to 12 to 15 minutes (1 minute for 120 to 170 ml) to minimize the period when the peritoneal cavity is almost empty and dialysis efficiency is markedly reduced. If a low drain alarm is triggered during the initial one or two exchanges, the patients are instructed not to prolong drain time but to bypass cycles, thus creating some sump volume in the peritoneal cavity. Low drain alarms usually do not occur during or after the third cycle unless the extension tubing is occluded. This technique, which is called IPD with restricted outflow time, is based on a principle that is fully optimized in a TPD technique (see below). Most patients use dialysis solution with a sodium concentration of 132 mEq/L. In a few patients, a sodium concentration of 120 to 126 mEq/L is used. For this purpose, 5 percent glucose solution (D5W) is mixed with peritoneal dialysis solution in an appropriate proportion to achieve the desired sodium concentration. For instance, 1 L of D5W added to 20 L of dialysis solution lowers the sodium concentration from 132 mEq/L to 126 mEq/L. Dilution of other electrolytes is of little significance. The use of an additional, little bag (1 L) increases the demand of the procedure and the risk of contamination. It would certainly be safer and more convenient to have premixed dialysis solutions with lower sodium concentrations for some NIPD patients.

Illustrative Case History

A case history of one of our early patients illustrates the evolution of NIPD throughout the years and common problems related to this therapy.

A white woman, born in 1960, with polycystic renal disease and Caroli disease, was started on hemodialysis in 1979; she tolerated the hemodialysis poorly and had difficulties in maintaining arteriovenous fistulas. Her left ventricular ejection fraction was 17 percent. She had frequent pulmonary congestion before dialysis and hypotension after dialysis. She had three unsuccessful kidney transplants in May 1980, November 1980, and August 1982 (all lost to acute rejections) and she became anuric. After her fourth blood access failed in December 1982, she decided to transfer to CAPD. In January 1983, a double-cuff Tenckhoff catheter was implanted. Shortly after starting CAPD she developed a pericatheter dialysate leak and was transferred to IPD for 40 hs/wk. This prescription yielded an inadequate creatinine clearance of 20 L/wk/1.73 m^2 body surface area (daily average, 2.9 L/1.73 m^2). The patient was switched to CAPD but developed an abdominal leak through a ventral hernia shortly thereafter and was admitted to the hospital for hernia repair. During 1983, she was hospitalized nine times for repairs of abdominal leaks and hernias. The patient refused attempts to create a new blood access and retry hemodialysis. A peritoneal equilibration test revealed a creatinine dialysate to plasma ratio of 0.54 at 4 hours dwell.

In January 1984, the patient started on NPD for 12 hours with 14 L of dialysis solution per treatment. Since the patient discontinued CAPD no abdominal leak or hernia developed, but initially the patient did not achieve adequate creatinine clearance. Table 4-8 portrays the most relevant laboratory and clinical data over 5 years of NIPD treatment. Because of uremic symptoms, increasing serum creatinine, and a suboptimal creatinine clearance, the volume of dialysis solution per treatment was increased to 20 L in January 1986. Outflow time was maintained at 20 minutes for 1,500 ml of drainage volume. The patient occasionally even used longer outflow times. Creatinine clearance was still unsatisfactory. In August 1986, dialysis time was shortened to 11 hours, but outflow time was shortened to 13 minutes for 1,600 ml of exchange volume. Since that change, the patient has clinically improved markedly and standardized creatinine clearance reached almost 5.7 L/d. Her recent left ventricular ejection fraction increased to 54 percent.

This patient has not been a good candidate for any dialysis modality except for peritoneal dialysis in the supine position. Standard intermittent peritoneal dialysis was inadequate because of low average peritoneal transport rates and complete anuria. NIPD proved to be the method of choice. The only two disadvantages were long treatment sessions and high treatment cost.

Current Status of Nighttime Intermittent Peritoneal Dialysis

Because of higher cost of dialysis compared with CCPD and CAPD, NIPD is not a viable alternative to CAPD or CCPD at present. NIPD is the best choice only in patients with complications related to elevated intra-

Table 4-8. Laboratory and Clinical Data on CAPD and NIPD in the Reported Case

	CAPD (12/83)	NIPD (01/86)	NIPD (08/86)	NIPD (01/89)
Treatment time (hr/d)	24	12	12	11
Exchange volume (L)	2	2	1.6	1.6
Dialysis solution dose (L/d)	8	14	20	20
Outflow time (min)	25	25	20	13
Body weight (kg)	54.8	56.5	56.9	63.2
Height (cm)	155	155	155	155
Blood pressure supine (mm Hg)	108/76	98/76	90/64	120/80
Hematocrit (%)	32.5	35.8	36.0	37.3
BUN (mg/dl)	63	77	72	52
Urea clearance[a]	7.7	9.2	10.4	10.9
Serum creatinine (mg/dl)	13.1	18.3	16.9	13.1
Creatinine clearance[a]	5.7	4.2	4.8	5.7
Serum potassium (mEq/L)	3.6	4.9	3.5	3.7
Potassium clearance[a]	7.9	7.9	8.5	8.6
Serum phosphorus (mg/dl)	5.6	5.6	5.6	3.7
Phosphorus clearance[a]	5.1	4.3	4.5	5.1

[a] All clearances in L/d 1.73 m^2 body surface area.

abdominal pressure and who cannot be on hemodialysis and in patients with high peritoneal transport rates resulting in poor ultrafiltration on CAPD or CCPD and excellent dialysis efficiency on NIPD (Figs. 4-1 and 4-4).

Future of Nightly Peritoneal Dialysis

In 1985, Scribner[91] postulated that "some form of nightly peritoneal dialysis, NPD, may prove as the best compromise of all [forms of peritoneal dialysis]." In fact, NPD is a promising dialysis prescription but its future depends on three improvements: the cost of dialysis must be decreased; dialysis solution compositions, particularly sodium concentration, must be easily adjusted to the patient needs; and the efficiency of dialysis has to be increased.

Cost of Dialysis

Cost of dialysis has to match that of CAPD. Designs of new machines for peritoneal dialysis have to be based on a reverse osmosis proportioning system (Fig. 4-6). Automated production of dialysis solution from pretreated water and concentrate would decrease the cost of dialysis.

Dialysis Solution

Some patients with low or low-average peritoneal transport rates and those with chronically low serum sodium concentrations require lower sodium concentrations in dialysis solution for NPD than that for CAPD or

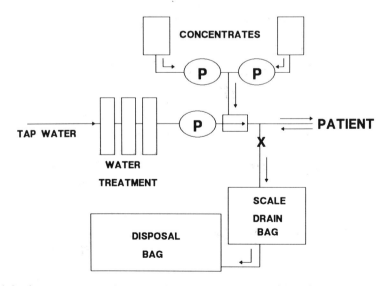

Fig. 4-6. A reverse osmosis proportioning system: a machine that produces dialysis solution from concentrates and treated water and also performs all functions of the cycler. Such a machine delivers more fluid at lower cost than the cycler. Because of low demand, these machines are not presently manufactured, but new interest in automated dialysis may revive this design. P, pump; X, occlusor.

CCPD. The concentrations between 120 and 132 mEq/L seem to be appropriate. It would be desirable to design peritoneal dialysis machines with the possibility of setting various sodium concentrations (e.g., 120, 123, 126, 129, or 132 mEq/L). Also, concentrations of other electrolytes may need adjustment. Such flexibility may be achieved with new peritoneal dialysis machines.

Efficiency of Peritoneal Dialysis

In the late 1960s and early 1970s, many attempts were made to increase IPD efficiency through modifications of continuous and intermittent flow techniques. A review of these modifications[61] indicated that the most promising seemed to be techniques explored by Di Paolo,[92] Finkelstein and Kliger,[93] and Kablitz et al.[49] Their techniques may be considered hybrids of continuous and intermittent flow techniques. Analogous to intermittent techniques, the fluid was delivered into and drained from the peritoneal cavity through a single catheter. However, the outflow and inflow followed each other without interruption; consequently, large quantities of fluid could be used for dialysis sessions. To avoid difficulties with fluid outflow, only a part of the dialysate was drained during each exchange, leaving some amount of sump volume in the peritoneal cavity throughout the dialysis session. An additional advantage of this sump (reserve) volume is the preservation of constant contact between the peritoneal membrane and the dialysate. This feature is important in increasing the efficiency of dialysis because in the intermittent technique, where dialysate is drained almost completely after each exchange, periods of minimal contact after an outflow and before the next inflow are associated with decreased solute transfer.

TIDAL PERITONEAL DIALYSIS

The efficiency of this technique has recently been reappraised and the technique was renamed tidal peritoneal dialysis (TDP).[61,94] Tidal peritoneal dialysis is a technique in which, after an initial fill of the peritoneal cavity, less than 50 percent of dialysate is drained and replaced by fresh dialysis fluid with each cycle, leaving the majority of dialysate in constant contact with the peritoneal membrane until the end of the dialysis session, when the fluid is drained as completely as possible. Assuming high and constant dialysate flow, there are at least two factors determining the efficiency of dialysis with this technique: the minimal volume of fluid in the peritoneal cavity assuring constant and full contact between the peritoneal membrane and dialysate (reserve volume), and proper mixing of fluid in the peritoneal cavity by a sufficiently high tidal exchange (stroke) volume. Mixing is better with a higher volume delivered into the peritoneal cavity with each tidal exchange, but the maximal tidal exchange volume is determined by the minimal reserve volume and maximum tolerable intraperitoneal fluid volume (which should not exceed 3 L).

Acute (Preliminary) Studies

Preliminary studies showed that the best efficiency of dialysis could be achieved with reserve and tidal volumes of 1.5 L, that tidal volumes of 1.2, 0.9, and 0.6 L yielded only minimally lower clearances, and that a tidal volume of 0.3 L yielded significantly lower clearances. Tidal peritoneal dialysis achieved creatinine clearances 20 percent better than intermittent flow peritoneal dialysis at the same overall dose of peritoneal dialysis solution. Eight-hour TPD provided creatinine clearances equal to 24-hour CAPD in patients with higher than average peritoneal permeability (dialysate to plasma creatinine at 4-hour dwell time > 0.65). In patients with lower than average peritoneal permeability, creatinine clearances over 8 hours of TPD were 10 to 20 percent lower than those of 24-hour CAPD. We concluded that for these patients, 9 to 10 hours of nightly TPD would be needed to match 24-hour CAPD creatinine clearance.[94]

Chronic Nightly Tidal Peritoneal Dialysis Study

This ongoing study is designed to test the conclusions of the acute study. Only stable peritoneal dialysis patients are eligible for the study. The patients are intended to remain on TPD for at least 4 months. TPD is performed on a modified PAC-X-2 cycler where the drain phase is regulated by a target volume. Clearances are measured at the beginning of chronic NTPD in all patients. The time of the dialysis session is adjusted to provide creatinine clearances similar to those on CAPD. Serum chemistries are followed monthly, and clearance measurements are repeated after 2 months of treatment. Every month the patient is assessed for clinical symptoms and signs of adequate dialysis. Three patients completed at least 3 months of study, including one patient who has continued on TPD for 17 months. All patients achieved clinically adequate dialysis and stable blood chemistries (Table 4-9). The mean time of TPD sessions to match CAPD creatinine clearance was 9 hours and 45 minutes in the three patients with low average peritoneal transport rates. Compared with CAPD, TPD of such duration yielded daily urea and potassium clearances 40 to 60 percent higher and phosphorus and protein 20 to 40 percent lower. One patient with high average peritoneal transport rates was recently commenced on TPD. This patient requires 8 hours and 35 minutes of nightly TPD to match CAPD creatinine clearance (Table 4-10).

Technical Problems

The technique requires uninterrupted dialysate drainage with an outflow rate of at least 150 ml/min in the supine position to assure delivery and drainage of the prescribed dose of dialysis solution in the specified time. Because of the constant presence of intraperitoneal reservoir volume, the difficulties with fluid outflow are rare. The cycler relies on gravity inflow and

Table 4-9. Results of Chronic Nightly Tidal Peritoneal Dialysis Study (Mean in Three Patients)

	CAPD (4 Months Before Study)	TPD (Initial)	TPD (After 3 Months)
Dialysis to plasma creatinine at 4-hour dwell	.59	.62	.58
Time of dialysis (hr)	24	9.15	9.72
Dialysis solution sodium (mEq/L)	132	132	125
Hematocrit (%)	25.3	27.8	26.6
BUN (mg/dl)	69.0	74.7	63.3
Urea clearance (L/d)	8.4	11.0	11.6
Serum creatinine (mg/dl)	12.6	13.0	13.3
Creatinine clearance (L/d)	6.6	6.5	6.6
Serum potassium (mEq/L)	4.2	4.1	5.2
Potassium clearance (L/d)	7.9	12.5	12.9
Serum phosphorus (mg/dl)	4.6	5.2	5.2
Phosphorus clearance (L/d)	7.2	5.6	6.2
Serum total protein (g/dl)	6.3	6.5	6.7
Protein clearance (L/d)	0.110	0.068	0.068

outflow; thus, the height of the bed is crucial for adequate flows. The best flow conditions are when the height of the patient is in the middle, between the heater and drainage bags (approximately 80 cm in both directions). The drainage problems occurred in patients with a low position of the bed. One patient had many times lower flow rates activating cycler alarms in spite of a proper position of the bed. Because of this problem, the patient could not complete the whole 4-month period of the study. A peritoneography[66] showed the catheter tip in the anterior paracolic gutter rather than in the pelvis. Only a small amount of fluid was seen around the tip. The patient had multiple adhesions due to previous severe peritonitis. Thus, when the patient drained in the supine position, the tip was far from the bulk of the fluid; consequently, the drainage flow rate was inadequate. Another patient had

Table 4-10. CAPD and NTPD Data in a Patient with High-Average Peritoneal Transport

	CAPD	TPD
Creatinine dialysis to plasma ratio at 4-hour dwell	0.79	
Dialysis time (hrs:min)	24:00	8:35
Dialysis solution dose (L/d)	8.0	30.0
Urea clearance (L/d)	9.9	12.5
Creatinine clearance (L/d)	8.3	8.7
Potassium clearance (L/d)	8.2	11.1
Phosphorus clearance (L/d)	9.7	7.6
Protein clearance (L/d)	0.117	0.120

relatively frequent cycler false alarms interrupting her sleep. The third patient felt much better on 9 hours and 15 minutes of nightly TPD than on CAPD; the study has been extended for this patient.

Prediction of ultrafiltration is important to assure that the reserve volume remains unchanged during dialysis. If ultrafiltration volume were overestimated, the reserve volume would become gradually depleted. If ultrafiltration volume were underestimated, the reserve volume would gradually increase, leading to abdominal discomfort. Contrary to our initial concerns, ultrafiltration predictions were easy and accurate within 300 ml.

CONCLUSION

The criteria of peritoneal dialysis adequacy are based mainly on clinical grounds. My experience indicates that clinically adequate dialysis may be achieved in anuric patients with weekly creatinine clearances of 40 to 50 L/1.73 m^2 body surface area. All peritoneal dialysis patients should receive individualized dialysis. The standardized peritoneal equilibration test is a valuable tool in optimizing the dialysis prescription. Continuous ambulatory peritoneal dialysis remains the most suitable dialysis regimen for most peritoneal dialysis patients. The CCPD patient population is growing rapidly. Nightly peritoneal dialysis is indicated in patients with high peritoneal transport and in patients with complications related to high intraabdominal pressure. Tidal peritoneal dialysis increases the efficiency of dialysis by approximately 20 percent compared with standard intermittent peritoneal dialysis with complete dialysate drainage of each exchange. Tidal peritoneal dialysis can render adequate dialysis for every patient provided the time of dialysis sessions is appropriate. This time most likely will not exceed 10 h/night, even in anuric patients with low peritoneal membrane transport rates. A new, fully automated peritoneal dialysis machine is needed for TPD to provide inexpensive dialysis solution of flexible composition in large quantities, as well as safe and false alarm-free dialysis sessions.

REFERENCES

1. Rosenak S, Siwon P: Experimentelle Untersuchungen über die Peritoneale Ausscheidung harnpflichtiger Substanzen aus dem Blute. Mitteilungen Grenzgebieten Med Chir 39: 391, 1926
2. Heusser H, Werder H: Untersuchungen über Peritonealdialyse. Bruns Beitrage klin Chir 141: 38, 1927
3. Balázs J, Rosenak S: Zur Behandlung der Sublimaturie durch peritoneale Dialyse. Wien Med Wochensch 47: 851, 1934
4. Wear JB, Sisk IR, Trinkle AJ: Peritoneal lavage in the treatment of uremia. J Urol 39: 53, 1938
5. Bliss S, Kastler AO, Nadler SB: Peritoneal lavage. Effective elimination of

nitrogenous wastes in the absence of kidney function. Proc Soc Exp Biol Med 29: 1978, 1932

6. Haam vE, Fine A: Effect of peritoneal lavage in acute uremia. Proc Soc Exp Biol Med 30: 396, 1932

7. Rhoads JE: Peritoneal lavage in the treatment of renal insufficiency. Am J Med Sci 196: 642, 1938

8. Odel HM, Ferris DO, Power MH: Peritoneal lavage as an effective means of extrarenal excretion. A clinical appraisal. Am J Med 9: 63, 1950

9. Legrain M, Merrill JP: Short-term continuous transperitoneal dialysis: a simplified technique. N Engl J Med 248: 125, 1953

10. Ascari S, Morales P, Hotchkiss RS: Peritoneal dialysis. NY State J Med 59: 1981, 1959

11. Maxwell MH, Rockney RE, Kleeman CR, Twiss MR: Peritoneal dialysis. I. Technique and applications. JAMA, 170: 917, 1959

12. Doolan PD, Murphy WP, Wiggins RA, et al: An evaluation of intermittent peritoneal lavage. Am J Med 26: 831, 1959

13. Boen ST: Kinetics of peritoneal dialysis. Medicine 40: 243, 1961

14. Teckhoff H, Ward G, Boen ST: The influence of dialysate volume and flow rate on peritoneal clearance. Proc Eur Dialysis Transplant Assoc 2: 113, 1965

15. Boen ST, Mulinari AS, Dillard DH, Scribner BH: Periodic peritoneal dialysis in the management of chronic uremia. Trans Am Soc Artif Internal Organs 8: 256, 1962

16. Tenckhoff H, Schechter H: A bacteriologically safe peritoneal access device. Trans Am Soc Artif Internal Organs 14: 181, 1968

17. Tenckhoff H, Shilipetar G, Van Paasschen WH, Swanson E: A home peritoneal dialysate delivery system. Trans Am Soc Artif Internal Organs 15: 103, 1969

18. Popovich RP, Moncrief JW, Decherd JF, et al: The definition of a novel portable/wearable equilibrium dialysis technique. Abstr Am Soc Artif Internal Organs 5: 64A, 1976

19. Popovich RP, Moncrief JW, Nolph KD, et al: Continuous ambulatory peritoneal dialysis. Ann Intern Med 88: 449, 1978

20. Oreopoulos DG, Robson M, Izatt S, et al: A simple and safe technique for continuous ambulatory peritoneal dialysis. Trans Am Soc Artif Internal Organs 24: 484, 1978

21. Twardowski ZJ: Peritoneal dialysis glossary. II. Peritoneal Dialysis Int 8: 15, 1988

22. Pendras JP, Erickson RV: Hemodialysis: a successful therapy for chronic uremia. Ann Intern Med 64: 293, 1966

23. De Palma JR, Abukurah A, Rubini ME: "Adequacy" of haemodialysis. Proc Eur Dialysis Transplant Assoc 9: 265, 1972

24. Twardowski Z: The adequacy of haemodialysis in treatment of chronic renal failure. Acta Med Pol 15: 227, 1974

25. Parker TF, Laird NM, Lowrie EG: Comparison of the study groups in the National Cooperative Dialysis Study and a description of morbidity, mortality, and patient withdrawal. Kidney Int 23: suppl 13, S-42, 1983

26. Twardowski ZJ, Nolph KD: Opinion: peritoneal dialysis—how much is enough? Semin Dialysis 1: 75, 1988

27. Ahmad S, Gallagher N, Shen FH: Intermittent peritoneal dialysis: Status reassessed. Trans Am Soc Artif Internal Organs 25: 86, 1979

28. Ghantous WN, Salkin MS, Adelson BN, et al: Limitations of peritoneal dialysis

(PD) in the treatment of ESRD patients. Trans Am Soc Artif Internal Organs 25: 100, 1979

29. Schmidt RW, Blumenkrantz MJ: IPD, CAPD, CCPD, CRPD—peritoneal dialysis: past, present and future. Int J Artif Organs 4: 124, 1981

30. Twardowski ZJ: Apparently inadequate peritoneal membrane function for solute removal. p. 134. Nissenson AR, Fine RN (eds): Dialysis Therapy. Hanley and Belfus, Philadelphia, 1986

31. Smeby LC, Wideroe TE, Jorstad S: Individual differences in water transport during continuous peritoneal dialysis. Am Soc Artif Internal Organs J 4: 17, 1981

32. Slingeneyer A, Canaud B, Mion C: Permanent loss of ultrafiltration capacity of the peritoneum in long-term peritoneal dialysis: an epidemiological study. Nephron 33: 133, 1983

33. Wideroe TE, Smeby LC, Mjaaland S, et al: Long-term changes in transperitoneal water transport during continuous ambulatory peritoneal dialysis. Nephron 38: 238, 1984

34. Faller B, Marichal JF: Loss of ultrafiltration in continuous ambulatory peritoneal dialysis: a role for acetate. Peritoneal Dialysis Bull 4: 10, 1984

35. Verger C, Larpent L, Dumontet M: Prognostic value of peritoneal equilibration curves in CAPD patients. p. 88. In Maher JF, Winchester JF (eds): Frontiers in Peritoneal Dialysis. Field, Rich and Associates, New York, 1986

36. Smeby LC, Wideroe TE, Mjaaland S, Dahl K: Changes in ultrafiltration and solute transport during CAPD. p. 68. In Maher JF, Winchester JF (eds): Frontiers in Peritoneal Dialysis. Field, Rich and Associates, New York, 1986

37. Spencer PC, Farrell PC: Solute and water kinetics in CAPD. p. 38. In Gokal R (ed): Continuous Ambulatory Peritoneal Dialysis. Churchill Livingstone, Edinburgh, 1986

38. Twardowski ZJ: Individualized dialysis for CAPD patients. Uremia Invest 8: 35, 1984

39. Babb AL, Strand MJ, Uvelli DA, et al: Quantitative description of dialysis treatment a dialysis index. Kidney Int 7: suppl 2, S-23, 1975

40. Gotch FA, Sargent JA, Klein ML, et al: Clinical results of intermittent dialysis therapy guided by ongoing kinetic analysis of urea metabolism. Trans Am Soc Artif Internal Organs 22: 175, 1976

41. Gotch FA, Sargent JA: A mechanistic analysis of the national cooperative dialysis study. Kidney Int 23: suppl 13, S-103, 1983

42. Johnson WJ, Schniepp BJ: Comparison of urea kinetic modeling with other approaches to dialysis prescription. Dialysis Transplant 10: 280, 1981

43. Teschan PE, Ginn HE, Bourne JR, et al: A prospective study of reduced dialysis. Am Soc Artif Internal Organs J 6: 108, 1983

44. Lysaght MJ, Pollock CA, Hallet MD, et al: The relevance of urea kinetic modeling to CAPD. ASAIO Trans (in press)

45. Boen ST, Haagsman-Schouten WAG, Birnie RJ: Long-term peritoneal dialysis and a peritoneal dialysis-index. Dialysis Transplant 7: 377, 1978

46. Frank HA, Seligman AM, Fine J: Further experiences with peritoneal irrigation for acute renal failure. Ann Surg 128: 561, 1948

47. Miller JH, Gipstein R, Margules R, et al: Automated peritoneal dialysis: analysis of several methods of peritoneal dialysis. Trans Am Soc Artif Internal Organs 12: 98, 1966

48. Pirpasopoulos M, Lindsay RM, Rahman M, Kennedy AC: A cost-effectiveness study of dwell times in peritoneal dialysis. Lancet 2: 1135, 1972

49. Kablitz C, Stephen RL, Duffy DP, et al: Technological augmentation of peritoneal urea clearance: past, present, and future. Dialysis Transplant 9: 741, 1980

50. Randerson DH: Continuous Ambulatory Peritoneal Dialysis—A Critical Appraisal. PhD Thesis, Sydney, Australia, University of New South Wales, 1980

51. Farrell PC, Randerson DH: Mass transfer kinetics in continuous ambulatory peritoneal dialysis. p. 34. In Lagrain M (ed): Continuous Ambulatory Peritoneal Dialysis. Excerpta Medica, Amsterdam, 1980

52. Pyle WK: Mass Trasfer in Peritoneal Dialysis. PhD Thesis, Austin, TX, University of Texas, 1981

53. Garred LJ, Canaud B, Farrell PC: A simple kinetic model for assessing peritoneal mass transfer in continuous ambulatory peritoneal dialysis. Am Soc Artif Internal Organs J 6: 131, 1983

54. Popovich RP, Moncrief JW, Pyle WK: Transport kinetics. p. 96. In Nolph KD (eds): Peritoneal Dialysis. 3rd Ed. Kluwer Academic Publishers, BV Dordrecht, 1989

55. Hiatt MP, Pyle WK, Moncrief JW, Popovich RP: A comparison of the relative efficacy of CAPD and hemodialysis in the control of solute concentration. Artif Organs 4: 37, 1980

56. Mactier RA, Twardowski ZJ: Influence of dwell time, osmolality, and volume of exchanges on solute mass transfer and ultrafiltration in peritoneal dialysis. Semin Dialysis 1: 40, 1988

51. Mactier RA, Khanna R, Twardowski Z, Nolph KD: Role of peritoneal cavity lymphatic absorption in peritoneal dialysis. Kidney Int 32: 165, 1987

58. Mactier RA, Khanna R, Twardowski Z, et al: Contribution of lymphatic absorption to loss of ultrafiltration and solute clearances in CAPD. J Clin Invest 80: 1311, 1987

59. Twardowski ZJ, Nolph KD, Khanna R, et al: Peritoneal equilibration test. Peritoneal Dialysis Bull 7: 138, 1987

60. Twardowski ZJ, Khanna R, Nolph KD: Peritoneal dialysis modifications to avoid CAPD dropouts. p. 171. In Khanna R, Nolph KD, Prowant B, et al (eds): Advances in Continuous Ambulatory Peritoneal Dialysis. Peritoneal Dialysis Bulletin, Toronto, 1987

61. Twardowski ZJ: New approaches to intermittent peritoneal dialysis therapies. p. 133. In Nolph KD (ed): Peritoneal Dialysis. 3rd Ed. Kluwer Academic Publishers BV, Dordrecht, 1989

62. Twardowski ZJ: Clinical value of standardized equilibration tests in CAPD patients. Blood Purif 7: 95, 1989

63. Mactier RA, Khanna R, Twardowski Z, Nolph KD: Ultrafiltration failure in continuous ambulatory peritoneal dialysis due to excessive peritoneal cavity lymphatic absorption. Am J Kidney Dis 10: 461, 1987

64. Verger C: Relationship between peritoneal membrane structure and its permeability. p. 87. In Khanna R, Nolph KD, Prowant B, et al (eds): Advances in Continuous Ambulatory Peritoneal Dialysis. Peritoneal Dialysis Bulletin, Toronto, 1987

65. Twardowski ZJ, Tully RJ, Nichols WK, Sunderrajan S: Computerized tomography in the diagnosis of subcutaneous leak sites during continuous ambulatory peritoneal dialysis (CAPD). Peritoneal Dialysis Bull 4: 163, 1984

66. Twardowski ZJ, Tully RJ, Ersoy FF, Dedhia NM: Computerized tomography with and without intraperitoneal contrast for determination of intraabdominal fluid distribution and diagnosis of complications in peritoneal dialysis patients. ASAIO Trans (in press)

67. Nolph KD, Lindblad AS, Novak JW: Current concepts: continuous ambulatory peritoneal dialysis. N Engl J Med 318: 1595, 1988

68. Diaz-Buxo JA, Walker PJ, Chandler JP, et al: Experience with intermittent peritoneal dialysis and continuous cyclic peritoneeal dialysis. Am J Kidney Dis 4: 242, 1984

69. Ahmad S, Shen FH, Blagg CR: Intermittent peritoneal dialysis as renal replacement therapy. p. 179.. Nolph KD (ed): Peritoneal Dialysis. 2nd Ed. Martinus Nijhoff Publishing, Boston, 1985

70. Nolph KD, Hano JE, Teschan PE: Peritoneal sodium transport during hypertonic peritoneal dialysis: physiologic mechanisms and clinical implications. Ann Intern Med 70: 931, 1969

71. Nolph KD, Sorkin MI, Moore H: Autoregulation of sodium and potassium removal during continuous ambulatory peritoneal dialysis. Trans Am Soc Artif Internal Organs 6: 334, 1980

72. Rubin J, Klein F, Bower JD: Investigation of the net sieving coefficient of the peritoneal membrane during peritoneal dialysis. Am Soc Artif Internal Organs J 5: 9, 1982

73. Boyer J, Gill GN, Epstein FH: Hyperglycemia and hyperosmolality complicating peritoneal dialysis. Ann Intern Med 67: 568, 1967

74. Miller RB, Tassistro CR: Peritoneal dialysis. N Engl J Med 281: 945, 1969

75. Twardowski ZJ, Nolph KD, Khanna R, (et al): Daily clearances with continuous ambulatory peritoneal dialysis and nightly peritoneal dialysis. ASAIO Trans 32: 575, 1986

76. Vas SI: Peritonitis. p. 261. In Nolph KD, (ed): Peritoneal Dialysis. 3rd Ed. Kluwer Academic Publishers BV, Dordrecht, 1989

77. Grodstein GP, Blumenkrantz MJ, Kopple JD, et al: Glucose absorption during continuous ambulatory peritoneal dialysis. Kidney Int 19: 564, 1981

78. Heide B, Pierratos A, Khanna R, et al: Nutritional status of patients undergoing continuous ambulatory peritoneal dialysis. Peritoneal Dialysis Bull 3: 138, 1983

79. Chan MK, Baillod RA, Tanner A, et al: Abdominal hernias in patients receiving continuous ambulatory peritoneal dialysis. B Med J 283: 826, 1981

80. Digenis GD, Khanna R, Mathews R, et al: Abdominal hernias in patients undergoing continuous ambulatory peritoneal dialysis. Peritoneal Dialysis Bull 2: 115, 1982

81. Diaz-Buxo JA: Continuous cyclic peritoneal dialysis. p. 169. In Nolph KD (ed): Peritoneal Dialysis. 3rd Ed. Kluwer Academic Publishers BV, Dordrecht, 1989

82. Bargman JM, Oreopoulos DG: Complications other than peritonitis or those related to the catheter and the fate of uremic organ dysfunction in patients receiving peritoneal dialysis. p. 289. In Nolph KD (ed): Peritoneal Dialysis. 3rd Ed. Kluwer Academic Publishers BV, Dordrecht, 1989

83. Twardowski ZJ, Khanna R, Nolph KD, et al: Intraabdominal pressure during natural activities in patients treated with continuous ambulatory peritoneal dialysis. Nephron 44: 129, 1986

84. Scribner BH: A current perspective on the role of intermittent vs. continuous ambulatory peritoneal dialysis. Proc North East Regional Meeting Renal Physicians Assoc 3: 76, 1979

85. Diaz-Buxo JA, Walker PJ, Farmer CD, et al: Continuous cyclic peritoneal dialysis—a preliminary report. Artif Organs 5: 157, 1981

86. Diaz-Buxo JA, Walker PJ, Farmer CD, et al: Continuos cyclic peritoneal dialysis. Trans Am Soc Artif Internal Organs 27: 51, 1981

87. Lasker N, McCauley EP, Passarotti CT: Chronic peritoneal dialysis. Trans Am Soc Artif Internal Organs 12: 94, 1966
88. Health Devices. Edited by ECRI. Plymouth Meeting, PA, 15: 31, 1986
89. Nissenson AR: Indications for CCPD in the adult. Perspect Peritoneal Dialysis 3: 46, 1985
90. Nolph KD, Twardowski ZJ, Khanna R: Clinical pathology conference: peritoneal dialysis. ASAIO Trans 32: 11, 1986
91. Scribner BH: Forward to second edition. p. XI. In Nolph KD (ed): Peritoneal Dialysis. Martinus Nijhoff Publishing, Boston, 1985
92. Di Paolo N: Semicontinuous peritoneal dialysis. Dialysis Transplant 7: 839, 1978
93. Finkelstein FO, Kliger AS: Enhanced efficiency of peritoneal dialysis using rapid, small-volume exchanges. Am Soc Artif Internal Organs J 2: 102, 1979
94. Twardowski ZJ, Nolph KD, Khanna R, et al: Tidal peritoneal dialysis. Proceedings of the IVth Congress of the International Society for Peritoneal Dialysis. Venice, June 29–July 2, 1987 (in press)

5

Peritoneal Dialysis Access

Ramesh Khanna

(Continues)

LONG-TERM RESULTS

INTRODUCTION

The Tenckhoff version of the silicone catheter[1] is still the most widely used catheter for peritoneal dialysis. Modifications of catheter design, placement techniques, meticulous postoperative care, and a standardized break-in procedure have contributed to overall better longevity, catheter function, and reduction in catheter-related complications such as catheter tip migration, dialysis solution leak, and exit site infection. Nevertheless, catheter exit site and tunnel infections are frequent in patients on continuous ambulatory peritoneal dialysis (CAPD) and are the major causes of increased morbidity, prolonged antibiotic therapy, recurrent peritonitis, and catheter failure. According to the National CAPD Registry, 12.4 percent of catheters are removed because of exit or tunnel infection.[2] This chapter will highlight and update information previously published in an even more extensive review.[3] We will review the requirements of an ideal catheter, the standard Tenckhoff catheter and its modifications, placement techniques, frequently observed complications and their management, and long-term catheter care in CAPD patients.

HISTORY OF CATHETER DEVELOPMENT

In the early years of peritoneal dialysis, access to the peritoneal cavity was improvised from available surgical equipment. Some of the materials used were metal trocars, surgical drains made of glass, gall bladder trocars, Foley catheters, perforated rubber and stainless steel tubing, and sump drains.[4-9] Although these devices allowed for adequate in-and-out flow, problems such as dialysis solution leak, infection, catheter occlusion by clot or omentum, pressure stress on tissues, constant suction of contaminated air into the peritoneal cavity, and inability to fix the tube to abdominal wall were frequent. Rosenak and Oppenheimer[10] were the first to develop an access specifically meant for peritoneal dialysis. Their access consisted of an upper rigid tube with an interchangeable flexible lower stainless steel coil extension. A straight inner tube extended from the outlet to the upper part of a flexible tube. This inner tube was connected to suction through a rubber tubing. This device permitted continuous inflow through the outer tube and outflow through the inner tube. There was an adjustable tie plate for fixation of the tube to skin. This device overcame some of the problems but did not become popular, because of inadequate drainage and because the metal tube was irritating to the peritoneum.

The next major progress was the introduction of polyvenyl chloride (PVC) and nylon rigid catheters[11-15] with multiple side perforations, slightly curved at the distal end with a solid rounded tip. The small perforations prevented omentum from entering the lumen during drainage. These catheters required the help of a trocar or stylet for their insertion into the peritoneal cavity. These devices improved catheter function considerably, but pericatheter dialysis solution leak and infections occurred at a high rate.

Implantation of an indwelling peritoneal teflon button in the abdominal wall was the next innovation.[16–18] A long rigid catheter was inserted inside the peritoneal cavity through these buttons. After each dialysis, the catheter was removed and the button was capped. Frequent episodes of peritonitis were a major problem. Because of frequent infections, Boen et al.[19] developed the intermittent puncture technique. Jacob and Deane[20] invented a teflon rod to keep the catheter hole patent between dialyses. At approximately the same time, subcutaneous access devices were designed and used with success.[21]

Palmer et al.[22] developed catheters made of polyethylene, polypropylene, and nylon. These catheters were relatively rigid; hence, they did not always make a good seal at the exit site. Also, these materials posed difficulties in creating a subcutaneous tunnel. Palmer et al. were looking for a catheter material that would be more biocompatible and less irritating to the peritoneum. The observations of Gutch[23] in both acute and chronic patients pointed out the remarkable compatibility of silastic with the peritoneal membrane. He found considerably lower protein losses in patients using silastic material compared with PVC. This finding led Palmer et al.[24] to develop the first permanent silicone catheter. This catheter had a long intramural segment. The intraperitoneal segment was coiled and had lead at the tip to prevent catheter migration. Halfway along the tube was a triflanged step for fixing the tube in the deep fascia and peritoneum. This catheter sealed properly at the exit site and, because of the long subcutaneous tunnel, prevented migration of bacteria to the peritoneal cavity. McDonald et al.[25] incorporated a Teflon velour skirt in the subcutaneous tissue and a Dacron-weaveknit sleeve from the skirt down to the peritoneum. Tenckhoff and Schechter[1] modified Palmer et al.'s catheter in several ways to adapt it for chronic use. For better mechanical fixation of the catheter to the abdominal wall tissue, they bonded felt Dacron cuffs to the catheter. To simplify the implantation procedure, they shortened the intramural tunnel segment. The intraperitoneal segment was kept open-ended and the sizes of the side holes were optimized to 0.5 mm to prevent tissue incarceration. For bedside insertion of the catheter, they developed the metal trocar that is still being used by many investigators. In CAPD patients, the use of the Tenckhoff catheter was associated with a high incidence of catheter tip displacement and poor solution drainage. To prevent such complications, several modified catheters were used in the subsequent years.[26–29]

REQUIREMENTS FOR OPTIMUM CATHETER FUNCTION

Catheter Material

Biocompatibility of the material used for catheters is a foremost requirement. Catheters made of polyethylene, polypropylene, and nylon were used extensively in the early days. These catheters were relatively rigid and did not always make a good seal at the exit site. Also, these materials posed difficulties in creating a subcutaneous tunnel. At about the same time, arteriovenous shunts made of silastic were found biocompatible for patients on hemodialysis. The observations of Gutch[23] on the remarkable compatibility of silastic for peritoneal use led to the development of the first permanent silicone catheter.[24] Because it is soft, flexible, atraumatic to the tissues, and biocompatible, silastic has remained the standard material for catheters. Catheters made of polyurethane have recently, been found to be biocompatible for human use.[30]

Role of the Catheter Cuff in the Tunnel

Catheter cuffs establish a mechanical bond with the surrounding tissues and provide a firm catheter anchorage. They also, prevent the formation of a fistulous communication between the exterior and peritoneum. Thus, cuffs create a mechanical barrier and prevent the entrance of external contaminants from entering the peritoneal cavity. Catheters are manufactured with either a single or double cuffs. When implanted, a single cuff catheter may have its cuff located either under the skin or at the peritoneal level. With a double cuff catheter implantation, a cuff is positioned under the skin and another is positioned at the preperitoneal level. In patients undergoing chronic intermittent peritoneal dialysis, single and double cuff catheters yield similar results.[31] However, in CAPD patients, the added benefit of one catheter over the other has not been clearly established.[32,33] In a retrospective survey of catheter complications in 395 patients, the tunnel infections were almost three times more frequent with single cuff than with double cuff catheters.[34] Also, in our experience, the exit infections tend to be more frequent and are significantly more resistant to treatment with single cuff catheters compared with double cuff catheters.[29] The discrepancy in the results reported may be partly due to variable implantation techniques. Nevertheless, personal preferences and biases based on experience seem to guide the individual center to use either of the catheters.

Material for the Cuff

The external cuff should promote quick mechanical binding with collagen fibers to provide a strong anchorage to the implanted catheter. Nonliving materials, such as a dacron cuff, have been used with success to provide a strong bond between it and collagen. In experiments on miniature pigs, Dacron velour, especially when wet with saline before implantation, provided the strongest collagen attachment with an excellent inhibition of epidermal down growth.[35] Twardowski's[36] observations of catheter cuffs removed from long-term CAPD patients indicated a profuse collagen tissue ingrowth between the Dacron felt cuff fibers providing a strong bondage between the two. However, in order to prevent sinus tract formation by promoting collagen ingrowth into the device, Dasse et al.[30] designed and used, with short-term success, catheters made of porous polyurethane material. Long-term outcomes with this material are still awaited. Paradoxic to these observations, the use of a polytetrafluoroethylene-covered right-angle catheter by Ogden et al.[37] resulted in a high rate of chronic exit site infections. Thus the saline-wetted Dacron velour presently seems to be the best material for the cuff.

Direction of Catheter Tunnel and Skin Exit

The direction of the tunnel and skin exit in relation to the long axis of the body may have significant influence on the frequency of exit infection and its management. A tunnel with an exit hole pointing cranially is prone to contamination by down-flowing sweat, water, and dirt on the skin surface. Whenever such an exit is infected, the pus tends to penetrate deep down into the tunnel and appears to be resistant to treatment because of poor pus drainage to the outside. As early as the late 1960s, and probably to facilitate pus drainage for the implantation of a straight Tenckhoff catheter, Tenckhoff and Schechter[1] recommended the creation of an arc tunnel with the skin exit pointing downward. Because of the catheter resilience, after a period of time such an arc tended to transform into a straight tunnel and caused cuff extrusion. Because of the high incidence of superficial cuff extrusion in CAPD patients, investigators preferred to create a straight tunnel with the exit pointing cranially. A retrospective analysis of our catheter experience showed that catheters with tunnels and skin exits directed downward tend to get infected less often and, when infected, were significantly less resistant to treatment than ones with tunnels and skin exits directed elsewhere.[29] Thus, in chronic peritoneal dialysis patients, creating a catheter tunnel and skin exit with a caudal direction might be conducive to less contamination, better drainage of necrotic material in the immediate postimplantation period, and, when infected, would drain better compared with other directions.

Catheter Tip Migration

The optimum conditions for free flow of dialysis solution are created when the catheter tip is positioned in the true pelvis. In the upright position, the pelvis is the most dependent part of the peritoneal cavity. Moreover, in the majority, the omentum does not reach all the way into the true pelvis. Twardowski et al.[29] observed that when a catheter was implanted with the tunnel and skin exit directed downward and the intraperitoneal entrance directed upward (either pointing to liver or spleen), even if the catheter tip was placed in the true pelvis, the tip invariably migrated to the upper abdomen. Because it is not anchored in the peritoneal cavity, the position of the intraperitoneal segment is influenced by the silastic resilience force. Therefore, to create favorable conditions for the catheter tip to remain deep in the pelvis, the intramural segment in the tunnel and the intraperitoneal segment in the peritoneal cavity must be implanted in such a way as to direct them toward the pelvis.

In order to satisfy the requirement of a tunnel with caudally directed skin exit and peritoneal entry, the catheter should be implanted in an arc tunnel. To implant catheters in such a manner and to avoid the unfavorable consequences of silastic resilience forces, the catheters should be manufactured with a molded curve in its intramural segment, as in the Swan Neck catheters.[29] A molded bend between cuffs eliminates the silastic resilience forces or the "shape memory" which tends to extrude the external cuff and displace the catheter tip from the pelvis.

Sinus Tract Length

The term sinus tract refers to that part of the tunnel from the skin exit to the margin of the nearest cuff. In CAPD patients, the sinus tract is covered by a continuous layer of epidermis only for 4 to 6 mm from the skin margin and the rest of the tract is covered by foreign body reaction tissue.[36] The epidermis covering the sinus tract undergoes a turnover that is probably similar to the normal epidermis with cell maturation and desquamation. If not expelled, the desquamated epidermal cells and dead inflammatory cells create a favorable milieu for bacterial growth. A long sinus tract may not be the most efficient for drainage of such debris, and may predispose to a higher incidence of infection.[38-40] Therefore, the sinus tract length should be as short as possible, preferably the length of the epidermal layer.

Pulling, twisting, and tugging forces applied unintentionally on the catheter during its daily use may cause recurrent tear and trauma, resulting in bleeding and external extrusion. A vector force, directed to the exterior, created by maturing epidermal basal cells in the sinus tract tends to extrude the implant.[38] The rate of implant migration due to this vector force has been calculated at 1 mm/mo in miniature pigs.[38] The resilience of the straight silastic catheter implanted in an arcuate tunnel undoubtedly plays a major role in cuff extrusion, but pulling and tugging forces applied on the catheter during its daily usage also contribute significantly to this complication.

Thus, in order to promote epidermal growth as close to the collagen in the vicinity of cuff, the sinus tract needs to be no longer than 4 to 6 mm; yet, a longer sinus tract length may be needed to avoid cuff extrusion. As a compromise, the cuff should be implanted approximately 1 cm from the exit. Resilience forces could be eliminated with a molded bent catheter, as in the Swan Neck catheters, which will be discussed below.

Uninterrupted Dialysis Solution Flow

When the peritoneal cavity is full of dialysis solution, the freely mobile small intestine and the active omentum tend to float over the fluid sump. During the drainage, fluid typically runs out at a rate of 200 ml/min, thus creating a negative suction due to a siphon effect, the force of which is determined by the difference in the height between the catheter tip and the empty dialysis bag. This force tends to pull the abdominal contents toward the catheter tip and side holes, occluding and preventing free drainage of dialysis solution. When the catheter tip is placed deep in the true pelvis, omentum is unable to reach the side holes and tip, allowing free fluid flow. Therefore, an ideal catheter design should include the means to stabilize the intraperitoneal portion of the catheter deep in the pelvis.

Tissue Reaction to a Foreign Body and Factors That Cause Early Infection and Delay Healing

The tissue reaction immediately after a break in the integument begins by forming a coagulum of clot and cellular debris at the site of injury. Polymorphonuclear leukocytes phagocytize invading bacteria. Together with the coagulum, cellular debris forms a scab. Healing starts with the formation of granulation tissue composed of new vessels, inflammatory cells, and fibroblasts enmeshed in the collagen fibers. Peripheral ingrowth of new epithelial cells begins to cover the granulation tissue. Based on animal experiments, it has been theorized that these cells stop spreading over the granulation tissue only if they meet cells from the opposite end or encounter collagen fibers attached to the foreign body (Dacron cuff in the case of peritoneal catheter), thus creating a sinus tract.[38] Twardowski's[36] of observations sinus tracts in humans removed several years after catheter insertion indicate that epidermal down growth stops 4 to 6 mm from the exit. The factors that stop the down growth of epidermis in the sinus tract of humans are unclear at this time. As the process of healing continues, part of the coagulum is absorbed and part of it, along with necrotic tissue, gradually drains from the sinus tract. Epidermal cells grow over the granulation tissue beneath the scab. If the scab is forcibly removed during cleansing, the epidermal layer is broken, thus prolonging the process of epidermization. The healing process is complete when the epidermis reaches its final depth (3 to 7 mm in humans) and the granulation tissue is replaced by the foreign body reaction tissue for the remaining distance to the outer cuff.

To promote free drainage of necrotic tissue and prevent skin sloughing, the sinus tract should be made sufficiently wide. Care should be taken to avoid creating too wide a tract because it would permit excessive movement of the catheter at the exit site. Mechanical stresses slow the healing process. To encourage unhindered healing, the catheter should be firmly anchored at the cuff and well-immobilized outside the tunnel, especially during the break-in period. Antibiotic penetration into the coagulum is poor; therefore, antibiotics should be present in sufficient concentration in the blood and tissue fluids before the coagulum is formed. This may be achieved if antibiotics are administered before implantation.

FREQUENTLY USED CATHETERS

An extensive survey by the National CAPD Registry of the National Institutes of Health revealed that a variety of catheters are being used by the surveyed centers.[2] Table 5-1 shows the types and numbers of each catheter used by the surveyed centers. Tenckhoff catheters in various modifications are still the most preferred type of catheters. Figure 5-1 shows frequently used catheters.

Tenckhoff Catheters (Straight, Coiled, Single, and Double Cuff)

The Tenckhoff catheter consists of a length of silicone rubber tube with a 2.6-mm internal diameter and a 5-mm external diameter with varying length and shape. The cuff is made of Dacron felt and is 1 cm long. The double cuff catheter has three segments: external, intramural, and intraperitoneal. The length of the intramural segment may vary between 5 and 7 cm. The length of the intraperitoneal segment can vary between 11 and 15 cm in both single and double cuff catheters. The intraperitoneal and intramural segments in pediatric double cuff catheters are 7 and 2 cm long. The intraperitoneal segment has multiple 0.5-mm perforations in the terminal 3 to 9 cm portion. The coiled Tenckhoff catheter differs from the straight catheter in that is has a longer perforated section that is molded to assume a coiled shape. The length of the coiled section is 18.5 cm. It is claim that the coil prevents migration and reduces the force of the inflowing dialysis stream.

Table 5-1. Number of Catheters and Their Survival Rates

	No. of Catheters Implanted	Months of Survival (%)			
		12	18	24	36
Straight intraperitoneal segment; double cuff	753	70	60	51	33
Straight intraperitoneal segment; single, inner cuff	116	60	44	33	22
Straight intraperitoneal segment; single, outer cuff	66	69	55	55	36
Curled intraperitoneal segment; double cuff	218	69	51	43	34
Curled intraperitoneal segment; single, inner cuff	73	70	64	49	6
Curled intraperitoneal segment; single, outer cuff	21	57	—	—	—
Toronto Western Hospital	94	69	52	35	22
Ash (Lifecath)	49	71	59	47	—
Gore-tex	28	57	41	—	—
Others and unknown	47				

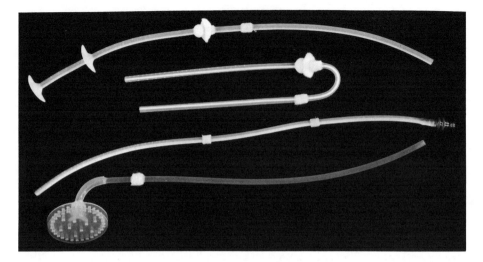

Fig. 5-1. Frequently used peritoneal dialysis catheters. (Top to bottom) Toronto Western Hospital catheter, Swan-Neck Missouri catheter, double cuff Tenckhoff catheter, Lifecath.

The Toronto Western Hospital Catheters

The main distinguishing features of the Toronto Western Hospital catheters[28] are the two flat silicone rubber discs on their intra-abdominal segment. They are available with a barium-impregnated radiopaque stripe to assist in the radiologic localization of the intra-abdominal section. Adult catheters are 41 cm long, whereas pediatric catheters are 35 cm long. The extra-abdominal section of the catheter is approximately 20 cm long and is identical in design to the Tenckhoff catheter. The long length of the extra-abdominal section allows easy handling and reserves enough length to permit trimming if a catheter split occurs at the connector site during its extended use. The distance between the cuffs is approximately 2 cm. A Dacron felt cuff 1 cm wide is bonded to the catheter by the manufacturer (Accurate Surgical Instruments Corporation, Toronto, Ontario, Canada) at the junction of the extra-abdominal section and the subcutaneous part. Except for the absence of a subcutaneous cuff, the Toronto Western II single cuff catheter is identical in design to the Toronto Western II double cuff catheter. The peritoneal end of the short intramural segment of the catheter is provided with another Dacron felt cuff identical to the subcutaneous cuff, and a Dacron disc 1 cm in diameter at the base of this cuff. One millimeter distal to the Dacron disc, an elastic bead or bubble is provided to create a groove on which peritoneum is tightly tied. These modifications are aimed at reducing the incidence of early and late dialysate leaks and the risk of incisional hernias. The fibrous tissue ingrowth bonds the catheter firmly to muscle and fascia to prevent its displacement. When the cuff is routed obliquely through the tissues, this bond will secure the intraperitoneal segment of the catheter in a direction pointing toward the pelvis. At the level of the Dacron cuff, tissue fibrosis in and around the peritoneum forms an effective seal preventing the occurrence of fluid leak. This design affords a good barrier against early or late dialysate leaks and later incision hernias. The intraperitoneal segment of this catheter is 15 cm long and is designed to provide an unrestricted flow of dialysis solution to and from the peritoneal cavity. With the objective of stabilizing the catheter tip deep in the true pelvis, Toronto Western catheters are provided with two flat silicone rubber disks that are 1 mm thick, 28 mm in diameter, and 5 cm apart on the intra-abdominal portion of the catheter. Because of their shape and design, two discs prevent the free mobility of the intra-abdominal section of the catheter in the peritoneal cavity.

Swan Neck Catheters

The noticeable feature of Swan Neck peritoneal dialysis catheters is the molded bend between the two cuffs. This catheter was designed so that the catheter could be implanted in an arcuate tunnel in an unstressed condition with both external and internal segments of the tunnel directed caudally.[29] The current prototype catheter, Swan Neck 2, is made with a 170° arc angle between the two cuffs and the distance between the cuffs is 5 cm.[36]

The Swan Neck catheters are available in three basic designs: the Missouri, Toronto, and Tenckhoff catheters. The Toronto type of Swan Neck catheter adapts the swan neck concept to the Toronto Western Hospital catheter.[41] It has a flange and bead just below the internal cuff. Unlike the Toronto Western Hospital catheter, the flange and bead are slanted approximately 45° relative to the axis of the catheter. When the slanted flange is positioned flat against the posterior rectus sheath, the desired direction of the catheter is maintained within the abdominal wall, with the intraperitoneal portion pointing in the desired caudal direction within the peritoneal cavity. Like Toronto Western Hospital catheters, the Toronto type of catheter is also provided with two intraperitoneal discs. The Missouri catheter is identical to the Swan Neck Toronto catheter except that it is not provided with the intraperitoneal discs. The Tenckhoff type of the Swan Neck peritoneal dialysis catheter differs from the double cuff Tenckhoff catheter only by being permanently bent between the cuffs. This type of catheter may be inserted at the bedside and does not require surgical insertion; however, a subcutaneous tunnel has to be created in the same way as for other Swan Neck catheters (see below).

For a lean person with a thin subcutaneous tissue layer, the distance between the cuffs is shortened to 3 cm (Swan Neck-3 catheter). Otherwise, this catheter, is identical to the Swan Neck-2 catheter. The catheters with longer intraperitoneal segments (22 cm) are suitable for patients who are tall or require the exit site to be placed above the belt line. The Swan Neck coiled catheters have a coiled intraperitoneal segment.

To facilitate recognition of right and left catheters the deep cuff in rectus muscle fascia usually lies medial to the superficial cuff), all Swan Neck catheters are provided with a radiopaque stripe in front of the catheter. The anterior location of the stripe is also helpful during insertion and postimplantation care, to facilitate recognition of catheter twisting. Right and left Swan Neck Tenckhoff catheters differ only with respect to the position of the stripe. Unlike Swan Neck Toronto and Missouri catheters, the Swan Neck Tenckhoff catheter is intended for either a right or left tunnel and can be interchanged. In such a case, the stripe would be positioned posteriorly. Nevertheless, to retain uniformity of the stripe position, it is recommended that Swan Neck Tenckhoff catheters be inserted with the stripe positioned anteriorly.

To aid proper implantation of the Swan Neck catheter with its shape undistorted, stencils have been developed for skin markings before surgery. Preinsertion marking of the site is important to avoid implantation of right for left or vice versa. In such mishaps, we have observed the intraperitoneal segment of catheter to inevitably migrate out of true pelvis because of unfavorable resilience forces. If the tunnel is created too short, the external cuff will inevitably extrude out of the skin exit or the catheter will kink in the tunnel, causing obstruction.

Lifecath Column Disc Catheter

The column disc catheter was developed by Ash et al.[42] Problems of slow outflow and one-way obstruction with the Tenckhoff catheter and its modification led Ash and coworkers to design a catheter that minimized omental involvement, eliminated catheter migration, and decreased fluid inlet velocity. The intra-abdominal end of the catheter is attached to a head made of two parallel discs, 5.1 cm in diameter, of silicone elastomer separated by 40 short pillars 6 mm long and anchored against the abdominal wall by a Dacron felt sleeve. Fixed to the anterior abdominal wall, the column disc catheter cannot drift down into the abdomen between bowel loops as can other catheters. Another Dacron felt sleeve served to stabilize the catheter and prevent exit site infection. Fluid inflow and outflow occur at the periphery of the large disc. Because of the large area of the disc, fluid inflow and outflow velocities are very low, resulting in less attraction of omentum toward the catheter. With the column disc catheter, outflow rate is equal to inflow rate throughout the drainage cycle. For a 2-L exchange, the abdomen could be drained completely within 300 seconds.

Polyurethane Percutaneous Access Device

The polyurethane percutaneous access device is constructed from porous polyurethane.[39] It is designed to encourage infiltration of dermal fibroblast and to promote deposition of collagen into interstices of the intercommunicating pores. The access consists of a small cylinder measuring approximately 1 cm in diameter which protrudes through the skin. This is attached to a thin disc approximately 2.5 cm in diameter which is positioned in a subdermal/subcutaneous plane. The surface of both these components are textured in such a way as to encourage tissue ingrowth. A 12-French (F) polyurethane tube passes through the access device. The tubing is identical to that found in the standard peritoneal dialysis catheters except that it is bent at a right angle as it enters and exits the access device and allows the disc to lie flat in the subdermal plane. An implantable cuff is also provided with the catheter for interfacing with the peritoneum. The cuff is supplied separately to facilitate the insertion of the device. By placing the cuff on the catheter after the access portion of the device is implanted, it can be positioned to account for differences in abdominal wall thickness.

CATHETER INSERTION

Practice of catheter insertion is variable from center to center and is highly influenced by local conditions. The most common insertion approach is either in an operating theater by a surgeon or at the bedside by an experienced nephrologist. The relative merits and demerits of different insertion techniques are summarized in Table 5-2.

Bedside Catheter Insertion Techniques

A rigid or Tenckhoff catheter may be inserted when the need to start peritoneal dialysis is urgent. Because of the ease of insertion at bedside and superior functional characteristics, many prefer Tenckhoff catheters over rigid catheters; many centers have almost abandoned the use of the rigid catheter, even for acute renal failure.[43] During insertion, extreme care

Table 5-2. Comparison of Catheter Insertion Techniques

Insertion Technique	Bedside	Peritoneo-scopic	Guidewire	Surgical
Access	Quick and convenient	Quick and convenient	Quick and convenient	Time-consuming
Incision	Small	Small	Small	Large
Hemostasis	Blind procedure	Good	Blind procedure	Good
Viscus perforation leak, poor flow	Higher	Very low	Higher	Very low
Hernias	Low	Low	Low	Higher
Cost	Low	Low	Low	High
Immediate use	Possible	Possible	Possible	Avoided

should be taken with patients who are extremely obese or who have had previous abdominal surgery, since abdominal adhesions increase the risk of inadvertent viscus perforation. Adherence to proper aseptic technique is an important part of the procedure. The details of the bedside insertion techniques for both rigid and Tenckhoff catheter and related complications have been previously published.[3]

Peritoneoscopic Insertion Technique

The use of peritoneoscopy for peritoneal catheter placement is still relatively new and is slowly becoming popular. In experienced hands, this procedure is relatively simple and devoid of any serious complications. This procedure allows for and ensures the placement of intraperitoneal catheter segments at the desired location, and a major surgical procedure is averted.

The technique reported by Ash and Daugirdas[44] is as follows. Prefilling the peritoneal cavity with dialysis solution is not necessary. After the appropriate local anesthesia, the abdominal wall is penetrated directly through the rectus muscle by a 2.2-mm minitrocar housed in a metal cannula. The cannula is in turn surrounded by an expandable thin plastic Quill cylinder. After penetration of the abdominal wall, the minitrocar is removed from the cannula and replaced with a small 2.2-mm Needlescope. When fully inserted, the sighted tip of the Needlescope is located exactly at the tip of the cannula. The intraperitoneal location of the cannula tip is thus confirmed under direct vision. The Needlescope is removed, and the abdomen is filled with micropore filter-sterilized air via the cannula. The Needlescope is now reinserted into the cannula and, under direct vision, both are advanced together down into the abdomen to the desired location, avoiding the adhesions and omentum that are identified. At this point, the Needlescope and cannula are both removed, leaving only the plastic Quill catheter guide in place. Next, the plastic guide is dilated to 6 mm using two dilators of graded diameter. A Tenckhoff catheter stiffened with an obturator is then inserted into the abdomen through the dilated Quill catheter guide, until the cuff is firmly positioned against the abdominal musculature. For the curled Tenckhoff, the catheter is advanced into the abdomen while holding the obturator in place. The plastic Quill catheter guide and obturator are carefully removed, leaving the catheter in place. The tunneler tool is inserted through a small skin exit site incision. The tool with the attached proximal end of the catheter is then pulled through the skin exit site. Swan Neck Tenckhoff and Swan Neck coil catheters may be inserted with this technique.

Catheter Insertion Through a Guide Wire

This technique can be used for insertion of a straight or curled Tenckhoff catheter and for Swan Neck Tenckhoff and Swan Neck coil catheters. The necessary equipment can be obtained through Cook Company, Bloomington,

IN. With this technique, the incidence of early leak is very low. However, high risks of viscus perforation and improper placement of the catheter are the drawbacks of this technique. Prefilling the abdomen with dialysis solution is essential for this technique of catheter insertion. The guide wire is inserted through the same needle or tubing that is used to fill the abdomen. A dilator, covered in a longitudinally perforated sheath, is then inserted over the guide wire. After the dilator sheath is inserted, the dilator is removed, leaving the sheath in place. The Tenckhoff catheter, stiffened by a soft, partially inserted obturator, is then directed down into the sheath. As the cuff advances, the sheath is split by pulling tabs on its opposing sides. Splitting the sheath allows the cuff to advance to a position next to the abdominal wall. By further splitting and retraction, the sheath is removed from its position around the catheter. The subcutaneous tunnel is then created by the standard procedure.

Surgical Insertion of Catheters for Chronic Dialysis

Preinsertion catheter preparation is essential to optimize catheter function and avoid early complications. To avoid contamination, the catheters should never be touched with bare hands. The unsterilized catheters are carefully withdrawn from the package, washed, drip dried, dried further on lint-free towels, inserted into labeled peel packs, then steam-sterilized at 270°F (132°C) and 30 pounds per square inch (PSI) (2.11 kg/cm^2) for a full cycle. Immediately before implantation, the catheter is removed from the sterile peel pack and immersed in sterile saline. Both the Dacron cuffs and flange are gently squeezed to remove air. When air is removed, the catheter sinks. Thoroughly wetted cuffs provide markedly better tissue ingrowth compared with unwetted, air-containing cuffs.

One day before surgery, abdominal hair should usually be removed with an electric shaver. I strongly recommend identifying and marking the catheter insertion site before surgery. The site chosen usually avoids the midline and belt line, and previous scars, if any. The belt line of the patient is identified, preferably in the sitting and/or standing position, with slacks and belt as usually worn. Depending on the size and shape of the abdomen, and taking into account the patient's preference, the tunnel site is marked. For those with a low belt line site, catheter insertion may be preferred above the belt line. In patients requiring catheter insertion high in the abdominal wall, it is necessary to use a catheter with a longer than standard intraperitoneal segment (approximately 20 cm). For those with a high belt line, the site chosen for insertion is usually below the belt line. In obese people with a pendulous abdomen, it is necessary to insert the catheter above the skin and fat fold; with the patient in the vertical position when the skin and fat fold sags, a lowly placed catheter would drag the intraperitoneal segment out of the pelvis.

In our own protocol, 1 g of vancomycin within 24 hours before surgery or a first-generation cephalosoporin 1 or 2 hours before surgery is given by slow intravenous infusion. Prior to operation, the patient is asked to empty the bladder and bowel and a tapwater enema is given if necessary. It is best to avoid general anesthesia because most patients require voluntary coughing and breathing exercises as a part of postoperative lung care. Additionally, a general anesthetic may promote vomiting and constipation during the postoperative period. Coughing, vomiting, and straining markedly increase intra-abdominal pressure[45] and may increase the risk of dialysis solution leak. With the simultaneous administration of a sedative and a local anesthetic agent, adequate patient relaxation should be obtained for catheter insertion.

Surgical Technique

After the standard surgical preparation of the abdominal wall and adequate local anesthesia with 1 percent lidocaine, a 3- to 4-cm lateral paramedian transverse incision is made through the skin and subcutaneous tissue. Once perfect hemostasis is achieved, an incision is made in the anterior rectus sheath; the rectus muscle fibers are then dissected bluntly in the direction of the fibers down to the posterior rectus sheath. A purse-string suture is placed through the posterior rectus sheath, the transversalis fascia, and the peritoneum. With extreme caution to protect the viscera, a 5-mm incision is made through the peritoneum. The catheter, stiffened with a wetted straight stylet, is introduced deep into the true pelvis until the patient feels some pressure on the bladder or rectum. The radiopaque stripe on the catheter is maintained in the anterior position. The stylet is withdrawn, leaving the catheter in place. After assuring the patency of the catheter with saline infusion, the internal cuff is fixed deep in the rectus muscle with an absorbable suture under direct vision. In the case of Swan Neck Missouri and Toronto Western Hospital catheters, the bead is placed in the peritoneal cavity, the flange is placed on the posterior rectus sheath, and the purse-string suture is tightened between them. The flange is sewn to the posterior rectus sheath with four sutures at the 12-, 9-, 6-, and 3-o'clock positions. The external segment of the catheter is drawn through the anterior rectus fascia.

A subcutaneous tunnel is made in the abdominal wall musculature with a "tunneller." The external cuff is positioned at lest 1 cm from the skin exit site, which should be determined during tunnelling. For Swan Neck catheters, a subcutaneous pocket is made at the level of skin marking to accommodate the bent portion of the catheter. The catheter is brought out to the exterior through a small stab wound in the skin threaded onto a trocar. Care is taken to keep the radiopaque stripe facing forward.

After attaching the titanium adapter and a sterile extension tube to the catheter, 1 L of sterile saline containing 1,000 U of heparin is infused and drained immediately. At least 200 ml of solution should drain within 1 minute. If good flow is obtained, the skin incision is closed with absorbable subcuticular sutures. The operative site is covered with several layers of gauze dressings and secured with microfoam surgical tape. Care is taken to keep the radiopaque stripe facing forward during the dressing.

Postoperative Care

The position of the intraperitoneal catheter segment is checked by a plain x-ray of the abdomen and the patient is sent to the ward. The catheter is anchored with several layers of microfoam tape and dressings which should be left in place for 1 week. Additional in and out 1-L exchanges are performed to check the patency of the catheter and to remove residual blood from the peritoneal cavity, if present. The exchanges are continued until the dialysis solution return is clear. If the position of the intraperitoneal catheter segment is not in the true pelvis, and even if the catheter is not functioning, no immediate correction of the position is attempted. Due to favorable resilience forces with the Swan Neck catheters, the intraperitoneal catheter segment usually translocates spontaneously into the true pelvis within a few days. Failure to function after a few days of observation would require surgical catheter repositioning. Drainage is usually slow (< 150 ml/min) if the catheter tip is not in the true pelvis. If the catheter tip is in the true pelvis but is nonfunctional, the omental wrapping is most likely and, for correction, omentectomy may be required. Analgesics with constipating side effects (opiates) should be avoided during the postoperative period.

Insertion Technique for the Lifecath Column Disc Catheter

The same general technique described above is followed for insertion with the exception of a few modifications. The peritoneal incision is larger (1.5 cm) and the catheter is inserted into the peritoneal cavity by folding the column disc. After placing traction on the catheter, the peritoneum is closed between the column disc and deep cuff.

Insertion Technique[46] for Polyurethane Percutaneous Access Device

The site selected for the skin button is marked with a template that describes the point for the terminal and circumference of the subdermal skirt. A circular coring knife is positioned over the central marking, and a core of tissue approximately 7 mm deep is removed. A # 11 blade is used to initiate dissection of a subdermal pocket for the skirt. This dissection is carried out radially from the margin of the core. The remainder of the subdermal pocket is created using sharp scissors. A transverse incision approximately 2 in long is made inferior to the exit site of the catheter and is carried down to the level of the peritoneum. The subcutaneous tissue at the dorsal margin of the incision is then dissected from the underlying fascia to create a plane superficial to skeletal muscle. This dissection is carried out to a level directly beneath the circular incision made by the coring knife. The floor of the superficial dermal plane is incised transversely so the two planes communicate. This dissection creates a path for the retrograde insertion of the device. A tunnel is then made for the catheter. The initial tunnel is in the subdermal plane. It then gently curves deeper as it leaves the margin of the skirt and exits in the subcutaneous tissue at the inferior incision above the level of the second plane of dissection. The system is inserted in a retrograde fashion. The internal conduit is then placed in the abdomen through a stab wound incision and the peritoneum is closed around it. All layers are closed with absorbable sutures. The patency is checked in the operating theater and left unused for a period of 2 weeks. A nonstick dressing is applied over the incision, and the catheter exit site is protected with a transparent dressing. During the period of non-use, the catheters are flushed with heparinized solution two to three times a week in an attempt to decrease the likelihood of obstruction due to fibrin accumulation within the device. The implant sites are visually examined on a routine basis for any evidence of sinus formation or infection around the terminal of the device.

Catheter Insertion in Children

Differences in size and nutritional status of children must be considered when choosing a peritoneal catheter. In general, adult catheters are used for children weighing over 30 kg, pediatric versions are used for children weighing 10 to 30 kg, and the neonatal catheter is reserved for infants weighing less than 10 kg.

The catheter is usually inserted through a midline subumbilical incision. For peritoneal closure, a slowly absorbable vicryl suture is used. The catheter is tunnelled subcutaneously for at least 5 cm, usually in a superolateral direction.

CATHETER BREAK-IN AND CARE

The break-in period for a peritoneal catheter is that which immediately follows catheter insertion. In order to achieve optimum long-term catheter function and low rates of complications, strict adherence to break-in procedures, as previously reported,[3] is essential. The purpose of the different steps suggested in the break-in procedure is to allow sufficient time for the incision to heal before it is subjected to high intraperitoneal pressure with standard CAPD. Therefore, it is desirable to delay CAPD for at lest 10 days after catheter implantation.

Usually, no break-in period is necessary after the bedside catheter insertion, although some prefer to use reduced volumes (500 ml, then 1,000 ml) for the initial four to eight exchanges before proceeding to the normal 2,000-ml exchange volume (in patients with small abdomens or with respiratory embarrassment, a reduced exchange volumes may be required indefinitely).

For an end-stage renal disease patient opting for CAPD, should acute dialysis be required, the newly inserted catheter could be used for dialysis with the patient in the supine position because the intra-abdominal pressure generated in this position with 2 L of solution is minimal and leakage is usually not a problem. Lower dialysis solution volumes are used with faster exchange time (1-L volume exchanged every 30 to 45 minutes) for the first supine dialysis. The usual cycler settings are 10 minutes of inflow, 10 minutes of dwell, and 12 minutes of outflow. Some set the exchange volume at 500 ml for the first four exchanges, 1,000 ml for the next four exchanges, then proceed to the desired exchange volume if tolerated. Heparin, 500 U/L, is added to each dialysis solution bag for at least the first 72 hours. Several sittings of supine dialysis may be given until the incision is well-healed and ready to commence standard CAPD.

When a catheter is replaced in a patient who is already on CAPD, it may be tempting to modify the break-in procedure to allow CAPD with lower volumes per exchange. However, such a practice may expose the patient to the risk of dialysis solution leak and delayed wound healing. It is our policy to provide peritoneal dialysis to such patients only in the supine position with a cycler until the incision is well-healed. Alternatively, hemodialysis is provided using a subclavian catheter as an access until standard CAPD can be resumed.

When a catheter is inserted at the time of another abdominal surgery, e.g., hernia repair or cholecystectomy, no change in break-in procedure is recommended except that standard CAPD be delayed longer than 15 days depending on the recommendation of the surgeon with respect to incision healing.

Subsequent Catheter Care

The important aspect of catheter care is to avoid trauma by minimizing movement at the skin exit site and always keeping it clean. The procedure practiced at our institution has been previously published.[3] In short, the procedure consists of removing the surgical dressing 1 week after the time of insertion. Care is taken to avoid catheter pulling or twisting. The exit and skin surrounding the catheter are cleansed with povidone-iodine scrub, rinsed with sterile water, patted dry with sterile gauze, covered with several layers of gauze dressings, and secured with microfoam surgical tape. Weekly dressing changes are continued until the healing process is completed. There are no data in humans with respect to the time needed for firm fibrous tissue ingrowth into the cuff and completion of epidermal growth into the sinus tract. We assume that it may take up to 6 weeks. The patient may shower only before the dressing change and must otherwise take sponge baths.

Protection of the catheter from mechanical stress seems to be extremely important, especially during break-in. The catheters should be anchored in such a way that the patient's movements are only minimally transmitted to the exit. The method of catheter immobilization is individualized, depending on exit location and abdomen shape. We think that better exit protection prevents infections in most patients.

After the healing process is completed, special care of the exit site, is essential to prevent infection. Routine exit site care includes examining the exit site and tunnel for signs of infection, cleaning the skin to remove dirt and decrease bacteria, and securing the catheter to avoid tension and tugging movements. Routine exit site care should be performed daily and at any time the exit site is red or dirty. Several methods of exit site care are currently practiced. The three commonly used methods are daily cleaning and leaving the exit site exposed, daily cleaning and topical application of povidone-iodine, or daily cleaning, topical application of povidone-iodine, and covering the exit site with a sterile gauze. The results of a prospective study[47] indicate that cleaning with soap and water is the least expensive procedure and tends to prevent infections better than application of povidone-iodine and cleaning with hydrogen peroxide.

Following a satisfactory healing (6 to 8 weeks after implantation), the patient may swim in the ocean or private swimming pools, preferably covering the exit site with a colostomy bag with the catheter spike and dialysate bag or capped spike within the same colostomy bag. Swimming in other surface waters, such as rivers, lakes, jacuzzis, public pools, and hot tubs, and scuba diving should be discouraged. Following swimming, the patient should shower to clean the exit site and should then cover it with a sterile dry dressing. The patient should avoid tub-bathing, but is allowed shower baths.

LATE CATHETER COMPLICATIONS

Exit Site Infection

A non-infected exit site should be clean, dry, and scab- and crust-free. A normal exit site is painless and not red. Scabs are found following trauma to exit sites when serous discharge drys. This usually falls off after healing. Crust, on the other hand, is dried drainage or debris at the exit site, usually due to infection. It should be gently removed during cleaning.

Problems of the exit site include inflammation and infection. Inflammation is indicated by redness with or without pain around the exit site. Induration, swelling, or purulent drainage indicates infection. Therapy of exit site infection should include daily frequent exit site care. Any one of the methods of exit site care described above would be satisfactory. If the infection is severe, care of the exit site more than once a day may be necessary. Systemic antibiotics are indicated if exit site care does not alleviate the infection. Choice of antibiotic would depend on the organism isolated from the exit site and its sensitivity. Antibiotics are given intravenously or intraperitoneally when patients are unable to take oral antibiotics. Topical application of antibiotics include local spraying of powder or injection in and around the exit site. In the majority of cases, the above measures would be adequate to control exit site infection. If resistance to therapy is encountered, longer courses of antibiotic therapy may be tried. If the infection persists, before removing the catheter, shaving the subcutaneous Dacron cuff may be tried. Under the appropriate antibiotic coverage and local anesthesia, the subcutaneous Dacron cuff, if it is not already extruded, is exposed through a small incision. With the help of fine scissors and/or scalpel blade, the Dacron felt is shaved off the catheter, taking care not to puncture the catheter during the procedure. It is important that the remaining catheter surface be smooth after cuff removal. If it is rough, it may cause irritation and inflammation of the skin due to constant friction and pulling movements at the exit site. As a last measure, the catheter may have to be removed if exit site infection persists. When a catheter is removed because of persistent skin exit infection, ideally, it should not be replaced by a new catheter at the same time but after 1 or 2 weeks. A new catheter is inserted at a site opposite to the removed one.

The usefulness of the superficial cuff is not yet clearly established. With the exception of hernias, some studies[33,34] show no significant differences between single and double cuff catheters with respect to their influence on early and late catheter-related complications, including exit site infection. Another study[29] although retrospective, showed a higher incidence of infection with single cuff catheters. There is no evidence to support the use of prophylactic antibiotics to reduce the incidence or frequency of exit site tunnel infections,[48,49] except the prophylactic use of cloxacillin for patients who experience a high incidence of staphylococcal infections.[50]

Dialysis Solution Leak

Dialysis solution leaks may occur months or even years after starting CAPD. Management of late leak is similar to that described for early leak. However, most cases of late leak are refractory to conservative therapy and require surgical repair.

Cuff Extrusion

The main cause of cuff extrusion is placement of the external segment of the catheter in any manner other than its natural shape. Due to the resilience force of the silastic, slowly over a period of months, the catheter tends to assume its original shape. During this process, the external cuff usually extrudes. If the cuff is not infected, it is left alone. However, cuff or catheter may have to be removed due to tissue trauma or infection. Infection is another cause of cuff extrusion. This aspect has been discussed in the section concerning exit site infection.

Indications for Catheter Removal

The need for catheter removal occurs under various conditions. These may be broadly categorized under two headings: catheter malfunction and complicating medical conditions with a functioning catheter.

Poor-functioning or Nonfunctioning Catheter

A poor-functioning or nonfunctioning may be seen under the following conditions: (1) intraluminal obstruction with blood or fibrin clot or omental tissue incarceration (the decision to remove the catheter is usually made only when conservative measures to dislodge the obstruction have failed); (2) catheter tip migration out of the pelvis with poor drainage; (3) a catheter kink along its course; or (4) a catheter tip caught in adhesions following severe peritonitis. In these situations, there are usually both inflow and outflow drainage problems.

Functioning Catheter With a Complication

Under the following conditions, catheters may have to be removed: (1) recurrent peritonitis with no identifiable cause, (2) peritonitis due to exit site and/or tunnel infection, (3) a catheter with persistent exit site infection, (4) tunnel infection and abscess, (5) late recurrent dialysate leak through the exit site or into the layers of the abdominal wall, (6) unusual peritonitis (i.e., tuberculosis, fungal, etc.), (7) bowel perforation with multiple organism peritonitis, (8) refractory peritonitis of other causes, (9) severe abdominal pain due to a catheter impinging on internal organs or during solution inflow, (10) catheter cuff erosion with infection, or (11) an accidental break in the continuity of the catheter.

Functioning Catheter That Is No Longer Needed

A catheter that is no longer needed is encountered after a successful renal transplantation or when peritoneal dialysis is discontinued because dialysis is no longer needed or the patient is transferred to another form of dialysis.

LONG-TERM RESULTS

The most exhaustive survey[2] of the current use of peritoneal dialysis catheters showed catheter survival rates at 12, 18, 24, and 36 months to be similar for all types of Tenckhoff catheters, TWH catheters, and Lifecath catheters (Table 5-1). In that survey, the Gore-tex catheter had the lowest survival result, mainly because of the unusually high incidence of exit site infections. The survey discussed the claimed advantages of catheters. The Toronto Western Hospital catheters, developed to prevent obstruction and dialysis solution leaks, were indeed associated with the lowest rates of these complications. Lifecath catheters were associated with the lowest rates of exit site and tunnel infections. For reasons not quite clear at this time, they failed more often than others during peritonitis (Table 5-3). Exit site infections were reported in proportionately more patients using a single subcutaneously placed cuff (13 percent) than for patients using a double cuff (7 percent).

Centers with larger experiences with Tenckhoff catheters[51–53] report 60 to 70 percent 1-year and 50 to 60 percent 2-year catheter survival rates. Exit site and poor flow due to catheter migration are the major drawbacks of these catheters. Coiled catheters seem to reduce these problems to some extent.[53]

Experiences with Toronto Western Hospital catheters[41,54–56] indicate survival rates almost comparable to Tenckhoff catheters, but considerably lower incidence of dialysis solution leaks and flow problems. Exit site infections are still a problem with the use of this catheter.

Preliminary experiences[36,57,58] with Swan Neck catheters disclose survival rates comparable to other currently used catheters. However, the major benefits of using Swan Neck catheters are the total elimination of the cuff extrusion problem. Dialysis solution leak and poor flow problems are practically eliminated. The incidence of exit site infections is lowered and, when infections do occur, they are amenable to therapy with antibiotics.

A multicenter experience using 89 column disc catheters was reported.[59] Twenty catheters were placed in patients who had previous failures using Tenckhoff catheters. Outflow failure was the most common cause of early failure and was less frequent after 1 month. Subcutaneous leak and herniation rarely occurred. Life table analysis revealed that compared with Tenckhoff catheters, the column disc catheter is more likely to fail in the early months, but over the long term is much less likely to fail.

Dasse et al.[30] reported their preliminary experience with the use of polyurethane percutaneous access devices in 19 patients for up to 8 months. Three of the 19 devices were implanted without an internal peritoneal cuff, two of which had pericatheter leakage that compromised healing. In contrast, excellent tissue ingrowth and healing has been observed in the remaining 16 patients, who had implantations of devices with a peritoneal cuff. One patient experienced an episode of peritonitis. Two of the 16 patients with catheters with a peritoneal cuff experienced transient cellulitis which subsequently healed. More recent experience indicates a high incidence of catheter amputation at the insertion site which is probably related to the design of the catheter and the insertion technique.

Table 5-3. Percent of Catheters Removed Due to Complications

Type of Catheter	Exit/Tunnel Infection	Peritonitis	Leak	Obstruction
Straight	13	19	3	6
Curled	12	21	3	5
Toronto Western Hospital	10	30	2	0
Ash	8	24	4	8
Gore-tex	39	21	7	7

REFERENCES

1. Tenckhoff H, Schechter H: A bacteriologically safe peritoneal access device. Trans Am Soc Artif Internal Organs 14: 181, 1968
2. Lindblad AS, Novak JW, Stablein DM, et al: Report of the National CAPD Registry of the National Institutes of Health. A publication of the National CAPD Registry of the National Institute of Diabetes and Digestive and Kidney Diseases, p. 10, 1987
3. Khanna R, Twardowski ZJ: p. 319. In Nolph KD (ed): Peritoneal Dialysis. Kluwer Academic Publishers, Dordrecht, 1989
4. Ganter G: Ueber die Beseitigung giftiger Stoffe aus dem Blute durch Dialyse. Mun Med Wochenschr, 70: 1478, 1923
5. Rosenak S, Siwon P: Experimentelle Untersuchungen uber die peritoneale Ausscheidung harnpflichtiger Substanzen aus dem Blute. Mitteilungen aus dem Grenzgebieten der Medizin und Chirurgie 39: 391, 1926
6. Engel D, Kerkes A: Beitrage zum permeabilitats Problem: Entgiftungsstudien mittels des lebenden Peritoneums als "Dialysator." Zeitschrift Fur die gesamte experimentalle Medizin 55: 574, 1927
7. Wear JB, Sisk IR, Trinkle AJ: Peritoneal lavage in the treatment of uremia. J Urol 39: 53, 1938
8. Reid R, Penfold JB, Jones RN: Anuria treated by renal decapsulation and peritoneal dialysis. Lancet 2: 749, 1946
9. Fine J, Frank HA, Seligman AM: The treatment of acute renal failure by peritoneal irrigation. Ann Surg 124: 857, 1946
10. Rosenak S, Oppenheimer GD: An improved drain for peritoneal lavage. Surgery 23: 832, 1948
11. Derot M, Tanzet P, Roussilon J, Bernier JJ: La dialyse peritoneale dans le traitement de luremie aigue. J Urol 55: 113, 1949
12. Legrain M, Merrill JP: Short term continuous transperitoneal dialysis. N Engl J Med 248: 125, 1953
13. Maxwell MH, Rockeny RE, Kleeman CR, Twiss MR: Peritoneal dialysis. J Am Med Assoc 170: 917, 1959
14. Doolan PD, Murphy WP, Wiggins RA, et al: An evaluation of intermittent peritoneal lavage. Am J Med 26: 831, 1959
15. Weston RE, Roberts M: Clinical use of stylet catheter for peritoneal dialysis. Arch Intern Med 115: 659, 1965
16. Boen ST, Mulinari AS, Dillard DH, Scriber BH: Periodic peritoneal dialysis in the management of chronic uremia. Trans Am Soc Artif Internal Organs 8: 256, 1962
17. Merrill JP, Sabbaga E, Henderson L, et al: The use of an inlying plastic conduit for chronic peritoneal irrigation. Trans Am Soc Artif Internal Organs 8: 252, 1962
18. Barry KG, Shambaugh GE, Goler D: A new flexible cannula and seal to provide prolonged access for peritoneal drainage and other procedures. J Urol 90: 125, 1963
19. Boen ST, Mion CM, Curtis FK, Shilipetar G: Periodic peritoneal dialysis using the repeated puncture technique and an automated cycling machine. Trans Am Soc Artif Internal Organs 10: 409, 1964
20. Jacob GB, Deane N: Repeated peritoneal dialysis by the catheter replacement method: description of technique and a replaceable prosthesis for chronic access to the peritoneal cavity. Proc Eur Dialysis Transplant Assoc 4: 136, 1967

21. Mallette WG, McPhaul JJ, Bledsoe F, et al: A clinically successful subcutaneous peritoneal access button for repeated peritoneal dialysis. Trans Am Soc Artif Internal Organs 10: 396, 1964
22. Palmer RA, Maybee TK, Henry EW, Eden J: Peritoneal dialysis in acute and chronic renal failure. Can Med Assoc J 88: 920, 1963
23. Gutch CF: Peritoneal dialysis. Trans Am Soc Artif Internal Organs 10: 406, 1964
24. Palmer RA, Newell JE, Gray EF, Quinton WE: Treatment of chronic renal failure by prolonged peritoneal dialysis. N Engl J Med 274: 248, 1966
25. McDonald HP, Gerber N, Mishra D, et al: Subcutaneous Dacron and teflon cloth adjuncts for silastic arteriovenous shunts and peritoneal dialysis catheters. Trans Am Soc Artif Internal Organs 14: 176, 1968
26. Goldberg EM, Hill W, Kabins S, Levin B: Peritoneal dialysis. Dialysis Transplant 4: 50, 1975
27. Stephen Rl, Atkin-Thor E, Kolff WJ: Recirculating peritoneal dialysis with subcutaneous catheter. Trans Am Soc Artif Internal Organs 22: 575, 1976
28. Oreopoulos DG, Izatt S, Zellerman G, et al: A prospective study of the effectiveness of three permanent peritoneal catheters. Proc Clin Dialysis Transplant Forum 6: 96, 1976
29. Twardowski ZJ, Nolph KD, Khanna R, et al: The need for a "Swan Neck" permanently bent, arcuate peritoneal dialysis catheter. Peritoneal Dialysis Bull 5: 219, 1985
30. Dasse KA, Dally BDT, Bousquet G, et al: A polyurethane percutaneous access device for peritoneal dialysis. p. 2435. In Khanna R, Nolph KD, Prowant BF, et al (eds): Advances in Peritoneal Dialysis. Peritoneal Dialysis Bulletin, Toronto, 1988
31. Tenckhoff H: p. 583. In Massry SG, Sellers AL (eds): Clinical Aspects of Uremia and Dialysis. Charles C Thomas, Springfield, 1976
32. Kim D, Burke D, Izatt S, et al: Single or double cuff peritoneal catheters? A prospective comparison. Trans Am Soc Artif Internal Organs 30: 232, 1984
33. Diaz-Buxo JA, Geissinger WT: Single cuff versus double cuff Tenckhoff catheter. Peritoneal Dialysis Bull 4: suppl. 3, S100, 1984
34. Smith C: CAPD: One cuff vs. two cuff catheters in reference to incidence of infection. p. 181. In Maher JF, Winchester JF (eds): Frontiers in Peritoneal Dialysis. Field, Rich and Associates, New York, 1986
35. Poirier VL, Daly BDT, Dasse KA, et al: Elimination of tunnel infection. p. 210. In Maher JF, Winchester JF (eds): Frontiers in Peritoneal Dialysis. Field, Rich & Associates, New York, 1986
36. Twardowski ZJ: Peritoneal catheter development: currently used catheters: advantages/disadvantages/complications, and catheter tunnel morphology in humans. Trans Am Soc Artif Internal Organs 34: 937, 1988
37. Ogden DA, Benavente G, Wheeler D, Zukoski CF: Experience with the Right Angle GORE-TEX® peritoneal dialysis catheter. p. 155. In Khanna R, Nolph KD, Prowant BF, et al (eds): Advances in Continuous Ambulatory Peritoneal Dialysis. Peritoneal Dialysis Bulletin, Toronto, 1986
38. Hall CW, Adams LM, Ghidoni JJ: Development of skin interfacing cannula. Trans Am Soc Artif Internal Organs 21: 281, 1975
39. Dally BDT, Dasse KA, Haudenschild CC, et al: Percutaneous energy transmission systems: long-term survival. Trans Am Soc Artif Internal Organs 29: 526, 1983
40. Kantrowitz A, Freed PS, Ciarkowski AA, et al: Development of a percutaneous access device. Trans Am Soc Artif Internal Organs 26: 444, 1980

41. Khanna R, Izatt S, Burke D, et al: Experience with the Toronto Western Hospital permanent peritoneal catheter. Peritoneal Dialysis Bull 4: 95, 1984
42. Ash SR, Johnson H, Hartman J, et al: The column disc peritoneal catheter. A peritoneal access device with improved drainage. ASAIO J 3: 109, 1980
43. Nolph KD: Placement of peritoneal catheters. Ann Intern Med 109: 989, 1988
44. Ash SR, Daugirdas JT: Peritoneal access devices. p. 194. In Daugirdas JT, Ing TS (eds): Handbook of Dialysis. Little, Brown, Boston, 1988
45. Twardowski ZJ, Khanna R, Nolph KD, et al: Intraabdominal pressure during natural activities in patients treated with continuous ambulatory peritoneal dialysis. Nephron 44: 129, 1986
46. Dally BDT, Dasse KA, Gould KE: A new percutaneous access device for peritoneal dialysis. Trans Am Soc Artif Internal Organs 32: 664, 1987
47. Prowant BF, Schmidt LM, Twardoswki ZJ, et al: A randomized prospective evaluation of three peritoneal exit site procedures. Peritoneal Dialysis Bull 7: 60, 1987
48. Low DE, Bas SI, Oreopoulos DG, et al: Randomized clinical trial of prophylactic cephalexin in CAPD. Lancet 2: 753, 1980
49. Churchill DN, Oreopoulos DG, Taylor DW, et al: Peritonitis in CAPD patients—a randomized clinical trial of trimethoprim-sulfamethoxazole prophylaxis. p. 97A. 20th Annual Meeting of the American Society of Nephrology (abstr.). Washington, 1988
50. Moriarty MV, Watson LJ: Prevention of *Staphylococcal aureus* peritoneal catheter related infections with prophylactic cloxacillin in CAPD patients. Peritoneal Dialysis Int (in press)
51. Slingeneyer A, Balmes M, Mion C: Surgical implantation of the Tenckhoff catheter inperitoneal dialysis. p. 133. In La Greca G, Biasioli S, Ronco C (eds): Peritoneal Dialysis. Wichtig Editore, Milano, 1983
52. Rubin J, Adair C: Peritoneal access using the Tenckhoff catheter. Perspect Peritoneal Dialysis 1: 2, 1983
53. Rottembourg J, De Groc F: Peritoneal access using the curled Tenckhoff catheter. Perspect Peritoneal Dialysis 1: 7, 1983
54. Grefberg N: Clinical aspects of CAPD. Scand J Urol Nephrol S72: 7, 1983
55. Hogg RJ, Coln D, Chang J, et al: The Toronto Western Hospital catheter in a pediatric dialysis program. Am J Kidney Dis 3: 219, 1983
56. Flanigan MJ, Ngheim DD, Schulak JA, et al: The use and complications of three peritoneal dialysis catheter designs: a retrospective analysis. Trans Am Soc Artif Internal Organs 33: 33, 1987
57. Bozkurt F, Keller E, Schollmeyer P: Swan Neck peritoneal dialysis catheter can reduce complications in CAPD patients. Abstracts of the IVth Congress of the International Society for Peritoneal Dialysis. Venice, Italy, June 29–July 2, 1987. Peritoneal Dialysis Bull, suppl. 7: S9, 1987
58. Baker WB, Pratt J, Stone K, et al: Peritonitis (P) and exit site infection (ESI) rates using single-cuff Tenckhoff (SCT) Missouri Swan-Neck peritoneal catheters (SNC). Peritoneal Dialysis Int, 1989 (in press)
59. Ash SR, Slingeneyer A, Scchardin KE: Peritoneal access using the column-disc catheter. Perspect Peritoneal Dialysis 1: 9, 1983

6

Clinical Results with Peritoneal Dialysis—Registry Experiences

Karl D. Nolph

WORLD POPULATION OF CHRONIC PERITONEAL DIALYSIS PATIENTS

Estimates from the industry suggest that as of early 1987 there were approximately 35,000 patients worldwide with end-stage renal disease (ESRD) maintained on chronic peritoneal dialysis.* For an estimated 90 percent or more of these patients, the peritoneal dialysis technique was continuous ambulatory peritoneal dialysis (CAPD). As of early 1987 in the United States, an estimated 750 dialysis facilities provided chronic peritoneal dialysis to nearly 15,000 patients (approximately 13,000 on CAPD).*

---

* Figures provided by Baxter Healthcare, Inc, Deerfield, IL.

Data from the Health Care Financing Administration (HCFA) summarizes the dialysis population in the United States as of December 31, 1987 (Table 6-1). Note that CAPD is by far the most common form of home dialysis therapy. The numbers of patients on CAPD are close to the industrial estimates. Smaller numbers are on home hemodialysis, home intermittent peritoneal dialysis (IPD), and continuous cyclic peritoneal dialysis (CCPD).

Table 6-2 summarizes industrial estimates of percentages of ESRD patients on chronic dialysis that are on peritoneal dialysis. These percentages are also estimates from early 1987. The values range from 4 to 74 percent and are most likely partly related to differences in the availability of hemodialysis facilities, geographic distances between dialysis facilities, and reimbursement policies.

Population characteristics and outcome measures have been monitored for patients maintained on chronic peritoneal dialysis by various registries. Four registries released their most recent information in late 1987 or early 1988. The highlights of these reports will be summarized and compared in this chapter.

The Eleventh Report of the Australia and New Zealand Dialysis and Transplant Registry was released in July 1988.[1] The registry requests input every 6 months from all known Australian and New Zealand dialysis and transplant units. Patients on all forms of renal replacement therapy, including kidney transplantation, are registered and followed. This registry follows the total population and has never failed to collect information on all patients known to all units by the end of the collection period. Data available through October 31, 1987 were analyzed in the 1988 report.

The Canadian Renal Failure Register released a report in 1987 covering analyses through 1986.[2] This registry commenced the collection of statistics on chronic renal failure in 1981. It also monitored all renal replacement therapies, including transplantation, in Canadian patients. This registry

Table 6-1. Dialysis in the United States as of December 31, 1987—Based on Data From the Health Care Financing Administration[a]

Hemodialysis	
Center	79,508
Home	3,580
IPD	
Center	441
Home	168
CAPD	12,995
CCPD	1,728
Total	98,420

[a] ESRD Information Analysis Branch, Division of Information Analysis, US Department of Health and Human Services.

Table 6-2. Percent of Dialysis
Population on CAPD or
CCPD (Industrial Estimates
as of June 1986)

Mexico	74
Venezuela	53
Finland	44
New Zealand	43
United Kingdom	42
Canada	39
South Africa	38
Columbia	36
Denmark	33
Australia	30
Israel	24
Switzerland	20
Brazil	16
United States	16
Italy	7
Japan	4
Germany	4

(Data from Baxter Healthcare, Inc, Deerfield, IL.)

was phased out as of April 1, 1988 since the Renal Failure Register will become part of the new Renal Dialysis and Multi-Organ Transplant Register.

Since 1965, the Registry of the European Dialysis and Transplant Association–European Renal Association (EDTA Registry) has collected data in an uninterrupted sequence of annual returns for all renal replacement therapy patients, including those with a kidney transplantation. A special chapter on peritoneal dialysis results in the EDTA Registry appears in the third edition of *Peritoneal Dialysis*.[3] This registry maintained a computerized database of 111,378 patients who were alive on dialysis or with a functioning transplant as of December 31, 1985. These data were analyzed through 1985 in the chapter.

The final report of the National Institutes of Health United States CAPD Registry was released in July 1988 and covered patient characteristics, selected outcome measures, and special topics for the period January 1, 1981 through January 31, 1988.[4] The National CAPD Registry sponsored by NIH has been responsible for developing information regarding a number of patients receiving CAPD and/or CCPD therapy, their characteristics, the extent of some of the more important treatment-related complications, and selected outcomes to the therapies. The Registry began operating in January 1981 as a voluntary registry. At the writing of the final report, 498 clinical centers had participated in the Registry, representing over half of those centers in the United States providing CAPD or CCPD. Unlike the other registries, the United States Registry only monitored patients on continuous forms of peritoneal dialysis. Also unlike the other registries, the United States Registry only monitored a portion of the peritoneal dialysis population, primarily because of the voluntary nature of the project. This registry was discontinued in July 1988; a total ESRD Registry in the United States, which will monitor experiences with all types of therapies in ESRD patients is planned.

Thus, at the time of writing this chapter, we have the unique opportunity to examine the results of four registries that have monitored patients on chronic peritoneal dialysis therapies during the rapid spread of CAPD since the late 1970s. Henceforth in this chapter, I will refer to the peritoneal dialysis populations as CAPD patients since the former are predominantly on CAPD. If I wish to comment on the particular characteristics or outcomes in IPD or CCPD patients (representing smaller fractions of peritoneal dialysis patients in the registries discussed in this chapter), I will name them specifically.

PERITONEAL DIALYSIS PATIENT
CHARACTERISTICS IN REGISTRY POPULATIONS

Table 6-3 shows a summary of the total peritoneal dialysis patients registered over different periods in each registry. Table 6-4 shows the latest reported end-year census in various registries at the end of the latest year for which data are available. The average number of patients registered per year by each registry is also indicated. The late 1970s and early 1980s was a period of increasing utilization of chronic peritoneal dialysis therapy, especially CAPD.

Increasing percentages of peritoneal dialysis patients have diabetic nephropathy as their primary renal disease. Table 6-5 summarizes the cumulative percentage of peritoneal dialysis patients with diabetic nephropathy in each registry as of the year indicated. The percentage of more recently registered patients with diabetic nephropathy is also indicated for each registry. These percentages are relatively high. For example, Table 6-6 shows the percentages of CAPD or CCPD patients in the United States Registry with diabetic nephropathy as their primary renal disease.[4] Table 6-6 also shows percentages of patients with other major primary diseases.

Table 6-3. Summary of Peritoneal Dialysis Registry Surveys in Australia-New Zealand, Canada, Europe, and the United States

	Period	Total No. of Peritoneal Dialysis Patients Registered	Average No. of Patients/Year
Australia-New Zealand	1983–87	1,566	313
Canada	1981–86	793	132
Europe	1976–85	38,723	3,872
United States	1981–87	26,554	3,793

Table 6-4. Latest Reported End-Year Census in Various Registries

	End-Year Census	Type of Peritoneal Dialysis	Year
Australia-New Zealand	730	CAPD	1987
Canada	1,538	All types	1986
Europe	7,377	CAPD	1985
	942	IPD	
United States	8,181	CAPD/CCPD	1987

The percentages of these primary diseases in the HCFA database (primarily hemodialysis) are also indicated. The higher percentage of patients with diabetic nephropathy in chronic peritoneal dialysis programs may relate to the option to use intraperitoneal insulin and the reduced risk of sudden hypotension in diabetic patients with cardiovascular instability.

Table 6-7 summarizes the percentage of patients on CAPD, CCPD, or in the total United States Registry by sex and race.[4] The distribution of the HCFA dialysis population (mainly hemodialysis) is also shown. There are higher percentages of black patients in the HCFA database, perhaps reflecting the increased prevalence of hemodialysis facilities in the urban areas and the preferential use of chronic peritoneal dialysis in the rural Midwest. Indeed, industrial sources estimate that 21.3 percent of dialysis patients are on peritoneal dialysis in the Midwest, compared with 13.6 percent, 15.3 percent, and 15.4 percent in the West, Northeast, and Southeast, respectively.

Table 6-8 summarizes the age distribution of patients on CAPD or CCPD, in the total United States registry, or in the HCFA database.[4] Note that 17 percent of the CCPD population is less than 20 years of age compared with 5 percent for CAPD patients and less than 3 percent for those in the HCFA database. This reflects the preferential use of CCPD by parents caring for children. The median age of the CAPD population is higher than that of the CCPD population. The median age of the HCFA population was not available. Comparing these age distributions with other registries is difficult because of various age category breakdowns in the different reports. Of new patients in 1987 in the Australia-New Zealand Registry, 36 percent were over 59 years of age; this is comparable to the 33 percent and 30 percent of patients over 59 years of age on CAPD and CCPD, respectively, in the United States. Also in the Australia-New Zealand Registry, 6 percent of these new

Table 6-5. Percent of CAPD Patients With Diabetic Nephropathy

	Cumulative	Recent
Australia-New Zealand	12% as of 1987	14% in 1987
Canada	22% as of 1986	24% in 1986
Europe	12% as of 1985	17% in 1985
United States	26% as of 1984	32% in 1987

Table 6-6. Primary Renal Disease Therapy (Percent of Patients)

	CAPD	CCPD	Total No. Registered	HCFA ESRD
Diabetes	26	27	26	20
CGN	17	16	17	23
Hypertension	15	11	15	23
Interstitial nephritis/ pyelonephritis	8	8	8	NA
Polycystic	6	5	6	NA

Abbreviations: CGN, chronic glomerulonephritis; NA, not available.
(Data from the 1988 United States Registry Report.)

Table 6-7. Sex and Race by Therapy (Percent of Patients)

	CAPD	CCPD	Total No. Registered	HCFA ESRD
No. of patients	21,807	1,629	23,436	99,101
Males	55	51	55	53
Females	45	49	45	47
White	76	74	76	63
Black	18	20	18	32
Other	6	6	6	5

(Data from the 1988 United States Registry Report.)

Table 6-8. Age and Type of Therapy (Percent of Patients)

Age (yr)	CAPD	CCPD	Total No. Registered	HCFA ESRD
<5	1	4	1	<1
5–9	1	4	1	<1
10–19	3	9	4	1
20–39	24	24	24	18
40–59	37	29	37	32
>59	33	30	33	48
Median age	53	47	53	NA

Abbreviation: NA, not available.
(Data from the 1988 United States Registry Report.)

1987 patients were less than 20 years of age; this is comparable to the 5 percent of CAPD patients less than 20 years of age in the United States Registry. Canada and Europe noted that 4 percent of new peritoneal dialysis patients registered in 1986 and 1985, respectively, were less than 15 years of age. Of those patients newly registered in Canada in 1986, 73 percent were over 44 years of age.

The United States CAPD Registry has compared characteristics of patients on chronic peritoneal dialysis for 3 or more years to those of patients that were on the same program less than 3 years (Table 6-9).[4] The long-term patients had lower percentages of patients with diabetic nephropathy. There were no striking differences in racial or age distributions.

The Australian-New Zealand Registry examined the percentages of the ESRD population maintained by various renal replacement therapies.[1] After 3 years, the percentage distributions in the overall ESRD population were 45 percent with functioning kidney transplants, 1 percent on IPD, 14 percent on CAPD, 17 percent on hospital hemodialysis, 16 percent on home hemodialysis, and 6 percent on self-care hemodialysis. The percentage of CAPD patients went from 27 percent at 1 year to 14 percent at 3 years. It is interesting to look at the impact of age on the choice of CAPD versus home hemodialysis in the Australian-New Zealand data. Table 6-10 summarizes the ratios of CAPD to home hemodialysis patients as a function of age and time on treatment. The highest ratio of CAPD to home hemodialysis patients is seen in the 60- to 85-year-old group at 1 year on treatment. This ratio is still 1:7 after 3 years. The ratio is relatively high in the 0- to 19-year-old group in the early years of treatment. Home hemodialysis patients outnumber CAPD patients in the 20- to 44-year-old group at all years on treatment. In all groups, the ratio decreases with time on treatment, reflecting the higher transfer rates from CAPD to other forms of therapy as compared with home hemodialysis.

Table 6-9. Patient Characteristics (Percent of Patients)

	On CAPD/CCPD 3 Years or More (N = 1,378)	On CAPD/CCPD Less Than 3 Years (N = 5,783)
Male	54	55
White	74	77
Black	18	17
Diabetic Nephropathy	18	27
CGN	22	17
Hypertension	15	15
CAPD	97	95
CCPD	3	5
<20 yr old	5	7
>20 yr old	95	93
Median age	52 (yr)	52 (yr)

Abbreviation: CGN, chronic glomerulonephritis.
(Data from the 1988 United States Registry Report.)

Table 6-10. Ratio of CAPD to Home Hemodialysis Patients Related to Age and Time on Therapy

Age (yr)	Years on ESRD Treatment		
	1	2	3
0–10	2.4	1.5	0.9
20–44	0.8	0.6	0.4
45–59	1.5	1.2	1.0
60–85	3.2	2.6	1.7

(Data from the Australia-New Zealand Registry, 1988.)

COMPLICATIONS

Table 6-11 summarizes the overall complication rates from the United States CAPD Registry for CAPD and CCPD.[4] The EDTA Registry reports recent overall peritonitis rates of 1.3 to 1.4 episodes per patient-year, similar to the cumulative rate in the United States, but a range of 0.52 to 3.29 from different countries.[3]

Table 6-12 summarizes peritonitis rates from selected European countries, modified from the data of Golper et al.[3] It is noted in the EDTA report that Belgium, Italy, and France extensively use the Y-set connection system. Many attribute lower peritonitis rates in these countries, at least in part, to the use of the Y-set.[5] Decreasing rates are very encouraging.

Table 6-13 summarizes the cumulative probabilities of the first complication with CAPD or CCPD over months on therapy with data from the NIH Registry.[4] These probabilities are very similar for the two therapies. In the study of long-term patients by the NIH Registry mentioned above, patients on CAPD or CCPD for 3 years or more differed from those on less than 3 years in the rate of peritonitis; peritonitis rates were 1.0 and 1.6 episodes per patient-year, respectively. Exit site infection and catheter replacement rates were similar. Those treated for 3 years or more had a 71 percent cumulative probability of developing their first episode of peritonitis by 2 years; for those

Table 6-11. Overall Complication Rates (Episodes Per Patient-Year)

	CAPD	CCPD
Patients	21,758	1,629
Patient-years	26,432	1,450
Peritonitis	1.4	1.3
Exit site infection	0.6	0.6
Catheter replacement	0.2	0.3

(Data from the 1988 United States Registry Report.)

Table 6-12. Peritonitis Rates in Selected European Countries

Country	Episodes Per Patient-Year	
	1984	1985
Belgium	0.77	0.69
France	1.29	0.77
Israel	2.71	1.50
Italy	1.05	0.63
Sweden	1.16	0.53

(Data from Golper et al.[3])

treated less than 3 years, the 2-year probability of first peritonitis was 83 percent. The median time to first peritonitis was 11.7 months in those treated 3 years or more; in those treated less than 3 years, the median time to first peritonitis was 7.3 months.

Table 6-14 summarizes CAPD complication rates by year of registration in NIH Registry patients of the 1-A category.[4] These so-called 1-A patients entered the Registry at the initiation of CAPD; CAPD was their first chronic replacement therapy. Rates are cumulative for each cohort. Note the consistent rates from cohort to cohort.

PATIENT AND TECHNIQUE SURVIVAL

Table 6-15 shows the cumulative percentage of patient and technique survival rates for the CAPD patients in the four registries. A CAPD death usually refers to death on therapy or within several weeks of any transfer.

Table 6-13. Cumulative Probability (Percent) of First Complications

	Months on Peritoneal Dialysis				
	6	12	18	24	36
Peritonitis					
CAPD	40	60	72	80	89
CCPD	37	56	67	78	84
Exit site infection					
CAPD	22	33	41	49	59
CCPD	21	30	40	48	63
Catheter replacement					
CAPD	10	18	25	32	43
CCPD	11	21	28	30	45
Any above[a]					
CAPD	53	73	83	89	95
CCPD	50	70	80	89	97

[a] Overall probabilities of developing any of the three complications listed in table.
(Data from the 1988 United States Registry Report.)

Table 6-14. CAPD Complication Rates by Year of Registration (Episodes Per Patient-Year in 1-A Patients)

	1981	1982	1983	1984	1985	1986	1987
Peritonitis	1.3	1.4	1.3	1.3	1.3	1.3	1.3
Exit site infection	0.6	0.7	0.5	0.5	0.6	0.6	0.8
Catheter replacement	0.2	0.3	0.3	0.3	0.2	0.2	0.3
Patients	177	679	854	1,310	1,553	1,709	1,301
Patient-years	342	1,206	1,326	1,909	1,948	1,573	485

(Data from the 1988 United States Registry Report.)

Readers interested in slight differences in these definitions should review the reports. The Australia-New Zealand and United States Registries reported overall survivals. The reports from Canada and Europe did not include overall survivals and survivals in large patient number subgroups are shown. The Canadian subgroup shown includes only patients starting peritoneal dialysis between 15 and 44 years of age who were nondiabetic. The European subgroup includes only 15- to 64-year-old patients (both diabetic and nondiabetic) who started CAPD as their first choice of therapy. It is well-known that age and diabetes have important effects on patient survival and this is clearly demonstrated in all of the reports. The higher patient survivals in the Canadian and European subgroups reflect these restrictions on age and/or diabetes. All of the reports, except the United States Registry report, provide information about hemodialysis survival. All of the reports that analyze both CAPD and hemodialysis therapies show similar patient survivals regardless of therapy for similar patient populations based on patient age, the presence or absence of diabetes, and other risk factors.

Table 6-15 also shows cumulative technique survivals at 3 years in these same patient groups from the four registries. For these analyses, death or kidney transplantation is considered a lost to risk, and technique failure usually represents transfer to hemodialysis. In the reports that include hemodialysis data, CAPD technique survivals tend to be lower than those for hemodialysis. For example, the Canadian report found cumulative 3-year technique survival rates of 72 percent and 57 percent on hemodialysis and peritoneal dialysis, respectively, in the 45- to 64-year-old nondiabetic patients.[2] In agreement with these findings, Gokal[6] has recently published the

Table 6-15. Patient and Technique Survivals (Percent at 3 Years) in Four Registries

	Patient Survival	Technique Survival
Australia-New Zealand (all patients)	60	45
Canada (15 to 44 years of age, nondiabetic)	88	40
Europe (15 to 64 years of age, first-choice therapy)	68	37
United States (all patients)	58	56

preliminary results of a prospective comparison of CAPD and hemodialysis patient and technique survivals. At 96 weeks, cumulative patient survivals were 85 percent for both therapies. At the same time on therapy, cumulative technique survival was 94 percent for hemodialysis and 80 percent for CAPD. Maiorca et al.[7] found similar patient survivals with CAPD and hemodialysis, but cumulative technique survival at 3 years was 85 percent for hemodialysis and 60 percent for CAPD. Reasons for higher transfer rates from CAPD to hemodialysis most likely relate to (1) frequent or severe peritonitis, (2) developing medical or psychosocial problems that interfere with self-care, (3) the ease by which CAPD can be attempted on a trial basis, (4) variations in facility experience and policy, and (5) failure to adjust dialysis recipes. The latter refers to the fact that some patients need a program with short cycles to generate adequate ultrafiltration and some patients of large size or with poor peritoneal transport need more frequent or larger volume exchanges to provide adequate dialysis, especially as renal function deteriorates.

Table 6-16 summarizes reasons for transfer from CAPD in the three registries that reported such transfers. The categories were not the same in the various reports. The United States report broke down the abdominal and CAPD problems into subclassifications of exit site infection, catheter problems, or hernias. Medical problems interfering with self-care were listed as other medical problems in the United States Registry, but were presumably included under "unable to cope" in the Canadian and European registries. The percentage of patients transferring from CAPD because of peritonitis is lower in North America, particularly the United States, than in Europe. The highest percentage of transfers because of inadequate dialysis or poor ultrafiltration was seen in the European report; in Europe, there have been more reports of losses of ultrafiltration and/or peritoneal sclerosis, often in association with solutions containing acetate as the buffer anion and/or the use of chlorhexadine as an antiseptic.[8,9]

Table 6-17 summarizes reasons for transfer to hemodialysis obtained from

Table 6-16. A Comparison of Reasons for Transfer From CAPD (Percent)

	Canada (N = 516)	Europe (N = 1,665)	United States (N = 1,455)
Peritonitis	36	52	27
Abdominal/CAPD problem	19	20	—
Exit site infections	—	—	9
Catheter problem	—	—	7
Hernia	—	—	2
Inadequate dialysis/poor ultrafiltration	12	14	8
Unable to cope	11	6	—
Patient/family request	16	7	15
Other	6	1	—
Medical	—	—	16
Nonmedical/unknown	—	—	16

Table 6-17. Reasons for Termination in 208 Patients After CAPD/CCPD for 3 or More Years

	Percent
Peritonitis	32
Other medical	16
Catheter complication	6
Exit site infection	6
Patient/family choice	6
Fluid/chemical control	4
Other	9
Unknown	21

(Data from the 1988 United States Registry Report.)

a special survey that appeared in the United States report.[4] For those patients who terminated CAPD or CCPD therapy after 3 or more years of treatments, the percentage breakdowns for reasons of transfer are similar to the overall experience.

In the United States report, a survey of causes of death revealed that 74 percent were unrelated to renal disease or peritoneal dialysis.[4] Twelve percent of the deaths were related to the renal disease and/or peritoneal dialysis therapy, 5 percent were related to renal and other problems, and 9 percent were of unknown cause. In 79 percent there were no peritoneal dialysis complications at the time of death, in another 10 percent there was a peritoneal dialysis complication but it was noncontributory, in 6 percent a peritoneal dialysis complication was considered of a minor contributory nature, and in 5 percent a peritoneal dialysis complication was considered major. Of those deaths unrelated to ESRD treatment, 45 percent were considered cardiovascular.

QUALITY OF LIFE

The Australian-New Zealand Registry report included a quality of life assessment of home CAPD patients (n = 701) and home hemodialysis patients (n = 561). In a variety of activity categories, 76 percent of the home CAPD patients and 85 percent of the home hemodialysis patients were considered capable of normal activities. Although the CAPD percentage is slightly lower, it is noteworthy that 43 percent of the CAPD patients were over 59 years of age compared with only 25 percent of the home hemodialysis patients. The findings in the Australian-New Zealand Registry are similar to recent findings by Morris and Jones.[10] Morris and Jones found that transplantation patients had the highest proportion of high life-satisfaction scores, followed by home hemodialysis and CAPD patients. There was a clear gap to center hemodialysis patients scores. Transplant patients had the greatest sense of control, followed by home hemodialysis patients and CAPD patients, with center hemodialysis patients far behind. CAPD patients contained a high proportion of widowed women. Morris and Jones concluded that "for older patients with ESRD, CAPD is surprisingly well tolerated and shows superiority over center hemodialysis." Thus, although there is a higher proportion of elderly CAPD patients than home hemodialysis patients, quality of life results do not lag far behind home hemodialysis.

GENERAL COMMENTS

CAPD has become the most common form of home dialysis therapy throughout the world. The proportion of CAPD patients to home hemodialysis patients is particularly high in young and elderly patients. Compared with hemodialysis, the percentage of CAPD patients with diabetic nephropathy is relatively high and seems to be increasing. In the United States, CAPD has a lower percentage of black patients as compared with hemodialysis.

Thus, the characteristics of CAPD patients and hemodialysis patients show different patterns. Comparisons of patient survivals, technique survivals, and other outcomes may simply reflect case mix differences rather than the choice of dialysis therapy. Adjustments for case mixes with statistical tools or comparisons of similar populations suggest that patient survivals on hemodialysis and CAPD are similar. In contrast, technique survival tends to be lower on CAPD, reflecting higher rates of transfer to other dialysis therapies, usually hemodialysis. Reasons for higher rates of transfer have been suggested. Decreasing peritonitis rates in countries using the Y-set, particularly in Europe, are encouraging, and if these trends continue, technique survivals of CAPD may improve. True comparisons of patient and technique survivals are not possible, however, without prospective randomized trials.

In spite of the problems with peritonitis and relatively high transfer rates, the use of CAPD has obviously enjoyed a rapid phase of growth. Registry analyses offer insight as to the types of patients that are being placed on CAPD and quantitations of survivals and complication rates. They also provide some information about life satisfaction and the locus of control, which explain some of the popularity of CAPD. Nevertheless, the registry studies do not tell the whole story. Home hemodialysis yields survivals and outcomes that are certainly as good, if not better, than those of CAPD. Why, then, has CAPD dominated home dialysis therapy?

Table 6-18 summarizes 25 reasons why CAPD may be so popular. Some of these reasons are reflected in the registry data and some are not. Let us examine some of the issues raised in Table 6-18.

Blood access clotting or infection are frequent cuases of hospitalization in hemodialysis patients. Needle punctures are painful and/or frightening experiences for some patients, particularly children. Although peritoneal dial-

Table 6-18. Advantages of CAPD Over Home Hemodialysis

No blood access, no needle punctures.
Shorter training period.
No systemic anticoagulant.
Usually no partner required.
No prolonged immobility.
Steady ultrafiltration.
Steady-state chemistries.
Higher β_2-microglobulin clearance.
Higher clearances of middle molecules.
No machine in the home.
No blood membrane interaction.
Allows use of intraperitoneal insulin.
Improved leukocyte functions (?).
Preservation of renal function (?).
Cardiovascular stability.
Low risk of life-threatening emergency.
Wilderness travel.
Caloric supplementation.
Aluminum removal, no deionizer
　needed.
Fewer dietary restrictions.
Immune to power failures.
Flexible schedules and locations.
Sepsis more likely with blood access
　infections than with peritonitis.
Transfer easily accomplished.
Peritonitis easily diagnosed.

ysis has the counterpart of catheter exit site infections, these are probably easier to manage and less stressful for patients. Blood access problems are, of course, avoided in chronic peritoneal dialysis patients. Although in some programs it is preferred to have a backup arteriovenous fistula in their chronic peritoneal dialysis patients, the frequent use of subclavian access for temporary hemodialysis has made this unnecessary.

Training for CAPD can often be accomplished in 5 to 10 training days. Training for home hemodialysis may take 5 to 6 weeks or more. This is one of the major reasons it is easier to use CAPD on a trial basis for a patient whose ability to succeed on a home program is doubtful for medical or psychosocial reasons. Trials of CAPD in patients whose techniques are destined to fail may also predispose to higher peritonitis rates. Thus, although the short training period is attractive to patients and the health care team and in part explains the high ratios of CAPD to home hemodialysis patients during the first year of dialysis therapy (as shown above from the Australian-New Zealand Registry), there is an unsurprising decrease in this ratio subsequent to many transfers from CAPD. On the other hand, many patients predicted to fail do succeed. Therefore, the short training and easy trial characteristics of CAPD can work to the advantage of some patients.

Anticoagulation is not routinely used during CAPD. Heparin may be added to solutions when fibrin clots are suspected in the peritoneal dialysis solution. Systemic effects of intraperitoneal heparin in the usual doses are negligible.

Home hemodialysis requires a partner to assist the patient. Since CAPD is a self-therapy for most patients, this factor has certainly been major in promoting home dialysis in the form of CAPD. For many patients, partners are not available or patients are reluctant to become dependent on another person.

Many patients, especially children, dislike being immobilized for hours at a time. Even during CAPD drainage, some mobility is possible. Disconnection from the filled drain bag and reconnection to a fresh bag take only a few moments.

The steady-state ultrafiltration and chemistries which are nearly achieved with CAPD are at least conceptually attractive for patients with cardiovascular instability and poor tolerance to sudden changes in blood pressure. At least modest disequilibrium symptoms are common with hemodialysis, and many patients who have changed from hemodialysis to CAPD find the lack of disequilibrium symptoms an attractive feature of CAPD.

On a weekly basis, clearances of molecules over 5,000 daltons in molecular weight are many times higher with CAPD than with standard hemodialysis.[11] The significance of this remains controversial. Currently, there is interest in the relatively higher removal rates of β_2-microglobulin. In a recent report, six patients had a serum concentration of β_2-microglobulin on hemodialysis of 59.4 ± 17.2 mg/L (mean $\pm$ SD) and after changing to CAPD, the levels decreased to 35.5 ± 4.5 mg/L.[12] Two of the six patients had dialysis arthropathy thought to be related to dialysis, associated amyloid. High levels of β_2-microglobulin may lead to the deposition of dialysis-associated amyloid, and this in turn may lead to dialysis arthropathy, recurrent carpel tunnel syndrome, and bone amyloid doses. On conversion to CAPD, both patients showed significant improvement in severity of pain and range of movement of the affected joints. Although this report is certainly anecdotal, it is mentioned only to exemplify the continued interest in CAPD clearances of larger molecules and the possible clinical implications related thereto.

Patients can be intimidated by the need for a hemodialysis machine in the home. Although on CAPD they still have to find storage space for solution bags and other equipment, the simplicity of the CAPD apparatus seems to be more acceptable. To many, life on a machine seems to be a step further removed from health than life that is dependent on solutions and bags.

Peritoneal dialysis is the only dialysis system that uses a human biologic membrane for the dialysis process. Peritoneal dialysis is the most blood-compatible dialyzer. Complement is not activated, there is no transient neutropenia, and, to our knowledge, there is no adherence of blood cellular elements to the membrane beyond that which occurs under physiologic conditions. The biocompatibility of the peritoneal membrane has been recently reviewed.[13] It is known, however, that inflammatory mediators are released from intraperitoneal leukocytes during peritonitis.[14]

The NIH Registry report shows the increasing percentages of diabetics on CAPD and this, in part, may reflect the opportunity to use intraperitoneal insulin.[4] Intraperitoneal insulin avoids the need for insulin injections and usually results in excellent blood sugar control.

Some reports suggest that cell-mediated immunity is better preserved in CAPD patients than in hemodialysis patients.[15] This needs additional confirmation.

Rottembourg et al.[16] suggested that residual renal function is better preserved in diabetics on CAPD than in diabetics on hemodialysis. This needs to be evaluated further. However, this possibility has led Rottembourg et al. to suggest that CAPD is the treatment of choice in patients in whom preservation of residual renal function and/or possible return of renal function is a feasible goal. The possibility that slow steady-state ultrafiltration and consistent blood pressure control maintain the lower glomerular capillary pressure is only speculative at this time, but of great interest.

Presumably low cardiovascular stress with CAPD has led many centers to place patients with severe angina on the therapy. CAPD has also been offered to many patients who have had recurring myocardial infarctions during hypotensive episodes on hemodialysis.

CAPD is a home therapy that is less frightening to many patients. Also, there is no shadow of the infrequent but serious life-threatening emergencies that can develop on home hemodialysis. These include (1) air embolus, (2) severe hypotension, (3) arrhythmias, (4) heater malfunction, (5) proportioning pump malfunction, (6) exsanguination, and (7) sepsis and/or endocarditis with access infection. Sepsis is a rare event with peritonitis. In a recent study of 304 blood access grafts infected over 7 years, the graft infection mortality rate was 17 percent and sepsis was the cause of 66 percent of the deaths.[17]

We have a patient whose hobby is hiking. She is a diabetic with advanced retinopathy. Nevertheless, on CAPD she has hiked over 3,000 miles in the past 3 years, including the Appalachian trail in 1987 and Alaska in 1988. Although hemodialysis is possible in campers, CAPD exchanges can be done under a variety of circumstances (hopefully with caution).

Although glucose absorption from peritoneal dialysis may contribute to weight gain and hyperlipidemia, caloric supplementation can have its advantages in some patients.

It is clear that peritoneal dialysis solutions contain low concentrations of aluminum and patients using aluminum-containing phosphate binders have some net removal of aluminum in their drainage bags.[18] Thus, CAPD is a low-aluminum water system that does not require a deionizer. Water purification is a problem for the manufacturer rather than the patient at home.

Continued dialysis and especially steady ultrafiltration allow some patients a little more flexibility in terms of dietary intakes of protein potassium, sodium, and fluid. Certainly, diets cannot be indiscriminate; however, accumulations of sodium and water can be adjusted on an hour to hour basis by monitoring weight, adjusting the osmolality of the solutions, and adjusting diet when necessary. Fluid accumulations and solute concentration increases between intermittent sessions require rapid removals during short treatment periods; these are features of intermittent therapies, but not of CAPD.

CAPD does not require electricity. The advantages of flexible schedules and locations, the reduced risk of sepsis, and the sometimes advantageous features of an "easy on–easy off" therapy overlap with some of the advantages mentioned above.

Finally, the most frequent and troublesome complication of peritonitis is a disadvantage, but fortunately can be easily diagnosed. Treatment can usually commence within hours of the first cloudy drainage. Drainage provides a window on what is happening in the peritoneal cavity. Although peritonitis is certainly an unattractive feature of CAPD, it is fortunate that this complication is so readily detected.

Thus, in understanding the phenomenon of CAPD, one can examine registry reports of demographics and outcomes, but this does not portray the entire story behind the growth and appeal of the therapy. The understanding of the entire picture is best reached through an integration of facts and figures coupled with a listing of the practical features of CAPD, which lends itself so readily to home therapy.

SUMMARY

I have focused on registry experiences from four populations based on three continents. The types of patients and the outcomes of the therapy as of early 1988 have been well-described. I have attempted to explain some of the features of registry data by listing some of the pragmatic characteristics of CAPD. All of this falls together to explain the growth and development of a dialysis therapy that is now the dominant form of home dialysis.

REFERENCES

1. Disney APS (ed): Eleventh Report of the Australia and New Zealand Combined Dialysis and Transplant Registry. Queen Elizabeth Hospital, Woodville, South Australia, 1988
2. Posen GA, Rappaport A, Lucas D (eds): The Canadian Renal Failure Register 1986 Report. Ottawa, Canada, 1987
3. Golper TA, Geerlings W, Selwood NH, et al (eds): Peritoneal dialysis results in the EDTA Registry. p. 414. In Nolph KD (ed): Peritoneal Dialysis. 3rd Ed. Kluwer Academic Publishers, Boston, 1988
4. Lindblad AS, Novak JW, Nolph KD, et al (eds): Final Report of the National CAPD Registry of the National Institutes of Health. EMMES Corporation, Potomac, MD, 1988
5. Maiorca R, Cantaluppi A, Cancarini GC, et al: Prospective controlled trial of a

Y-connector and disinfectant to prevent peritonitis in continuous ambulatory peritoneal dialysis. Lancet 2:642, 1983

6. Gokal R: Worldwide experience, cost effectiveness and future of CAPD—its role in renal replacement therapy. p. 349. In Gokal R (ed): Continuous Ambulatory Peritoneal Dialysis. Churchill Livingstone, Edinburgh, 1986

7. Maiorca R, Kencarini G, Manili L, et al: Life table analysis of patient and method survival in continuous ambulatory peritoneal dialysis and hemodialysis after six years experience. p. 27. In Khanna R, Nolph KD, Prowant B, et al (eds): Advances in CAPD (Proceedings of the Sixth Annual CAPD Conference, Kansas City, MO). University of Toronto Press, Toronto, 1986

8. Nolph KD: A survey of ultrafiltration in continuous ambulatory peritoneal dialysis (an international cooperative study with 40 participating centers). p. 79. In Khanna R, Nolph KD, Prowant B, et al (eds): Advances in Continuous Ambulatory Peritoneal Dialysis (Proceedings of the Fifth Annual CAPD Conference, Kansas City, MO). University of Toronto Press, Toronto, 1985

9. Junor BJR, Briggs JD, Forwell MA, et al: Sclerosing peritonitis. Role of chlorhexidine in alcohol. Peritoneal Dialysis Bull 5:101, 1985

10. Morris PLP, Jones B: Transplantation versus dialysis: A study of quality of life. Transplant Proc 20: 23, 1988

11. Nolph KD, Popovich RP, Moncrief JW: The theoretical and practical implications of continuous ambulatory peritoneal dialysis. Nephron 21:117, 1978

12. Sethi D, Brown EA, Gower PE: CAPD, protective against developing dialysis–associated amyloid? Nephron 50:85, 1988

13. Nolph KD: Comparison of continuous ambulatory peritoneal dialysis and hemodialysis. Kidney Int 33:S123, 1988

14. Crozzi S, Nasini MG, Lamperi S: Cellular and humoral defense mechanisms in peritoneal dialysis. p. 91. In LaGreca G, Chiaramonte S, Fabris A, et al (eds): Peritoneal Dialysis (Proceedings of the Third International Course on Peritoneal Dialysis, Vicenza, Italy, 1988). Wichtig Editorie, Milan, 1988

15. Goldstein CS, Bomalaski JS, Zurier RB, et al: Analysis of peritoneal macrophages in continuous ambulatory peritoneal dialysis. Kidney 26:733, 1984

16. Rottembourg J, Issad B, Poigenet JL, et al: Residual renal function and control of blood glucose levels in the insulin-dependent diabetic patients treated by CAPD. p. 339. In Keen H, Legrain M (eds): Prevention and Treatment of Diabetic Nephropathy. MTP Limited, Lancaster, 1983

17. Dietzek A, Wilkins S, Cohen JR: The management of infected arteriovenous ePTFE grafts. Dialysis Transplant 17:422, 1988

18. Sorkin M, Nolph KD, Anderson H, et al: Aluminum mass transfer during continuous ambulatory peritoneal dialysis. Peritoneal Dialysis Bull 1:91, 1981

Peritonitis: Risk Assessment and Management

7

E. Dale Everett

INTRODUCTION

Substantial strides in the reduction of the number of episodes of peritonitis per patient-year associated with continuous ambulatory peritoneal dialysis (CAPD) have been made since our first report in 1980.[1] Despite a reduction to approximately 1.4 episodes per patient-year, peritonitis remains the Achilles heel of CAPD and accounts for approximately 30 to 50 percent of the dropouts. This chapter will deal with the current understanding of the pathogenesis, prevention, detection, treatment, and complications of CAPD-associated peritonitis.

145

PATHOGENESIS

There are many opportunities for the introduction of microbials into the peritoneum of patients undergoing CAPD. These may include exogeneous contamination from breaks in technique, accidental disconnections, cracks in tubing and catheters, airborne skin scales, or contaminated dialysate. Endogenous infection of the peritoneum may occur from inflamed or perforated abdominal viscera, transmural migration of microorganisms across the gut, hematogenously from other infected foci, from the female genital tract, and perhaps from transient bacteremias that occur frequently in individuals. Furthermore, when the permanent peritoneal catheter is inserted, two major factors that affect host defense take place: a localized area of a major host defense mechanism is destroyed i.e., the skin, and a foreign body is introduced. Both of these promote colonization with microorganisms and may lead to infection. While maneuvers such as keeping the area clean, using double cuffed catheters, and tunneling of the catheter before perforation in the peritoneal cavity may reduce infection, one must remember that the problem involves macroscopic defects in the setting of microorganisms.

It is known that the uremic state alters the immune status of the host, particularly cell-mediated immunity. Some of these parameters improve with CAPD, but evidence is accumulating that the local defenses within the peritoneal cavity are significantly impaired. Peritoneal macrophages are thought to be the first line defense against microbial contamination, followed shortly by polymorphonuclear cells. Evidence is available from in vitro studies using zymosan particles that the dialysate itself may suppress macrophage and leukocyte phagocytosis in the absence of loss of viability of the cells. This tends to be present for the first 2 hours of the dwell cycle.[2] Others have shown that low levels of IgG or C_3 are present in dialysis effluent and that in vitro studies using normal leukocytes and effluent demonstrate suboptimal or inadequate phagocytosis and killing.[3,4] Coles et al.[5] have been able to show that low levels of IgG, C_3, and C_4 may be used to predict those patients who are likely to develop *Staphylococcus epidermidis* peritonitis.

Finally, there has been considerable interest in the role of biofilms on the catheter in the pathogenesis of peritonitis. It has been well-established that both Gram-positive and -negative bacteria can form an extensive exopolysaccharide glycocalyx that is attached to the catheter[6] and contains trapped viable bacteria. Despite these phenomena, it has been difficult to prove an association between episodes or relapses of peritonitis and the presence of biofilm.[7]

Overall, it is thought that approximately 50 percent of the cases of CAPD-associated peritonitis are due to extrinsic contamination; however, this has been difficult to document with certainty.[8,9] Based on the species of organisms causing peritonitis and the reduction of peritonitis rates by certain interventions, this is probably a reasonable estimate. Nevertheless, the pathogenesis of CAPD-associated peritonitis is multifactorial, including contamination, foreign bodies, and defects in host defense mechanisms. Current and future attempts at reducing episodes of peritonitis will need to focus on these multiple facets of pathogenesis.

PREVENTION OF PERITONITIS

Several avenues of approach aimed at the reduction of peritonitis episode have been used or are undergoing trials. Most of the preventive measures have involved changes of the mechanical apparatus used for dialysis or attempts at sterilization of inadvertant contamination. Clearly one advancement, at least in the United States, was the conversion from bottled to bagged dialysate with a resultant two- to three-fold reduction in peritonitis rates. Modification of connector devices, incorporation of an antiseptic into connector devices, use of a double bag technique, ultraviolet irradiation of the spike-bag junction, heat produced by microwaves, and placement of in-line millipore filters have all been reported to be successful in reducing peritonitis rates. While it might be expected that such devices may have some impact on peritonitis rates, the reports have been largely anecdotal, noncomparative trials that either involved small numbers of patients or were shown to be effective in centers that were having high peritonitis rates compared with well-established, large CAPD programs. For example, in a randomized multicenter trial of ultraviolet irradiation, no benefit was found,[10] while a reduction in peritonitis rates occurred[11] in another uncontrolled study. However, the latter study incorporated a lever-operated assist device for removal and insertion of the spike.

The most promising mechanical device change for the prevention of peritonitis since the advent of bagged dialysate is the introduction of the "Y" connector with indwelling antiseptic, namely, sodium hypochlorite. This innovation was first reported by Maiorca et al. in 1983.[12] In their controlled trial, institution of this connector reduced peritonitis rates from one episode every 11.3 patient-months to one episode every 33 patient-months. Less well-controlled trials[13,14] and unpublished controlled data confirm the findings of Maiorca et al. Anecdotal data suggest that flushing the Y-connector with fresh dialysate may obviate the use of indwelling antiseptic.[15] A comparative trial between the flush and the indwelling antiseptic technique is needed.

Other nonmechanical means have been tried in an attempt to prevent peritonitis. These include prophylactic antimicrobial agents and the instillation of γ-globulin into the peritoneal cavity. Two randomized controlled trials of prophylactic antimicrobials have been published. In one study, 500 mg of cephalexin administered orally every 12 hours was unsuccessful in the prevention of peritonitis.[16] The other placebo-controlled study used 160 to 800 mg of orally administered trimethoprim/sulfamethoxazole once daily.[17] The results of this study showed a statistically insignificant reduction in peritonitis rates and an unacceptable number of side effects in patients receiving the drug.

In patients designated as "high peritonitis incidence CAPD patients," a report of diminished rates occurred in a subset of patients who were able to maintain high levels of IgG in the peritoneum after infusion of a total of 12 g of immune globulin at 3-week intervals. The responders appeared to be a subset of patients whose peritoneal macrophages had normal numbers of fc receptors on their surface.[18]

While there have been significant advances in the prevention of peritonitis in CAPD, more work is still required, especially toward exit site-associated episodes of peritonitis.

DIAGNOSIS

Clinical Symptoms and Signs

Peritonitis denotes inflammation of the peritoneum with a resultant increase in numbers of cells. One of the clinical hallmarks of peritonitis is the return of cloudy fluid after dwelling in the peritoneal cavity. Almost all patients with peritonitis will manifest cloudy effluent. While noninfective causes of cloudy effluent exist, it should be assumed to be secondary to infection until proven otherwise. In addition to cloudy effluent, the majority of patients will complain of abdominal pain and exhibit tenderness. Other accompanying symptoms may include nausea, vomiting, constipation, fever, and chills. In contrast to surgical peritonitis, systemic symptoms and toxicity are uncommon and fever is often low-grade or absent.

Based on the above clinical observations, once the diagnosis of peritonitis is entertained, expeditious steps should be taken to establish the etiologic diagnosis and to institute therapy. As with all patients, initial evaluation should include a history and careful physical examination to assess the patient status. Particular emphasis should be placed on the examination of the exist site and the tunnel. Of course, under some circumstances (e.g., when the patient is at home and cannot report immediately to a medical center), this may not be possible.

Laboratory Evaluation

After initial assessment, fluid should be obtained for examination. If at home, the patient should be instructed to save the bag of dialysate and to transport it to the nearest laboratory as soon as is feasible. Otherwise, an aliquot of fluid, preferably the entire bag, should be submitted to the laboratory. Minimal examination should include a cell count, differential, Gram stain, and culture of the effluent.

The cell count is useful for detecting peritoneal inflammation. Normal cell counts from effluent of uninfected CAPD patients vary from 0 to $50/\mu l$, with a predominance of mononuclear cells.[1,19] In infected patients, the counts are almost always $\geq 100/\mu l$ and the differential white blood cell count shows a predominance of neutrophils with uncommon exception.

Gram stains of centrifuged sediments are of low sensitivity with reports of positivity varying from 9 to 42 percent.[1,20–22] However, since it can be easily and rapidly performed and may give valuable information, staining should be done. The Gram stain can be useful in guiding initial therapy, in the early detection of unusual organisms such as budding yeast, or in the detection of organisms that do not grow, suggesting fastidious or anaerobic microorganisms. Because of the low sensitivity of the Gram stain method, others have tried alternate methods for early detection of microorganisms, such as staining with acridine orange. Acridine orange binds to the nucleoprotein of microorganisms and when viewed through a fluorescent microscope, bacteria emit a reddish-orange fluorescence. This method increases the sensitivity of organism detection,[22] but has a drawback in that it does not allow one to distinguish gram-positive from gram-negative bacteria.

Identification of the etiologic agent by culture techniques remains the most important aspect in the diagnosis of CAPD-associated peritonitis. Solidly establishing the etiology allows for tailoring of therapy, may have prognostic implications in relation to catheter removal, can precipitate early surgical exploration of the abdomen, reduces the number of ancillary laboratory and radiologic studies, and diminishes the anxiety of the patient and treating physician.

Over the past several years, a number of techniques have been used for isolation of microorganisms in an attempt to improve the yield of positive cultures. Currently, there are several acceptable methods that produce a high yield of organisms but they may not be available in all laboratories processing effluent cultures.

One of the most common and simple methods is centrifugation of an aliquot of fluid and then culturing a loopful (0.01 ml) onto several media and into broth. Some controversy exists as to what volume of effluent to centrifuge. Existing evidence indicates that the yield from a 50-ml volume is equivalent to 1,000 ml.[23] Vas and Low[24] found that culturing the sediment of a 10-ml aliquot resulted in essentially the same yield as that from a 100-ml sample. In addition, others have found in a comparative study of a millipore filter method (Addi-Check), a blood culture bottle technique (BACTEC), and the 10-ml centrifugation method that isolation of organisms were comparable.[25] In another study, Ryan and Fessia[26] compared centrifugation of 20 ml of effluent with a modified Millipore filtration technique and injection of 20 ml of dialysate into a commercial blood culture system (Septi-Check). Their results showed the Millipore filter and the Septi-Check system to be far superior to the centrifugation method in the recovery of organisms (91 percent, 93 percent, and 51 percent, respectively).

A recent study has compared two commercially available blood culture systems, BACTEC and "The Isolator." Both systems were highly and equally sensitive for detection of organisms. Specific identification of organisms and antimicrobial susceptibilities were available approximately 24 hours earlier with "The Isolator."[27]

Other methods that are reported to increase the yield of microbials have been a total volume method in which concentrated media is added to the bag of effluent[28] or a method in which chemical or physical disruption of the cells in 15 ml of effluent is carried out before culture.[29]

Each method to isolate organisms has some disadvantages, such as being labor intensive, having the potential for contamination, being of questionable sensitivity, being cumbersome, or being costly. While there is some conflict in the data, particularly regarding the simple centrifugation method followed by culturing, I recommend that if the centrifugation method is used, 50 ml of effluent should be used as the volume, and that if the technology is present in the hospital, one of the newer blood culture systems should be used (i.e., Septi-Check, BACTEC, or The Isolator. Also, I find Millipore systems are satisfactory and have excellent yield, but they are labor-intensive and can be fraught with technical problems, particularly with fluids that have large numbers of cells and fibrin debris.

In the future, DNA probes may become practical for detecting the etiologic agents of CAPD-associated peritonitis.

In patients with persistent peritonitis unresponsive to therapy for gram-positive and gram-negative organisms, other infectious and noninfectious cases should be sought. This may require coordination with the laboratory to process fluid anaerobically and/or for fungi and acid-fast bacilli. If the patient is receiving antibiotics, processing the cultures through resin-binding devices to remove antimicrobials may be advantageous. Other studies to help define the inflammatory response may include special staining of cells to better detect eosinophils and testing for endotoxin with the Limulus assay.

ETIOLOGY OF PERITONITIS

A host of organisms have been identified as causes of peritonitis. gram-positive cocci, mainly *S epidermidis* and *Staphylococcus aureus,* are consistently the most common infectious causes, but gram-negative rods cause a clinically important number of cases. A compilation of the common causes of CAPD-associated peritonitis is listed in Table 7-1. Table 7-2 depicts uncom-

Table 7-1. Common Infectious Causes of CAPD-Associated Peritonitis[30,31]

Microorganism(s)	Percentage of Cases
S epidermidis	32–45
S aureus	9–24
α-Streptococci	2–21
Enterococci	2–11
Diphtheroids	1.6
Escherichia coli	0–15
Pseudomonas sp	0–8
Klebsiella sp	1–6
Enterobacter sp	1.6
Acinetobacter sp	2.4

Table 7-2. Uncommon Infectious Causes of Dialysis-Associated Peritonitis

Bacteria	Fungi	Mycobacteria
Actinomyces israelii[32]	*Alternaria* sp[49]	*Mycobacterium tuberculosis*[68,69]
Agrobacterium sp[33]	*Aspergillus* sp[44,50,51]	*M chelonei*[70]
Bacillus sp[34]		*M avium intracellulare*[71]
Bacteroides sp[24]	*Candida albicans*[43,44,52]	*M fortuitum*[70]
Bordetella bronchiseptica[35]		*M chelonei*-like organisms[72]
Campylobacter sp[36,37]	*Candida glabrata*[53] *Candida parapsilosis*[43,44]	*M gordonae*[73]
Corynebacterium sp[38,39]	*Candida tropicalis*[43,52]	
Flavobacterium sp[40]		
Hemophilus influenzae[41]	*Cephalosporium acremonium*[54]	
Listeria monocytogenes[42]		
Neisseria sp[41]	*Coccidioides immitius*[55]	
Nocardia asteroides[43,44]	*Cryptococcus neoformans*[56]	
Pasteurella multocida[30,45]	*Dreschlera spicifera*[57,58]	
Pseudomonas mesophilica[46]	*Exophiala jeanselmei*[58]	
	Fusarium sp[59,60]	
Group Ve-2[47]		
Vibrio alginolyticus[48]	*Mucor* sp[61]	
	Paecilomyces sp[41]	
	Penicillium sp[62,63]	
	Pityrosporon sp[64]	
	Prototheca wickerhamii[65]	
	Rhodotorula rubra[66]	
	Trichoderma viridae[67]	
	Trichosporon sp[64]	

mon agents that have been etiologic of dialysis-associated peritonitis. It also lists references providing further information, since many of these agents are discussed in case reports.

Noninfectious causes of peritonitis are also known to occur. These include endotoxin,[74] ovulation and menstruation,[75] drugs,[76] and eosinophils.[40,77,78] Other less well-substantiated postulates include chemicals, disinfectants, pH, and osmolarity as causes for peritonitis.

TREATMENT OF PERITONITIS

There have been many regimens used in the therapy of the CAPD-associated peritonitis, including oral, intravenous (IV), and intraperitoneal (IP) delivery of antimicrobial agents. Lavaging the peritoneal cavity followed by interrupting CAPD for 48 hours without the use of antimicrobial agents in mild cases of peritonitis has also been reported to be a successful means of treatment.[79]

Despite approximately 12 years' experience with CAPD, there have been no well-controlled trials of comparative studies of various regimens which show the superiority of one treatment modality over another. Most therapeutic experience has been with the use of a variety of cephalosporins, aminoglycosides, and vancomycin, often in combination, for the treatment of bacterial peritonitis. Much less data are available for the management of fungal, mycobacterial, and the more unusual bacterial causes of infectious peritonitis.

Bacterial Peritonitis

Oral Therapy

Oral therapy of bacterial CAPD-associated peritonitis has undergone limited trials. In 1982, Knight et al.[80] reported on the use of oral antimicrobial agents in 43 episodes of peritonitis. Thirty-seven of these patients received 500 mg of oral cephradine every 6 hours for 7 days, then were reassessed at 2 to 7 days following therapy. The remaining episodes were treated with a variety of oral agents. Overall, the cure rate was 79 percent. Six episodes from which cephradine-resistant organisms were isolated recovered with cephradine therapy. Similar results were reported by Searle and Raman[81] in 29 episodes of peritonitis treated by a single intramuscular (IM) dose of 500 mg cephradine followed by 500 mg orally four times a day for 7 days with a subsequent follow-up to 10 days. Response rate was 66 percent. In this latter study, response rate was equivalent to IM cefuroxime followed by IP cefuroxime for 7 days. Relapse rates were not clearly defined in either study.

Another trial of cephradine using a 500-mg oral loading dose followed by 250 mg orally at the time of each exchange resulted in a 75 percent response rate in 88 episodes. In this study, patients with gram-negative rods on Gram stain were excluded and only an additional 60 percent of episodes were cured. The investigators found that patients with methicillin-resistant *S epidermidis* strains initially responded to cephradine but relapsed within 2 weeks, thus resulting in the discrepancy between response and cure.[82] Duration of therapy varied in this study, but averaged approximately 10 days.

Recently, an interest in oral therapy has been rekindled by the advent of a group of potent oral antimicrobial agents, designated fluoroquinolones. A brief report indicated that oral ciprofloxacin was successful in treating ten of ten patients.[83] A more detailed report showed that ofloxacin used at a loading dose of 400 mg followed by 300 mg daily for 10 days resulted in cure of 16 of 18 episodes with no relapse over a 1 to 2-month follow-up. This series included three patients with Gram-negative rod infections. Side effects were minimal despite achieving rather high levels of ofloxacin in serum.[84] While these preliminary data are encouraging, more patients need to be treated. In addition, many renal failure patients receive aluminum-containing ant-acids. Evidence is available that ciprofloxacin is absorbed less well in the presence of antacids, resulting in reduction of intraperitoneal levels of drug.[85] Whether this is true of other quinolones remains to be determined.

Intravenous Therapy

While a large number of antimicrobial pharmacokinetics have been stud-ied following IV administration and during peritoneal dialysis, there are few reports of their therapeutic efficacy. Most antimicrobials achieve therapeutic levels in the peritoneum when given IV, but because of the inconvenience of administration, the requirement for multiple doses, the need for supplemen-tation of doses following dialysis, and the easy access to the IP route, therapy by way of the IV route is seldom used. An exception has been vancomycin, which has a prolonged half-life and an excellent activity against gram-positive cocci that have made IV therapy reasonably practical.

A report by Krothapalli et al.[86] disclosed that IV vancomycin, 1 g/wk for 4 weeks, resulted in the cure of 82 percent of 62 episodes of gram-positive peritonitis. Failures were associated with tunnel infections. An additional report has confirmed the report of Krothapalli et al. in a smaller number of patients. In the latter study, there were two failures with IV vancomycin. One patient responded to the addition of rifampin and the other responded to the use of IP streptokinase.[87] While mention is made concerning loading doses of IV and IM antibiotics followed by IP antibiotics or oral antibiotics and continuation of parenteral antimicrobials after catheter removal, no large series exists in which other IV antibiotics were used as the sole therapy during continuation of CAPD.

Intraperitoneal Therapy

Like IV antimicrobial drugs, many classes of these agents have undergone pharmacokinetic investigations but most have not been subjected to orga-nized, well-documented trials.

In the absence of a clear-cut, positive Gram stain or with home initiation of therapy, patients are treated empirically on a statistical likelihood of the causitive agents. This has resulted in therapy aimed at gram-positive cocci, namely, *Staphylococcus* sp, *Streptococcus* sp, and aerobic gram-negative rods. Many centers have therefore chosen a first-generation cephalosporin plus an aminoglycoside or vancomycin plus an aminoglycoside as initial therapy before knowing culture results.

While the cephalosporin-aminoglycoside regimen has been used exten-sively, particularly early in the development of CAPD as a technique for treatment of renal failure, I have been unable to find a detailed analysis of the expected results from such therapy. More recently, because of the bioac-tivity of vancomycin against gram-positive cocci and the increasing reports of *S epidermidis* resistant to methicillin and cephalosporins, vancomycin plus an aminoglycoside has been recommended and widely used. Gruer et al.[33] have reported on this combination. Using a regimen of 500 mg vancomycin IV followed by 15 mg/L of vancomycin and 8 mg/L of tobramycin per exchange for 12 days, they were able to cure 32 of 38 (84 percent) episodes of peritonitis. Most of the failures were due to gram-negative rods, while only one of 24 (4 percent) coagulase-negative staphylococci failed to respond. Antibiotics were tailored to a single drug if positive cultures were obtained.

Cefuroxime administered IP has been used extensively but because of suboptimal response rates and high relapse rates, it has been largely abandoned.[33,77,81]

Other reported successful regimens include netilmicin-vancomycin in 90 percent of ten episodes of peritonitis,[88] trimethoprim-sulfamethoxazole for 4 weeks in 85 percent of 45 episodes,[89] and ceftazidime plus vancomycin for 7 to 14 days in 32 of 33 (96 percent) culture-positive episodes.[90]

Three recent publications have addressed the treatment of uncomplicated gram-positive peritonitis with once weekly vancomycin. Two reports involved small numbers of patients, eight and ten patients, respectively, who were given 30 mg/kg of vancomycin in one 6-hour dwell weekly for 2 and 3 weeks, respectively.[91,92] A second report by Bastani et al.[93] involving 24 episodes of gram-positive or "sterile" peritonitis showed a 96 percent success rate with this method of vancomycin administration. Each of the other reports showed 100 percent cure rates with this regimen.

A recently introduced antibiotic, teicoplanin, with a spectrum similar to vancomycin has been used in a randomized trial. Twelve patients were randomized to receive either vancomycin or teicoplanin IP for 6 days. Results indicated that teicoplanin and vancomycin were equivalent in this small group of patients.[94]

A listing of drugs and their suggested dosages based on pharmacokinetic studies are presented in Table 7-3.

Duration of Therapy

No prospective studies exist as to the optimum duration of therapy. General recommendations have been 7 to 10 days for gram-positive and 10 to 14 days for gram-negative organisms causing peritonitis. Others have suggested continuation of therapy for 5 days after the effluent becomes clear or for 7 days after the last positive culture. Most have found these recommendations to be satisfactory. However, in a retrospective analysis, Golper et al.[96] found a high incidence (23 percent) of relapse within 3 weeks of a 10 to 14-day course of IP treatment. In this analysis, several antibiotic regimens were used and it is not possible to say if recurrences were the same with all regimens. Some have been treated for up to 4 weeks, depending on the route of therapy and the interval of antimicrobial dosages.[86,89]

Mycobacterial and Fungal Peritonitis

Mycobacterial infection of the peritoneum has been uncommonly reported during CAPD. Both tyical tuberculosis and atypical mycobacterial infections have been described (see Table 7-2). The general setting has been continued

Table 7-3. Drugs That May Be Used in Dialysis-Associated Peritonitis[30,31,84,93,95]

	Dose[a]	
	Initial (mg/2-L Bag)	Maintenance (mg/2-L Bag/Exchange)
Aminoglycosides		
Amikacin	350–500	30–50
Gentamicin	120	8–16
Netilmicin	140	8–16
Tobramycin	120	8–16
Cephalosporins		
Cefamandole	1,000	250
Cefazolin	500–1,000	250
Cefoperazone	2,000	500
Cefotaxime	2,000	500
Cefoxitin	1,000	250
Ceftazidime	1,000	250
Ceftizoxime	1,000	250
Ceftriaxone	1,000	250
Cefuroxime	1,500	400
Cephradine	500	250
Cephalexin	1,000 orally	500/6 h orally
Penicillins		
Ampicillin	1,000	100
Azlocillin	2,000	500
Aztreonam	1,000	500
Ticarcillin	2,000	500
Miscellaneous		
Vancomycin	2,000/wk × 2	NA
Vancomycin	1,000	30–50
Ciprofloxacin	750 orally	750/12 h orally
Ofloxacin	400 orally	300/24 h orally
Trimethoprim-sulfamethoxazole	—	80–400
Metronidazole	500 orally/IV	500 orally/8 h
Rifampin	—	600 orally/24 h

[a] Doses are for adults and vary somewhat with between studies. All doses IP unless otherwise stated.

symptoms of peritonitis and cloudy fluid, negative routine cultures, and failure to respond to therapy for common organisms that cause peritonitis. The findings in peritoneal fluid cell counts have been variable, with either neutrophilic or mononuclear response. Smears for acid-fast bacilli are occasionally positive, as are myobacterial cultures of effluent. Cases are often diagnosed at laparotomy. Successful therapy generally involves removal of the catheter and antituberculous drugs. Atypical mycobacteria, especially *Mycobacterium chelonei* and *Mycobacterium fortuitum*, are often resistant to the classic antituberculous agents but respond to other antimicrobials, such as trimethoprim-sulfamethoxazole, cefoxitin, amikacin, doxycycline, or erythromycin.

A large number of species of fungi and algae have been isolated from CAPD patients with peritonitis (see Table 7-2). *Candida* sp predominate the causes, with most other fungi being sited as etiologies in case reports. In a review of the literature and a report of 11 of their own patients, Eisenberg et al.[97] found the following characteristics of fungal peritonitis: (1) the signs and symptoms are indistinguishable from bacterial peritonitis; (2) approximately 70 percent of patients had received a course of antimicrobial therapy before onset of the fungal infection; (3) cell counts and differentials were no different from those of bacterial infections; (4) of those reported, 50 percent had a positive Gram stain for yeast or hyphae; (5) the majority of patients have positive effluent cultures; (6) therapeutic regimens were highly variable, but only 26 percent responded without removal of the catheter; and (7) no deaths ocurred in 15 patients who had early removal of catheters. Since this review, three additional series with numbers of cases varying between five and 17 have been reported.[43,52,98] These reports have dealt primarily with therapy. Struijk et al.[98] reported cure of six of nine episodes of *Candida* sp peritonitis treated with IP amphotericin B and 5-fluorocytosine. Rubin et al.[43] found successful therapy by catheter removal and administration of a total dose of 500 mg of amphotericin B. Five episodes of *Candida* peritonitis treated with IP fluorocytosine failed to respond without catheter removal in the study of Eisenberg et al.[52]

Miscellaneous Infections

Failure to eradicate the infectious agent with initial therapy or relapse after what appears to be successful therapy are two of the more commonly encountered complications of peritonitis. Failure with initial therapy occurs most commonly with gram-negative rod infections, especially those caused by *Pseudomonas aeruginosa,* and with fungi.

Krothapalli et al.[99] were the first to point out the high degree of refractoriness to medical therapy of *P aeruginosa* infections. In their report, nine of nine patients with *P aeruginosa* infections failed to respond to IP aminoglycosides active against the organism following 10 to 14 days of treatment. Patients responded after catheter removal and continuation of antibiotics. Other investigators have had similar experiences.[100] In contrast to the universal failures reported by the above investigators, Nguyen et al.[101] and Bernardini et al.[102] have reported successful therapy for some cases of *Pseudomonas* sp infections with antimicrobials and without catheter removal. From analysis of these studies, the presence of evidence for an exit site and/or tunnel infection appears to predict failure.

Relapsing peritonitis, arbitrarily defined as a recurrence of peritonitis due to the same organism within 2 to 4 weeks and after a response to initial therapy, also represents a problem. Such recurrences may be due to poor patient technique or a tunnel infection (occult at times), and may also be postulated to derive from bacteria which escape antimicrobial action by virtue of being trapped in fibrin debris. Recommendations such as prolonging antimicrobial therapy for 4 weeks rather than the customary 7 to 14 days or adding rifampin to a vancomycin regimen for gram-positive peritonitis have been made but remain untested as to success rates. Another adjunct to therapy that has been successful in a few patients is the addition of streptokinase to the antibiotic regimen. Details of administration are outlined in a report by Norris et al.[103] Another ploy for relapsing peritonitis is to interrupt CAPD, administer antibiotics for 14 to 21 days, then resume CAPD.[104]

Perforation of a viscus is an uncommon but serious complication during CAPD. Its presentation is similar to the more common nonperforation peritonitis. It often occurs secondary to a perforated diverticulum of the colon in the older population. Clues to the diagnosis include isolation of more than one organism from the effluent and/or anaerobic bacteria. Therapy is with antibiotics active against aerobes and anaerobes and early laparotomy with removal of the catheter. Therapy with amphotericin may also be necessary in that yeast are often a part of the bowel flora.

A possible complication of peritonitis, particularly multiple episodes of peritonitis, is sclerosing peritonitis. However, not all patients who develop sclerosing peritonitis have a history of infectious peritonitis. Signs and symptoms of this disease process include progressive loss of the ultrafiltration capacity of the peritoneum, nausea, vomiting, abdominal cramping, intestinal obstruction, and an occasional mass.[105] Occasionally, patients may develop calcification of the peritoneum.[106]

While clinical observations may suggest the diagnosis, absolute diagnosis requires laporatomy with biopsy. Computerized tomography of the abdomen may be used and may be highly suggestive of the diagnosis by disclosing loculated ascites, adherent bowel loops, narrowing of the lumen of the bowel, and thickening of the peritoneal membrane.[107] While the etiology of sclerosing peritonitis remains incompletely resolved, infection, antiseptics such as chlorhexidine, and certain types of dialysates are suspect.[105,108] Repeated injections of providone-iodine into the peritoneal cavity of rats has produced changes in the peritoneal membrane similar to those seen in sclerosing peritonitis.[109] At present, no satisfactory treatment is available for sclerosing peritonitis except changing to another form of dialysis.

Other complications include those that occur secondary to therapy. These are the usual reactions to drugs and, in addition and more specifically, vestibular/ototoxicity secondary to aminoglycosides and *Clostridium difficile* pseudomembranous colitis secondary to antibiotics, especially cephalosporins.[110] Denominator data related to the frequency of ototoxicity are lacking but are mentioned in various reviews.[1,111] Avoidance of such toxicity has not been systematically examined, but there are suggestions of how to do so, such as measuring serum concentrations to assure trough levels less or equal to 2 mg/L in serum intermittently during therapy, reduction of aminoglycoside doses, and giving larger doses at less frequent intervals.

Catheter Removal and Reinsertion

Some patients with peritonitis fail to respond to appropriate therapy or have repeated relapses. A response to therapy generally occurs when the foreign body is removed. This may occur with any organism, but *S aureus,*

P aeruginosa, and fungal infections are the most common causes for catheter removal.

No hard data exist as to the appropriate times for catheter removal and insertion. It is known that with bacterial peritonitis a clinical response and reduction in inflammatory indices in the effluent occurs within 48 hours in most patients receiving appropriate therapy. Because of the fear of loss of the peritoneum as a means of dialysis and occasional mortality, some have recommended removal of the catheter at 96 hours if there is no clear-cut response to therapy.[95] This seems a reasonable recommendation unless further studies show differently.

Some have had success with immediate replacement of the catheter with an alternate exit site,[112] while others have opted to allow an arbitrary time of 2 to 3 weeks to pass before reinsertion (Everett, unpublished data). In the report of Paterson et al.,[112] gram-positive and gram-negative peritonitis as well as aseptic peritonitis were successfully treated with replacement. On the other hand, Krothapalli et al.[99] noted reinfection of catheters replaced within 1 week in patients with pseudomonas peritonitis. More published data are needed before routine immediate catheter replacement can be recommended.

SUMMARY

Peritonitis associated with CAPD continues to cause significant morbidity and adds to the cost of the care of such patients. Steps have been taken that have reduced the incidence of peritonitis, such as the introduction of bagged dialysate and the recent introduction of the Y-connector in conjunction with indwelling antiseptic. Future improvement of peritonitis rates will need further technologic improvements, better management of exit sites, and perhaps change of the host defense mechanisms in the peritoneal cavity.

When a patient develops peritonitis, every effort should be made to isolate the causitive agent. A number of sensitive techniques are suitable for culturing, and the method chosen depends on its availability in the laboratory. These include the Isolator technique, BACTEC, Septi-Check, Millipore filter techniques, and centrifuging 50 ml of effluent and culturing the sediment. When unusual organisms are suspected, consultation with the microbiology laboratory and/or an infectious disease specialist should be done.

After material has been obtained for laboratory examination, the patient should be started on antimicrobial agents. There are several routes of delivery of drugs and possible regimens. At present, if the Gram stain is negative or unavailable, such as in home therapy, I recommend IP vancomycin plus an aminoglycoside. Other possible alternatives could be ceftazidime or aztreonam plus vancomycin, but these are more expensive and have less clinical experience to support their use. If gram-positive organisms are isolated, it appears that the regimen of IP vancomycin once weekly is an effective means of therapy. Gram-negative rod peritonitis should be treated based on the susceptibility of the organisms. At this point, most cases of fungal peritonitis, mainly yeast, should be treated by early catheter removal followed by a course of IV amphotericin B to a total dosage of 300 to 500 mg. Oral therapy with fluoroquinolones appears to be promising, but more data need to be accumulated before their routine usage can be recommended. Therapy for 10 to 14 days is adequate for most cases.

The option of immediate catheter replacement after removal for infection needs to be subjected to a large randomized trial.

REFERENCES

1. Rubin J, Rogers WA, Taylor HM, et al: Peritonitis during continuous ambulatory peritoneal dialysis. Ann Intern Med 92:7, 1980
2. Alobaidi HM, Coles GA, Davies M, Lloyd D: Host defense in continuous ambulatory peritoneal dialysis: the effect of the dialysate on phagocytic function. Nephrol Dial Transplant 1:16, 1986
3. Harvey DM, Sheppard KJ, Morgan AG, Fletcher J: Effect of dialysate fluids on phagocytosis and killing by normal neutrophils. J Clin Microbiol 25:1424, 1987
4. McGregor S, Brock JH, Briggs JD, Junor BJR: Relationship of IgG, C-3 and transferrin with opsonising and bacteriostatic activity of peritoneal fluid from CAPD patients and the incidence of peritonitis. Nephrol Dial Transplant 2:551, 1987
5. Coles GA, Alobaidi H, Topley N, Davies M: Opsonic activity of dialysis effluent predicts those at risk of *Staphylococcus epidermidis* peritonitis. Nephrol Dial Transplant 2:359, 1987
6. Dasgupta MK, Ulan RA, Bettcher KB, et al: Effect of exit site infection and peritonitis on the distribution of biofilm encased adherent bacterial microcolonies (BABM) on Tenckhoff (T) catheters in patients undergoing continuous ambulatory peritoneal dialysis (CAPD). p. 102. In Khanna R, Nolph K, Prowant B, et al (eds): Advances in Continuous Ambulatory Peritoneal Dialysis. Peritoneal Dialysis Bulletin, Toronto, 1986
7. Holmes CJ, Evans RC, Spinowitz BS: Biofilm in CAPD: an update. p. 256. In Khanna R, Nolph K, Prowant B, et al (eds): Advances in Continuous Ambulatory Peritoneal Dialysis. Peritoneal Dialysis Bulletin, Toronto, 1988
8. Goodship T, Heaton A, Rodger R, et al: Factors affecting development of peritonitis in continuous ambulatory peritoneal dialysis. Br Med J 289:1485, 1984
9. Prowant B, Nolph K, Ryan L, et al: Peritonitis in continuous ambulatory peritoneal dialysis: analysis of an 8-year experience. Nephron 43:105, 1986
10. Nolph KD, Prowant B, Serkes KD: A randomized multicenter clinical trial to evaluate the effects of an ultraviolet germicidal system on peritonitis rate in continuous ambulatory peritoneal dialysis. Peritoneal Dialysis Bull 5:19, 1985
11. Zappacosta AR, Perres ST: Reduction of CAPD peritonitis rate by ultraviolet light with dialysate exchange assist device. Dialysis Transplant 17:483, 1988
12. Maiorca R, Cantaluppi A, Cancarini G, et al: Prospective controlled trial of a Y-connector disinfectant to prevent peritonitis in continuous ambulatory peritoneal dialysis. Lancet 2:642, 1983
13. Buoncristiani U, Quintaliani G, Cozzari M, Carobi C: Current status of the

Y-set. p. 165. In Khanna R, Nolph K, Prowant B, et al (eds): Advances in Continuous Ambulatory Peritoneal Dialysis. Peritoneal Dialysis Bulletin, Toronto, 1986

14. Cantaluppi A, Scalamogna A, Castelnovo, C, Graziani G: Long term efficacy of a Y-connector and disinfectant in continuous ambulatory peritoneal dialysis. p. 182. In Khanna R, Nolph K, Prowant B, et al (eds): Advances in Continuous Ambulatory Peritoneal Dialysis. Peritoneal Dialysis Bulletin, Toronto, 1986·

15. Ryckelynck J, Verger C, Cam G, et al: Importance of the flush effect in disconnect systems. p. 282. In Khanna R, Nolph K, Prowant B, et al (eds): Advances in Continuous Ambulatory Peritoneal Dialysis. Peritoneal Dialysis Bulletin, Toronto, 1988

16. Low DE, Vas SI, Oreopoulos DG, et al: Prophylactic cephalexin ineffective in chronic ambulatory peritoneal dialysis. Lancet 2:753, 1980

17. Churchill DN, Taylor DW, Vas SI, et al: Peritonitis in continuous ambulatory peritoneal dialysis (CAPD) patients: a randomized clinical trial of cotrimazole prophylaxis. Peritoneal Dialysis Int 8:125, 1988

18. Lamperi S, Carozzi S, Nasini MG, et al: Response to intraperitoneal (i.p.) immunoglobulin (Ig) therapy in high peritonitis incidence CAPD patients. p. 181. In Khanna R, Nolph K, Prowant B, et al (eds): Advances in Peritoneal Dialysis. Peritoneal Dialysis Bulletin, Toronto, 1988

19. Williams P, Pantalowy D, Vas S, et al: The value of dialysate cell count in the diagnosis of peritonitis in patients on CAPD. Peritoneal Dialysis Bull 1:59, 1981

20. Males B, Walshe J, Amsterdam D: Laboratory indices of clinical peritonitis: total leukocyte count microscopy and microbiologic culture of peritoneal dialysis effluent. J Clin Microbiol 25:2367, 1987

21. Gould I, Casewell M: The laboratory diagnosis of peritonitis during continuous ambulatory peritoneal dialysis. J Hosp Infect 7:155, 1986

22. Cocanour B, Fessia S, Ryan S: Improved methods for detecting peritonitis causing microorganisms in peritoneal dialysate. p. 118. In Khanna R, Nolph K, Prowant B, et al (eds): Advances in Continuous Ambulatory Peritoneal Dialysis. Peritoneal Dialysis Bulletin, Toronto, 1986

23. Hachler H, Vogt K, Binswanger U, Von Graevenitz A: Centrifugation of 50 ml of peritoneal fluid is sufficient for microbiological examination in continuous ambulatory peritoneal dialysis (CAPD) patients with peritonitis. Infection 14:102, 1986

24. Vas SI, Low L: Microbiological diagnosis of peritonitis in patients on continuous ambulatory peritoneal dialysis. J Clin Microbiol 21:522, 1985

25. Males BM, Walshe J, Grarringer L, et al: Addi-Chek filtration, BACTEC, and 10 ml culture methods for recovery of microorganisms from dialysis effluent during episodes of peritonitis. J Clin Microbiol 23:350, 1986

26. Ryan S, Fessia S: Improved method for recovery of peritonitis causing microorganisms from peritoneal dialysate. J Clin Microbiol 25:383, 1987

27. Forbes BA, Frymoyer PA, Kopecky RT, et al: Evaluation of the lysis centrifugation system for culturing dialysates from continous ambulatory peritoneal dialysis patients with peritonitis. Am J Kidney Dis 11:176, 1988

28. Dawson MS, Harford AM, Garner BK, et al: Total volume culture technique for the isolation of microorganisms from continuous ambulatory peritoneal dialysis patients with peritonitis. J Clin Microbiol 22:391, 1985

29. Taylor PC, Poole-Warren LA, Grundy RE: Increased microbiol yield from con-

tinuous ambulatory peritoneal dialysis peritonitis effluent after chemical or physical disruption of phagocytes. J Clin Microbiol 25:580, 1987

30. Report of a Working Party of the British Society for Antimicrobial Chemotherapy: Diagnosis and management of peritonitis in continuous ambulatory peritoneal dialysis. Lancet 1:845, 1987

31. Peterson PK, Matzke G, Keane WB: Current concepts in the management of peritonitis patients undergoing continuous ambulatory peritoneal dialysis. Rev Infect Dis 9:604, 1987

32. DiSancto N, Attucci P, Giandano C: Actinomyces peritonitis associated with dialysis. Nephron 16:236, 1976

33. Gruer LD, Turney JH, Curley J, et al: Vancomycin and tobramycin in the treatment of CAPD peritonitis. Nephron 41:279, 1985

34. Biasioli S, Chiaramonte S, Fabris A, et al: *Bacillus cereus* as an agent of peritonitis during peritoneal dialysis. Nephron 37:211, 1984

35. Byrd L, Anama L, Gutkin M, Chmel H: *Bordetella bronchiseptica* peritonitis associated with continuous ambulatory peritoneal dialysis. J Clin Microbiol 14:232, 1981

36. Wens R, Dratwa M, Potvliege C, et al: Campylobacter septicemia after peritonitis complicating peritoneal dialysis. Arch Intern Med 144:653, 1984

37. Pepersack F, D'Haene M, Toussaint C, Schoutens E: *Campylobacter jejuni* peritonitis complicating continuous ambulatory peritoneal dialysis. J Clin Microbiol 16:739, 1982

38. Pierard D, Lauwers S, Mouton M, et al: Group Jk Corynebacterium peritonitis in a patient undergoing CAPD. J Clin Microbiol 18:1011, 1983

39. Morris A, Henderson G, Bremner D, Collins J: Relapsing peritonitis in a patient undergoing continuous ambulatory peritoneal dialysis due to *Corynebacterium aquatium*. J Infect 13:151, 1986

40. Chan MK, Chow L, Lam SS, Jones B: Peritoneal eosinophilia in patients on continuous ambulatory peritoneal dialysis: a prospective study. Am J Kidney Dis 11:180, 1988

41. Swartz R, Campbell D, Stone D, Dickenson C: Recurrent polymicrobial peritonitis from a gynecologic source as a complication of CAPD. Peritoneal Dialysis Bull 3:32, 1983

42. Myers J, Peterson G, Rashid A: Peritonitis due to *Listeria monocytogenes* complicating continuous ambulatory peritoneal dialysis. J Infect Dis 148:1130, 1983

43. Rubin J, Kirchner K, Walsh D, et al: Fungal peritonitis during continuous ambulatory peritoneal dialysis: a report of 17 cases. Am J Kidney Dis 10:361, 1987

44. Arfania D, Everett ED, Nolph KD, Rubin J: Uncommon causes of peritonitis in patients undergoing peritoneal dialysis. Arch Intern Med 141:61, 1981

45. Paul RV, Rostand SG: Cat-bite peritonitis: *Pasteurella multocida* peritonitis following feline contamination of peritoneal dialysis tubing. Am J Kidney Dis 10:318, 1987

46. Rutherford PC, Narkowicz JE, Wood CJ, Peel MM: Peritonitis caused by *Pseudomonas mesophilica* in a patient undergoing continued ambulatory peritoneal dialysis. J Clin Microbiol 26:2441, 1988

47. Silver M, Felegie T, Sorkin M: Unusual bacterium, group Ve-2 causing peritonitis in a patient on continuous ambulatory peritoneal dialysis. J Clin Microbiol 21:838, 1985

48. Taylor R, McDonald M, Russ G, et al: Vibrio alginolyticus peritonitis associated with ambulatory peritoneal dialysis. Br Med J 283:275, 1981

49. Horisberger J, Bille J, Wauters J: Fungal eosinophilic peritonitis due to alternaria in a patient on continuous ambulatory peritoneal dialysis. Peritoneal Dialysis Bull 4:255, 1984

50. Carpenter J, Foulks C, Weiner M: Peritoneal dialysis complicated by *Aspergillus flavus* peritonitis: a role for fungal antigen serodiagnosis. Nephron 32:258, 1982

51. Prewitt K, Lockard J, Rodgers D, Hasbargen J: Successful treatment of *Aspergillus* peritonitis complicating peritoneal dialysis. Am J Kidney Dis 13:501, 1989

52. Eisenberg ES: Intraperitoneal flucytosine in the management of fungal peritonitis in patients on continuous ambulatory peritoneal dialysis. Am J Kidney Dis 11:465, 1988

53. Rahko P, Davry P, Wheat J, Bartlett M: Treatment of *Torulopsis glabrata* peritonitis with intraperitoneal amphotericin B. JAMA 249:1187, 1983

54. Landay M, Greenwald J, Stemer A, Ashbach D: *Cephalosporium* (*acremonium*) in dialysis-connected peritonitis. J Indiana State Med Assoc75:391, 1982

55. Ampel NM, White JD, Varanasi UR, et al: Coccidioidal peritonitis associated with continuous ambulatory peritoneal dialysis. Am J Kidney Dis 11:512, 1988

56. Smith JW, Walson CA: Cryptococcal peritonitis in patients on peritoneal dialysis. Am J Kidney Dis 11:430, 1988

57. O'Sullivan F, Stuewe B, Lynch J, et al: Peritonitis due to *Drechslera spicifera* complicating continuous ambulatory peritoneal dialysis. Ann Intern Med 94:213, 1981

58. Kerr C, Perfect J, Craven P, et al: Fungal peritonitis in patients on continuous ambulatory peritoneal dialysis. Ann Intern Med 99:334, 1983

59. Fabris A, Biasioli S, Borin D, et al: Fungal peritonitis in peritoneal dialysis: our experience and review of treatments. Peritoneal Dialysis Bull 4:75, 1984

60. McNeely D, Vas S, Dombros N, Oreopoulos D: Fusarium peritonitis: an uncommon complication of CAPD. Peritoneal Dialysis Bull 1:94, 1981

61. Khanna R, Oreopoulos D, Vas S, et al: Treating fungal infections. Br Med J 280:1147, 1980 (letter)

62. Locci R, Romagnoni M, Beccari S, et al: Massive colonization of in-dwelling catheter by *Penicillium pinophilum* without peritonitis. Peritoneal Dialysis Bull 4:243, 1984

63. Pearson J, McKinney T, Stone W: Penicillium peritonitis in a CAPD patient. Peritoneal Dialysis Bull 3:20, 1983

64. Mion C, Slingeneyer A, Canaud B: Peritonitis. p. 163. In Gokal R (ed): Continuous Ambulatory Peritoneal Dialysis. Churchill Livingstone, Edinburgh, 1986

65. West LM, Golper TA, Hatch J, Rashad AL: Algae peritonitis misdiagnosed as fungal. p. 163. In Khanna R, Nolph K, Prowant B, et al (eds): Advances in Continuous Ambulatory Dialysis. Peritoneal Dialysis Bulletin, Toronto, 1987

66. Eisenberg E, Alpert R, Weiss R, et al: *Rhodotorula rubra* peritonitis in patients undergoing continuous ambulatory peritoneal dialysis. Am J Med 75:349, 1983

67. Loeppky C, Sprouse R, Carlson J, Everett E: *Trichoderma viridae* peritonitis. South Med J 76:798, 1983

68. Kluge G: Tuberculous peritonitis in a patient undergoing chronic ambulatory peritoneal dialysis (CAPD). Peritoneal Dialysis Bull 3:189, 1983

69. Khanna R, Fenton S, Cattran D, et al: Tuberculous peritonitis in patients undergoing continuous ambulatory peritoneal dialysis (CAPD). Peritoneal Dialysis Bull 1:10, 1981

70. Poisson M, Bermiade V, Falardeau P, et al: *Mycobacterium chelonei* peritonitis in a patient undergoing continuous ambulatory peritoneal dialysis (CAPD). Peritoneal Dialysis Bull 3:86, 1983

71. Pulliam J, Vernon D, Alexander S: Non-tuberculosis mycobacterial peritonitis associated with continuous ambulatory peritoneal dialysis. Am J Kidney Dis 2:610, 1983

72. Band J, Ward J, Fraser D, et al: Peritonitis due to *Mycobacterium chelonei*-like organisms associated with intermittent chronic peritoneal dialysis. J Infect Dis 145:9, 1982

73. London RD, Damsker B, Neibart EP, et al: *Mycobacterium gordonae*—an unusual peritoneal pathogen in a patient undergoing continuous ambulatory peritoneal dialysis. Am J Med 85:703, 1988

74. Karanicolas S, Oreopoulos DG, Izatt I: Epidemic of aseptic peritonitis caused by endotoxin during chronic peritoneal dialysis. N Engl J Med 296:1136, 1977

75. Poole CL, Read DL, Westervelt FB: Aseptic peritonitis associated with menstruation and ovulation in a peritoneal dialysis patient. p. 134. In Khanna R, Nolph K, Prowant B, et al (eds): Advances in Continuous Ambulatory Peritoneal Dialysis. Peritoneal Dialysis Bulletin, Toronto, 1986

76. Piraino B, Bernardini J, Johnston J, Sorkin M: Chemical peritonitis due to intraperitoneal vancomycin (Vancoled). Peritoneal Dialysis Bull 7:156, 1987

77. Gokal R, Ramos JM, Ward MK, et al: "Eosinophilic" peritonitis in continuous ambulatory peritoneal dialysis (CAPD). Clin Nephrol 15:328, 1981

78. Nolph KD, Sorkin M, Prowant B, et al: Asymtomatic eosinophilic peritonitis in CAPD. Dialysis Transplant 11:309, 1982

79. Pagniez DC, McNamara E, Hober D, et al: Treatment of mild CAPD peritonitis using natural defenses of the peritoneal cavity. VIII Annual CAPD Conference. Peritoneal Dialysis Int 1988 (abstr. 124)

80. Knight K, Crump J, Polak A, Maskell R: Laboratory diagnosis and oral treatment of CAPD peritonitis. Lancet 2:1301, 1982

81. Searle M, Raman GV: Oral treatment of peritonitis complicating continuous ambulatory dialysis. Clin Nephrol 23:241, 1985

82. Boeschoten EW, Rietra P, Krediet RT, et al: CAPD peritonitis: A prospective randomized trial of oral versus intraperitoneal treatment with cephradine. J Antimicrob Chemother 16:789, 1985

83. Scott AC, Fleming LW, Stewart WK: Efficacy of ciprofloxacin in treatment of CAPD peritonitis. Eur J Clin Microbiol 6:599, 1987

84. Chan MK, Chau PY, Chan WWN: Oral treatment of peritonitis in CAPD patients with two dosage regimens of ofloxacin. J Antimicrob Chemother 22:371, 1988

85. Golper TA, Hartstein AI, Morthland VH, Christensen JM: Effects of antacids and dialysate dwell times on multiple dose pharmacokinetics of oral ciprofloxacin in patients on continuous ambulatory peritoneal dialysis. Antimicrob Agents Chemother 31:1787, 1987

86. Krothapalli RK, Scnekjian HO, Ayus JC: Efficacy of intravenous vancomycin in

the treatment of Gram-positive peritonitis in long-term peritoneal dialysis. Am J Med 75:345, 1983

87. Obermiller LE, Tzameloukas AH, Leymon P, Avasthi PS: Intravenous vancomycin as initial treatment for Gram-positive peritonitis in patients on chronic peritoneal dialysis. Clin Nephrol 24:256, 1985

88. Mistry CD, Salgia P, Manos J, et al: Netilmicin and vancomycin in the treatment of peritonitis in patients on continuous ambulatory peritoneal dialysis (CAPD). p. 127. In Khanna R, Nolph K, Prowant B, et al (eds): Advances in Continuous Ambulatory Peritoneal Dialysis. Peritoneal Dialysis Bulletin, Toronto, 1986

89. Glasson P, Favre H: Treatment of peritonitis in continuous ambulatory peritoneal dialysis patients with co-trimoxazole. Nephron 36:65, 1984

90. Gray HH, Goulding S, Eykn SJ: Intraperitoneal vancomycin and ceftazidime in the treatment of CAPD peritonitis. Clin Nephrol 23:81, 1985

91. Bastani B, Freer K, Read D, et al: Treatment of Gram-positive peritonitis with two intraperitoneal doses of vancomycin in continuous ambulatory peritoneal dialysis patients. Nephron 45:283, 1987

92. Morse GD, Nairn DK, Walshe JJ: Once weekly intraperitoneal therapy for Gram-positive peritonitis. Am J Kidney Dis 10:300, 1987

93. Bastani B, Sherman RA, Freer K, et al: Further experience with two intraperitoneal vancomycin loading doses for treatment of Gram-positive or sterile peritonitis in CAPD patients. Peritoneal Dialysis Int 8:27, 1988

94. Bowley JA, Pickering SJ, Scantlebury AJ, et al: Intraperitoneal teicoplanin in the treatment of peritonitis associated with continuous ambulatory peritoneal dialysis. J Antimicrob Chemother 21:suppl A, 133, 1988

95. Keane WF, Everett E, Fine R, et al: CAPD related peritonitis management and antibiotic therapy recommendations. Peritoneal Dialysis Bull 7:55, 1987

96. Golper TA, Hartstein AT: Analysis of the causative pathogens in uncomplicated CAPD-associated peritonitis: duration of therapy, relapses and prognosis. Am J Kidney Dis 7:141, 1986

97. Eisenberg ES, Leviton I, Soeiro R: Fungal peritonitis in patients receiving peritoneal dialysis: experience with 11 patients and review of the literature. Rev Infect Dis 8:309, 1986

98. Struijk DG, Krediet RT, Boeschoten EW, et al: Antifungal treatment of *Candida* peritonitis in continuous ambulatory peritoneal dialysis patients. Am J Kidney Dis 9:66, 1987

99. Krothapalli RK, Duffy B, Lacke C, et al: Pseudomonas peritonitis and continuous ambulatory peritoneal dialysis. Arch Intern Med 142:1862, 1982

100. Juergensen PH, Finkelstein FO, Brennan R, et al: Pseudomonas peritonitis associated with continuous ambulatory peritoneal dialysis: a six year study. Am J Kidney Dis 11:413, 1988

101. Nguyen V, Swartz RD, Reynolds J, et al: Successful treatment of pseudomonas peritonitis during continuous ambulatory peritoneal dialysis. Am J Nephrol 7:38, 1987

102. Bernardini J, Piraino B, Sorkin M: Analysis of continuous ambulatory peritoneal dialysis-related *Pseudomonas aeruginosa* infections. Am J Med 83:829, 1987

103. Norris KC, Shinaberger JH, Reyes GD, Kraut JA: The use of intracatheter instillation of streptokinase in the treatment of recurrent bacterial peritonitis in continuous ambulatory peritoneal dialysis. Am J Kidney Dis 10:62, 1987

104. Kant KS, Goetz D, Marzluff C, Motz D: Relapsing peritonitis in continuous ambulatory peritoneal dialysis: treatment by interruption of CAPD and prolonged antibiotic therapy. Peritoneal Dialysis Int 8:155, 1988

105. Slingenneyer A, Mion C, Mourad G, et al: Progressive sclerosing peritonitis: A late and severe complication of maintenance peritoneal dialysis. Trans Am Soc Artif Internal Organs 29:633, 1983

106. Marichal JF, Faller B, Brignon P, et al: Progressive calcifying peritonitis: a new complication of CAPD. Nephron 45:229, 1987

107. Korzets A, Korzets Z, Peer G, et al: Sclerosing peritonitis. Am J Nephrol 8:143, 1988

108. Oules R, Challah S, Brunner FP: Case-control study to determine the cause of sclerosing peritoneal disease. Nephrol Dial Transplant 3:66, 1988

109. Mackow RC, Argy WP, Winchester JF, et al: Sclerosing encapsulating peritonitis in rats induced by long-term intraperitoneal administration of antiseptics. J Lab Clin Med 112:363, 1988

110. Gokal R, Ramos JM, Francis D, et al: Peritonitis in continuous ambulatory peritoneal dialysis. Lancet 2:1388, 1982

111. Oreopoulos DG, Williams P, Khanna R, Vas S: Treatment of peritonitis. Peritoneal Dialysis Bull 1:517, 1981

112. Paterson AD, Morgan AG, Bishop MC, Barden RP: Removal and replacement of Tenckhoff catheter at a single operation: successful treatment of resistant peritonitis in continuous ambulatory peritoneal dialysis. Lancet 2:1245, 1986

8

Experiences with the Y-System

Rosario Maiorca
Giovanni C. Cancarini

INTRODUCTION

The Y-system has significantly improved the prophylaxis of peritonitis in continuous ambulatory peritoneal dialysis (CAPD), but outside Italy has had an unjustifiably low diffusion. One possible explanation might be a certain reluctance for using a disinfectant in line because of the real possibility that it may accidentally enter the peritoneal cavity. Although this has been demonstrated to happen only rarely and is not dangerous, there may still be a psychological barrier. More recently, the persuasive effect of the reported good results seems to have reduced resistances: in 1988, 2,500 patients worldwide were using some kind of Y-system.[1]

In this review, the principles of the method and the results obtained so far will be illustrated. We believe that better knowledge should facilitate the larger application of the Y-system in CAPD.

THE PROBLEM

Studies of the pathogenesis of peritonitis in CAPD have led to the conclusion that the largest number of peritoneal infections are due to transluminal (intraluminal) contamination.

Etiologic agents enter the system when it is open (i.e., during the bag exchange) due to touching or to airborne (coughs, sneezes) contamination. It follows from this that any attempt to prevent this contamination must (1) avoid germ entrance, (2) kill germs already present before they reach the peritoneum, (3) wash out germs already in the system, or (4) regularly put disinfectants or antibiotics into the dialysis fluid.

All of these recommendations have been tried, in addition to experimentation with new connectors and devices, but the results have not always been satisfactory.

The first method, avoiding germ entrance, implies that the bag is exchanged in absolute asepsis, which means using a sterile room, clothes, mask, gloves, etc., or devices that make any contamination impossible. However, asepsis is practically impossible to obtain in the usual conditions of home treatment, with patients having a limited knowledge of the meaning and procedures. In fact, even with the best training programs, the incidence of peritonitis has not been better than one episode per year. Attempts to avoid bacterial entry by putting bacteriologic filters on line have been made.[2-11] Unfortunately, in these devices bacteria proliferate upstream,[12] and the filter lets through endotoxins and other bacterial products, which stimulate peritoneal macrophages to produce cytokines and other mediators able to induce fibroblast proliferation and peritoneal chronic inflammation. In the long run, this might favor a loss of permeability or even a sclerosing encapsulating peritonitis.[13-16] This method is rarely used today.

The second method, germ killing, can be chemical or physical, but it does not avoid the entrance of killed bacteria and their products into the peritoneal cavity, reproducing the same inconvenience as bacteriologic filters.

The third method, removal of bacteria already in the system, is to flush the connector. Y-shaped connectors are the more convenient for this: the washout is done with a small quantity of fresh dialysis fluid and/or the peritoneal effluent just before filling the peritoneal cavity (the "flush before fill" concept). This method will be treated more extensively below, but doubts persist concerning its ability to wash out all kinds of bacteria, especially those able to adhere to the plastic tubing.

The fourth method, placing disinfectants or antibiotics into the dialysis fluid has many unwanted effects: the continuous introduction of foreign substances can cause chronic peritoneal inflammation, with dangerous effects on solute clearance or water ultrafiltration. Continuous introduction of antibiotics might select resistant strains of bacteria or facilitate fungal infections.

Based on these premises, the ideal connection system should (1) prevent or effectively limit touch contamination; (2) kill germs entering the system at the time of connection; (3) prevent proliferation of germs entering the connector after bag exchange; (4) wash out germs and germ products; and (5) prevent regular introduction into the peritoneal cavity of potentially dangerous substances.

The Y-system has these characteristics and in open and controlled studies, has been demonstrated capable of significantly reducing the frequency of peritonitis. In Italy, where the method was devised, more than 90 percent of patients treated by 24 centers in the Italian CAPD Cooperative Study Group (ICSG), corresponding to approximately 50 percent of all CAPD patients in the country, were using Y-systems at the end of 1987 (ICSG, unpublished data).

THE Y-SYSTEM

Basic Composition

The Y-connector was first used by Grollman et al.[17] for intermittent peritoneal dialysis. Its application in the CAPD technique is a convincing demonstration of how useful it is to remember old inventions when devising new ideas.

The Y-system was first described by Buoncristiani et al.[18] and named the "Perugia system"; the name is derived from the Italian city where the system was devised. Subsequently, Y-set and Y-system were the terms more broadly used. A clearcut distinction should be made between Y-set (synonymous with Y-connector) and Y-system. The term Y-system indicates the use of a Y-set, *together with a disinfectant,* maintained in line during the entire dwell-time and washed out as a first step in bag exchange.

The Y-set

One of the three branches of the Y-set is connected to the catheter through a titanium luer-lock adaptor; the other two branches are not connected and are covered by a cap during the dwell-time. In our practice, the connector is maintained in-site for 2 months. This makes it inexpensive and it can be changed in true asepsis by a trained nurse during the patient's check-up in the CAPD center. At bag exchange, the second branch of the Y-set is connected to the new bag and the third branch is connected to an empty bag or to a glass or plastic container to collect and measure the outflowing dialysate. In the original Perugia system, the drainage tube of the new, full bag was long enough to be connected directly to the branch of the Y-set. Since this kind of bag was initially produced by only one manufacturer, to use the method with widely available standard bags, the design of the Y-set was modified, making the inlet branch long enough to be easily connected to the new bag (Fig. 8-1). Another modification of the Y-connector introduced elsewhere is the "O-set," which has a "Y" configuration during use, but assumes an "O" shape between bag exchanges by connection of two of the branches of the Y.[1]

The Disinfectant

The disinfectant is introduced into the Y-set at the end of the bag exchange and fills the set for the entire dwell time. At the beginning of a new bag exchange, the disinfectant is washed out with 100 to 200 ml of fresh dialysis fluid, followed by draining the dialysate from the peritoneal cavity.

Summarizing the effect of the method, it washes out germs entering the set at connection and kills and washes out germs entering at the time of bag exchange. The use of the Y-system is diagrammed in Figure 8-2. All steps of our current procedure are discussed in depth in the appendix to this chapter.

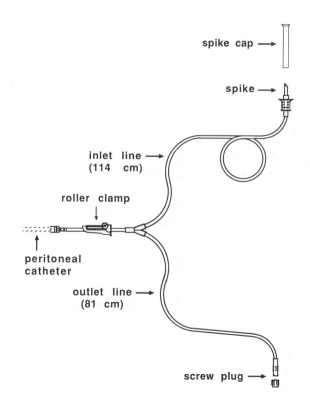

spike cap →

spike →

inlet line →
(114 cm)

roller clamp

peritoneal
catheter

outlet line →
(81 cm)

screw plug →

Fig. 8-1. The Y-Solution Transfer Set

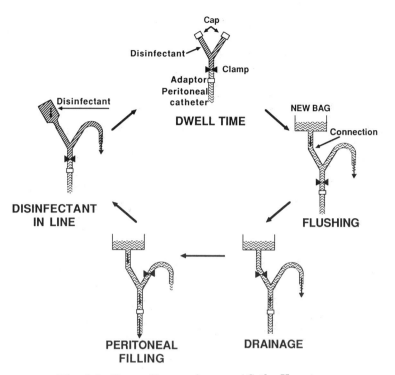

Fig. 8-2. Steps of bag exchange with the Y-system.

The Flushing

In Vitro Studies

Wash-out of bacteria entering the line during the bag exchange is important for the prevention of peritonitis. The ideal goal is to remove all bacteria, but it is probably sufficient to greatly reduce the bacterial load, with the residual germs eliminated by the peritoneal defense mechanisms.

Several studies have demonstrated the effectiveness of flushing in reducing bacterial contamination. After contaminating a Y-set branch before bag connection with 2,000 colony-forming units (CFU) of *Pseudomonas aeruginosa,* flushing with 5 ml of fresh dialysate removed up to 50 percent of the bacteria, and flushing with 110 ml removed all of the bacteria.[19] In a simulated peritoneal dialysis with an "O-set," only 0.2 to 2 percent of all *Staphylococcus epidermidis* inoculated into the connecting end of a branch reached the "peritoneal cavity" after the wash out.[20] In another study, flushing with 100 ml of fluid alone removed up to 10^4 CFU of bacteria. Increasing the volume of flushing from 100 to 500 ml increased the efficacy of wash out. Immersion of the connecting ends of the set in sodium hypochlorite also increased the efficacy of flushing, eliminating up to 94 percent of contamination by 10^3 to 10^7 CFU of several microbial species (*Escherichia coli,*

P aeruginosa, Staphylococcus aureus, S epidermidis, Streptococcus sangui-nis, Difteroid bacillus, Candida albicans).[21]

The efficay of flushing for removing bacteria is heavily influenced by the adherence of microorganisms. Washing with 100 ml of fluid immediately after inoculation removed 100 percent of *S epidermidis* inoculated at a concentration of 10^3 CFU, but removed only 60 percent of *S aureus* and 30 percent of *P aeruginosa*. If flushing was done 9 hours after contamination, its efficacy was still 100 percent for *S epidermidis*, but was reduced to 0 for *S aureus* and *Pseudomonas* organisms.[22] In another study, similar results were obtained.[29]

In Vivo Studies

The efficacy of washing alone for preventing peritonitis has been demonstrated in a multicenter prospective controlled trial, unfortunately published only in abstract form.[24] Forty-three new patients who were never on CAPD were randomized into two groups, one (20 patients; cumulative follow-up, 244 months) using a conventional system, the other (23 patients; follow-up, 268 months) using a Y-set without disinfectant. Frequency of peritonitis was one episode every 7.9 patient-months in the conventional group and one episode every 61 patient-months in the Y-set group. In earlier studies of the same group,[25-27] it had also been found that soaking the connecting ends of the set in providone-iodine does not further reduce the incidence of peritonitis. However, the disinfectant was not introduced in line and it is known that when povidone-iodine is used for few minutes, as in this work, it has poor disinfectant activity. In another prospective controlled study including 50 new patients,[28] the frequency of peritonitis for a Y-set without disinfectant was one episode every 23 patient-months (follow-up, 220 patient-months), whereas it was one episode every 12 patient-months for the standard connector (follow-up, 290 patient-months). In the same study, another 14 patients were switched from a standard connector to the Y-set and changed from one peritonitis episode per 10 patient-months to one episode per 24 patient-months. Fifty-five additional patients going on a standard connector had, in a follow-up of 800 patient-months, one episode every 12 patient-months. Other favorable results obtained with the flushing have also been reported.[29]

The Disinfectant

Is It Necessary?

As stated above, both in vitro and in vivo studies clearly demonstrate the importance of flushing for prophylaxis of peritonitis; the question is whether or not disinfection in line adds something to the positive effects of flushing.

In clinical practice, most peritonitis episodes are caused by *S epidermidis*, which should be easily washed out by flushing. Moreover, the bacterial load coming from touch contamination should not be very large. The number of bacteria in normal skin, although variably estimated by different techniques, should approximate 10^3 to 10^4 microorganisms/cm^2,[30] a concentration not exceeding the possibility of washing out by flushing alone.[21] However, the situation is not so good for contamination by *S aureus* or gram-negative bacteria. The in vitro studies of connector contamination in simulated peritoneal dialysis seem to indicate that flushing alone is insufficient for bacteria able to adhere to plastic surfaces, such as *S aureus* or *Pseudomonas* sp., even more so if present in heavy loads.[21,22,24]

On the other hand, the results in vivo might be different from those in vitro. Donald et al.,[31] using the "O" system, which includes 0.5 percent sodium hypochlorite in line, obtained a peritonitis rate of one episode per 23.2 patient-months in 89 patients followed for a total of 765 patient-months, a result consistent with those (one episode per 22 patient-months) obtained by other investigators for 171 patients followed for 1,413 patient-months with the same system.[1] In the report of Donald et al.,[31] using the same "O" system but without disinfectant, eight additional patients developed peritonitis within 2 months, mostly with environmental saprophytes. According to the investigators, these results demonstrate that simple flushing of the connectors is inadequate to prevent infection and that organisms may multiply in the tubing between exchanges.

Of course, only well-designed clinical trials comparing flushing alone with flushing plus disinfectant in line will be able to solve this problem. So far, clinical results obtained with the Y-set *plus* disinfectant (see below) support the suggestion that disinfection in line further improves the results of flushing.

Which Disinfectant?

The ideal disinfectant for this particular use should have the following characteristics.

1. Very quick and intense antibacterial activity
2. Active against spores and viruses
3. Not inactivated by dialysis fluid
4. Not dangerous to peritoneal or other tissue cells
5. Lacks acute or chronic toxicity in case of accidental introduction into the peritoneal cavity
6. Not corrosive to plastic lines
7. Not sediment-producing
8. Not expensive
9. Colored to help the patient remember to wash it out before a bag exchange
10. Stable

The disinfectants that best fulfill these requisites are the chlorinated preparations, which are characterized by broad, intense, and quick bactericidal activity, simple use, low toxicity, and low cost.

In the original Y-system, the antiseptic used is sodium hypochlorite obtained by partial electrolysis of hypertonic sodium chloride (Amukin), used undiluted or at a 50 percent concentration. In this product, up to 18 g/dl of the sodium chloride remains as such in the solution, together with traces of hypochlorous acid, which easily permeates bacterial membranes, and 1.1 percent of free, available chlorine.[32] The pH of Amukin is lower than that of sodium hypochlorite alone and this facilitates its antibacterical activity. Of course, it is not the ideal disinfectant; it can be inactivated by organic material,[33] corrodes metals, cannot be colored, and causes sharp pain if introduced intraperitoneally at high concentrations (25 to 100 percent). However, in clinical practice it has given good results. It has been demonstrated to be well-tolerated by animals[34] and humans,[35] and when injected locally in concentrations of 2 to 5 percent, it has been successful in curing intraperitoneal or retroperitoneal abscesses.[36] In a comparison with Dakin's solution, Amukin showed similar bacteriologic effectiveness but greater stability.[32] Stored, it is stable for 4 years.[37] In an in vitro study, 5×10^9 CFU of *P aeruginosa* were sterilized in less than 30 seconds by 5 ml of a 4.5 percent concentration, and in 5 minutes by a 0.7 percent concentration of Amukin.[19] In a comparative study in rats of long-term effects of a daily intraperitoneal injection of 10 percent Amukin, Dakin's solution, or alkyldimetilammonium chloride (Ampercide), none caused mesothelial lesions after up to 12 weeks. In contrast, povidone-iodine at similar concentrations causes intestinal adhesions, mesothelial thickening, and sclerosis, a picture simulating human sclerosing encapsulating peritonitis.[34]

On rare occasions, the disinfectant can be accidentally introduced into the peritoneal cavity. In a large experience with the "O" set, this occurred with a frequence of one episode every 33.6 patient-months (i.e., one episode per 4380 bag exchanges).[1] In our experience, it has occurred with an incidence of approximately one episode every 7,500 bag exchanges (one episode per 62.4 patient-months). In these cases, the patient feels an abdominal burning pain that disappears after a few quick washes of the peritoneal cavity with fresh dialysis solution. In our experience, we observed neither subsequent alterations of blood chemistry nor early or late modifications of peritoneal permeability to water or solutes. Table 8-1 shows the results of ultrafiltration

Table 8-1. Results of 4-Hour Equilibration/Ultrafiltration Test Performed With 2 L of Dianeal Solution 4.25%

	Patients With Previous Amukin Introduction Into Peritoneal Cavity	Patients Without Previous Amukin Introduction Into Peritoneal Cavity	*P* Value
No. of patients	11	51	
Peritoneal drainage	2,852 ± 192	2,686 ± 238	NS
Dialysate to plasma creatinine	0.76 ± 0.10	0.74 ± 0.12	NS
Dialysate end/start dwell-time glucose	0.20 ± 0.10	0.20 ± 0.10	NS

studies with populations of patients who did or did not have accidental introduction of Amukin into the peritoneal cavity. No differences were observed between the two groups. Figure 8-3 illustrates the case of a patient who had repeated Amukin introduction. No reduction in peritoneal creatinine clearance or in ultrafiltration was observed over time.

CLINICAL RESULTS WITH THE Y-SYSTEM

Controlled and Open Studies

The first clinical results with the Y-system were obtained by Buoncristiani et al.[38] in an open study. The incidence of peritonitis was one episode every 42-patient months. However, only those cases that gave rise to bacterial growth in cultures were considered peritonitis episodes. Since in the literature variable percentages, from 10 to 25 percent, of peritonitis episodes indicate "no growth," it is probable that the real frequency of peritonitis was higher, but surely much lower than that obtained with standard connectors.

A bicenter prospective controlled study comparing the Y-system (Y-solution Transfer Set with Amukin) and the standard connection technique of Oreopoulos et al.[39] was reported by Maiorca et al. in 1983.[40] Sixty-two new CAPD patients were randomly allocated to the standard method (group A, 30 patients) and to the Y-system (group B, 32 patients). The two groups were comparable for age, dialysis duration, and a number of bags exchanged per day. The diagnosis of peritonitis was based on the presence of two of the following three findings: abdominal pain, dialysate white blood cell counts over $100/mm^3$, and positive dialysate cultures. During a cumulative follow-up of 351 months in group A, there were 31 peritonitis episodes in 17 patients (57 percent) (i.e., one episode every 11.3 patient-months) and in a 363-month follow-up in group B, there were 11 peritonitis episodes in ten patients (31 percent) (i.e., one episode every 33 patient-months). The risk of developing peritonitis was significantly different for the two methods (life-table analysis, $P < .001$). Further experiences of these centers have been reported for several open studies.[41-48] In our center, the positive results obtained with the Y-system have been confirmed and also improved. The Y-system also proved to be effective in reducing the frequency of peritonitis in patients with high peritonitis rates on the standard system (Fig. 8-4). The frequency of peritonitis was not significantly different between diabetics and non-diabetics (Table 8-2), although other investigators[49] have reported a higher incidence in diabetics.

On the basis of the above results, many Italian centers have adopted the Y-system, and several open studies have been reported.[50-54] Data for the Perugia system have been published by Buoncristiani et al.[38,55,56] Some recent results are summarized in Table 8-3. Other favorable results, usually obtained with the O-system but also with other variants of the Y-system, have been obtained outside Italy.[1,31,57-59]

A new multicenter controlled study of the efficacy of the Y-system for

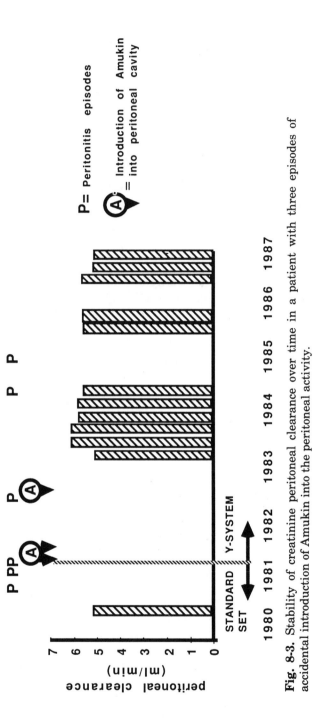

Fig. 8-3. Stability of creatinine peritoneal clearance over time in a patient with three episodes of accidental introduction of Amukin into the peritoneal activity.

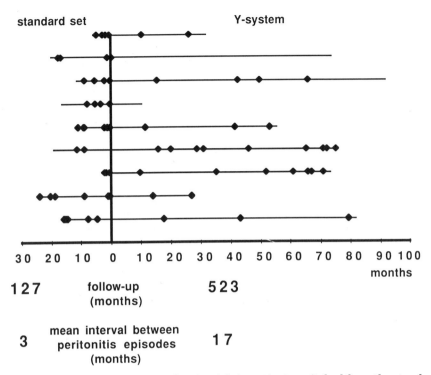

Fig. 8-4. Reduction of incidence of peritonitis in patients switched from the standard set to the Y-system because of high frequency of peritonitis.

preventing peritonitis has been recently reported.[6] Eight hospitals in six Canadian cities participated in the study. Sixty-one new CAPD patients were allocated to the Y-system, and 63 were assigned to the standard system. There were 21 episodes of peritonitis in 15 Y-system patients (one episode per 21.5 patient-months) and 47 episodes in 30 standard connector patients (one episode per 9.9 patient-months). There were no differences in the exit site infection rates. Accidental intraperitoneal infusion of disinfectant occurred in 15 of 61 Y-system patients on 22 occasions (i.e., one per 2,500 exchanges). The probability of developing peritonitis by 1 year was 0.53 for Y-system patients and 0.74 for standard system patients. In the Y system group, peritonitis due to *S epidermidis* was greatly reduced (1/21 peritonitis for the Y-system group and 16/47 for standard-system group). These results definitively confirm the efficacy of the Y-system in preventing peritonitis.

Table 8-2. Incidence of Peritonitis in Diabetic and Nondiabetic Patients

	Follow-up (Patient-Months)	Peritonitis Episodes	Mean Interval Between Peritonitis Episodes (Months)
Diabetics	645	26	26
Nondiabetics	3,537	104	34

Table 8-3. Clinical Studies of the Efficacy of the Y-System

Reference	Follow-up (Patient-Months)	Mean Interval Between Peritonitis Episodes (Months)
Dozio et al.[52]	665	32
Scalamogna et al.[48]	3133	37
Catizone et al.[53]	232	46
Maiorca et al.[44]	457	57
Buoncristiani et al.[55]	717	42

Center Effect

Interesting results have been obtained by the Italian CAPD Cooperative Study Group (ICSG), which has gathered data since 1981 from a minimum of 13 to a maximum of 34 centers. The percentage of patients on the Y-system changed from 32 percent in 1983 to 90 percent in 1987. One interesting aspect of the ICSG is the variability of results from center to center.[61] It seemed that the use of a method more effective in preventing peritonitis amplified, instead of reduced, this "center effect." In a first study in 1983,[62] the influence of the Y-set on the frequency of peritonitis appeared weak, whereas other factors were either beneficial in reducing the peritonitis rate, such as a greater experience of the center or the frequency at which the patient took showers, or detrimental, such as the presence of exit site infections, urinary tract infections, or visual/motor inability. It must be stressed, however, that even minor differences in technique among centers might influence the results (e.g., the Y-set without titanium adaptor gave worse results in our experience).

More recently in the ICSG, in addition to the extension of the use of the Y-system up to 66 percent of overall exposure time, better results have been obtained, and the positive influence of the Y-system has become even more evident.[61] However, the differences in incidence of peritonitis among centers have remained remarkable and have promoted a case-control study.[63] The basic hypothesis was that the peritonitis events were dependent on two sets of variables. One, "center-dependent," included the quality of training offered by each center and the carefulness of getting the patient informed and monitored. The other, "patient-dependent," included patient dexterity and compliance with the instructions, characteristics of domestic milieu, etc.

After a 2-month feasibility study, two physician-monitors who were experienced in CAPD and suitably trained, monitored on the spot for 6 months, moving from one of the 24 centers to another, the possible causes of each peritonitis episode. In a center in which a peritonitis episode had occurred, another patient, comparable for type of connector, sex, age, and CAPD treatment duration, was evaluated ("in-center control" to evaluate "patient-dependent" variables); another comparison was made with well-matched patients from another center with a different peritonitis rate ("out-center control"). In conclusion, the results of this study confirmed what seemed initially probable, that the "center-effect" is only partially dependent on differences in particular kinds of patients, but is largely dependent on the quality of training offered by the center.

The different results among the centers should not be surprising. It is evident that in centers in which the training is insufficient, with a lack of attention to apparently minor details of the technique, the results will not be good. For example, details such as the right handling of the clamp on the outlet port, the correct use of a mask, attention to avoiding drafts, etc. (see Appendix), if not sufficiently understood and assimilated by the patient or the partner, can significantly influence the final peritonitis rate. Also, the decision whether to train only the patient or partner, to train them both, or to train more than one relative can influence the results. On the whole, one can say that the Y-system improves the results in every center, but the improvement is correlated with the degree of staff skill in training the patients or their partners.

Even inside each single center it is possible to have fluctuations in the peritonitis rate, depending on the standard of self efficiency or other factors. In our center, we have documented a transitory worsening of results in coincidence with the substitution of a nurse or of the leading physician of the CAPD staff. Another period of less acceptable results coincided with the decision to use Amukin at a concentration of 25 percent instead of the 50 percent used up to then. (This is another reason why we believe in the importance of disinfectant in the Y-system.) In the long run, however, our results have followed the trend of continuous improvement, thanks to the small modifications in the technique suggested by patient mistakes and the staff's collective experience. Figure 8-5 shows this trend in terms of intervals between peritonitis episodes. The very low incidence in 1987 was not obtained in 1988; but in 1988, the results were better than in 1986 and previous years. It must be stressed that there has not been any positive selection over time; the number of patients at risk has continuously increased, but the percentage of patients dropping out of the method because of peritonitis has remained stable.

Recent Personal Results

In 1988 in our center, 89 patients using the same Y-set (Y-solution Transfer Set) and Amukin for a cumulative period of 858 patient-months had 20 episodes of peritonitis, with an incidence of one episode every 43 patient-months. Seventy-five patients (84 percent) did not develop peritonitis, 11 patients (12 percent) had one episode, and three patients (4 percent) had three episodes. Table 8-4 provides information about the patients who developed peritonitis, such as length of treatment and episodes of peritonitis in their global follow-up on the Y-system. There is also information concerning patients who had been on other connector-systems. The last column refers to the number of peritonitis episodes in 1988. Results of dialysate cultures are

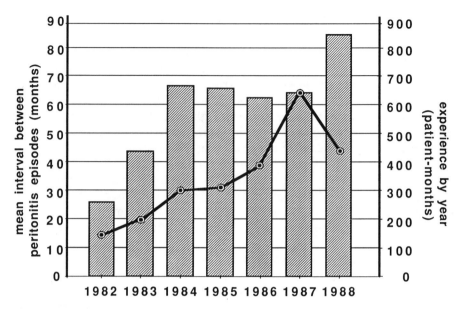

Fig. 8-5. Frequency of peritonitis over time with the Y-system. Line indicates mean intervals between peritonitis episodes. Bars indicate yearly experience at our center. Only patients treated with the Y-Solution Transfer Set are included.

Table 8-4. Peritonitis Episodes in 14 Patients Who Used the Y-Solution Transfer Set in 1988 and Developed Peritonitis Episodes[a]

	CAPD			Other Connectors			Y-System			Peritonitis Episodes in 1988
		Peritonitis Episodes			Peritonitis Episodes			Peritonitis Episodes		
Patient	Months	No.	Incidence	Months	No.	Incidence	Months	No.	Incidence	
CF	95	11	1/9	19	2	1/9	76	9	1/8	3
AL	98	8	1/12	16	5	1/3	82	3	1/27	1
BL	93	1	1/93	—	—	—	93	1	1/93	1
FG	90	3	1/30	36	2	1/18	54	1	1/54	1
ZE	80	6	1/13	—	—	—	80	6	1/13	1
BB	76	10	1/8	3	3	1/1	73	10	1/8	3
SC	68	1	1/68	—	—	—	68	1	1/68	1
CM	61	5	1/12	—	—	—	61	5	1/12	1
RD	51	1	1/51	—	—	—	51	1	1/51	1
GL	46	5	1/9	26	4	1/6	20	1	1/20	1
TV	13	1	1/13	—	—	—	13	1	1/13	1
MB	5	3	1/2	—	—	—	5	3	1/2	3
PS	79	1	1/79	43	0	—	36	1	1/36	1
CU	29	1	1/29	—	—	—	29	1	1/29	1

[a] The remaining 75 patients using the Y-Solution Transfer Set in 1988 did not develop peritonitis.

given in Table 8-5. Patients with three episodes of peritonitis were at high risk of developing peritonitis. One of these patients who had been on hemodialysis for 12 years and on CAPD for 8 years, always had gram-negative cultures: he abused laxatives and eventually died from bowel perforation. The second patient, has a duodenal diverticulum and episodes of peritonitis were preceded by exacerbation of related symptoms and were caused by gram-negative bacteria. In the third patient, two of three episodes were associated with a tunnel infection. In all other cases, which had only one episode of peritonitis, excluding those associated with tunnel infection, gram-positive bacteria were present in only three cases. The important reduction of gram-positive infections that we obtained further confirms the efficacy of the Y-system in preventing intraluminal infections. At the same time, our data point out the importance of the remaining problems (i.e., exit site and tunnel infections).

Table 8-5. Culture Results and Risk Factors in Patients Presented in Table 8-4

Patient	Peritonitis Episodes in 1988	Cultured Bacterium	Comments
CF	1st	*Pseudomonas putida*	On CAPD after 12 years of hemodialysis
	2nd	*E coli*	
	3rd	*Citrobacter freundi* and *Bacteroides* species	See text
AL	1st	*S aureus*	
BL	1st	Negative culture	After biliary colic
FG	1st	*Streptococcus viridans*	The patient used a perforated bag
ZE	1st	*E coli*	Some diverticula in colon and sigmoid
BB	1st	*Morganella morganii*	
	2nd	*Pseudomonas* species	Diverticulum duodenalis
	3rd	*Klebsiella* species and *E coli*	
SC	1st	*S aureus*	Tunnel infection (same bacterium)
CM	1st	*P aeruginosa*	Tunnel infection (same bacterium)
RD	1st	*E coli*	Cirrhosis
GL	1st	*S aureus*	Tunnel infection (same bacterium)
TV	1st	*Streptococcus β*-emol group D	
MB	1st	*E coli*	Diabetic. Tunnel infection (*S aureus*)
	2nd	*S aureus*	Tunnel infection
	3rd	*S aureus*	Tunnel infection (same bacterium)
PS	1st	*E coli*	
CU	1st	*Staphylococcus albus*	

ADDITIONAL ADVANTAGES OF THE Y-SYSTEM

Besides its important efficacy in reducing the frequency of peritonitis, the Y-system has additional advantages. It leaves the patient free of the bag during the dwell-time or when the abdomen is left empty, during the night, for example, as is possible or necessary in several cases. The possibility of changing the set only every 2 to 4 months makes it very inexpensive. At the same time, it can be changed in the center, in real asepsis, with more chances of avoiding catheter contamination, while not overburdening the center. The apparatus is simple and does not require electricity or technical assistance.

Some improvements have been recently introduced. The size has been reduced, to minimize patient discomfort and to limit the disinfectant content, which reduces the concentration of it in the peritoneal cavity in case of accidental introduction. The connection of the set to a new bag is made through a luer-lock instead of a spike. It is also possible to collect the dialysate in a sterile bag.

In a multicenter study[64] after a follow-up period of 246 patient-months, the peritonitis frequency was one episode per 61 patient-months. This frequency is low, but not yet different from that obtained for the controls using the former Y-system.

REFERENCES

1. Villano R: Multicenter registry of patients using the "O" set system of CAPD. p. 304. In Khanna R, Nolph KD, Prowant B, et al (eds): Advances in Continuous Ambulatory Peritoneal Dialysis 1988. Peritoneal Dialysis Bulletin, Toronto, 1988

2. Slingeneyer A, Liendo-Liendo C, Mion C: Continuous ambulatory peritoneal dialysis with a bacteriological filter on the dialysate infusion line. p. 59. In Legrain M (ed): Continuous Ambulatory Peritoneal Dialysis. Proceedings of the International Symposium on CAPD. Excerpta Medica, Amsterdam, 1980

3. Sarles HE, Lindley JD, Fish JC, et al: Peritoneal dialysis utilizing a millipore filter. Kidney Int 9:54, 1976

4. Slingeneyer A, Mion C, Despaux E, et al: Use of bacteriologic filter in the prevention of peritonitis associated with peritoneal dialysis: long term clinical results in intermittent and continuous ambulatory peritoneal dialysis. p. 301. In Atkins RC, Thomson NM, Farrel PC (eds): Peritoneal Dialysis. Churchill Livingstone, Edinburgh, 1981

5. Slingeneyer A, Mion C: Peritonitis prevention in continuous ambulatory peritoneal dialysis: long term efficacy of bacteriological filters. p. 388. In Davison AM, Guillou PJ (eds): Proceedings of the European Dialysis Transplant Association. Vol. 19. Pitman Books Limited, London, 1983

6. Slingeneyer A, Mion C, Ponsot JF, Rossi P: Peritonitis prevention in CAPD: A comparison of 3 models of connecting devices with an in-line bacteriological filter. Peritoneal Dialysis Bull 4:suppl. 2, S60, 1984

7. Winchester JF, Ash SR, Bousquet G, et al: Successful peritonitis reduction with an unidirectional bacteriologic CAPD filter. p. 611. In Schreiner GE, Balow JE,

Winchester JF, Mendelson BF (eds): Transactions of the American Society For Artificial Internal Organs. Vol. 29. Charbray Printers, Lovettsville, 1983

8. Ash SR, Winchester JF: Effect of the Peridex Filter on peritonitis rate in a CAPD population. Peritoneal Dialysis Bull 4:S118, 1984

9. Rotellar C, Winchester JF, Ash SR, et al: Long-term use of unidirectional bacteriologic filters to reduce peritonitis frequency in CAPD. p. 203. In Maher JF, Winchester JF: Frontiers in Peritoneal Dialysis. Field, Rich and Associates, New York, 1986

10. Morgan B, Dale A, Foulks C, Singh S: Efficacy of the Peridex filter in reducing peritonitis rates in CAPD patients. p. 73. In Khanna R, Nolph KD, Prowant B, et al (eds): Advances in Continuous Ambulatory Peritoneal Dialysis 1985, Proceedings of the Fifth Annual CAPD Conference, Kansas City. Peritoneal Dialysis Bulletin, Toronto, 1985

11. Boeschoten EW, Southwood J, Struijk DG, et al: Prevention of peritonitis: filter or UV system? Contrib Nephrol 57:158, 1987

12. Tranaeus A, Lindholm B, Myrback KE, Flink O: Bacteriological filter in CAPD—unfavourable clinical and laboratory results. Peritoneal Dialysis Bull 7: suppl. 2, S77, 1987

13. Shaldon S: Future trend in biocompatibility aspects of hemodialysis and related therapies. Clin Nephrol 26: suppl. 1, S13, 1986

14. Shaldon S, Kock KM, Quellhorst E, Dinarello CA: Pathogenesis of sclerosing peritonitis in CAPD. p. 193. In Schreiner GE, Winchester JF, Rakowski TA, et al (eds): Transaction of the American Society for Artificial Internal Organs. Vol. 30. Charbray Printers, Lovettsville, 1984

15. Du JT, Foegh M, Maddox Y, Ramwell PW: Human peritoneal macrophages sintesize leukotrines B4 and C4. Biochem Biophys Acta 753:159, 1983

16. Davies SJ, Ogg CS, Cameron JS: Evidence for T-cell activation and B-cell recruitment in continuous ambulatory peritoneal dialysis peritoneal lymphocyte populations. Nephr Dial Transplant 2:452, 1987

17. Grollman A, Turner LB, McLean JA: Intermittent peritoneal lavage in nephrectomized dogs and its application to the human being. Arch Intern Med 87:379, 1951

18. Buoncristiani U, Bianchi P, Cozzari M, et al: A new safe simple connection system for CAPD. Int J Nephrol Urol Androl 1:50, 1980

19. Buoncristiani U, Bianchi P, Barzi AM, et al: An ideal disinfectant for peritoneal dialysis (highly efficient, easy to handle and innocuous). Int J Nephrol Urol Androl 1:45, 1980

20. Schmid E, Augustin R, Kuhlmann U, et al: Quantitative in vitro contamination and recovery studies: the flush principle in CAPD. Contrib Nephrol 57:185, 1987

21. Orange GV, Henderson IS, Marshall EA: Effectiveness of the flush technique in CAPD disconnect system. Int J Artif Internal Organs 10:185, 1987

22. Verger C, Luzar MA: In vitro study of CAPD in-line systems. p. 160. In Khanna R (ed): Advances in Continuous Ambulatory Peritoneal Dialysis 1987. Peritoneal Dialysis Bulletin, Toronto, 1987

23. Luzar MA, Slingeneyer A, Cantaluppi A, Peluso FP: In vitro study of the flush effect in two reusable CAPD disconnect systems. Peritoneal Dialysis Int 9:169, 1989

24. Verger C, Faller B, Ryckelinck JPH, et al: Efficacy of CAPD Y-line systems without disinfectant and standard systems on peritonitis prevention: a multicentre prospective controlled trial. Peritoneal Dialysis Int 8:104, 1988 (abstr)

25. Ryckelynck JPH, Verger C, Cam G, et al: Role of the antiseptic in the efficacy of disconnect systems: a prospective controlled trial. Peritoneal Dialysis Bull 7:suppl., S66, 1987
26. Verger C, Faller B, Ryckelinck JPH, et al: Comparison between the efficacy of CAPD Y-lines without disinfectant and standard systems: a multicenter prospective controlled trial. Peritoneal Dialysis Bull 7: suppl., S82, 1987
27. Ryckelinck JPH, Verger C, Cam G, et al: Importance of the flush effect in disconnect systems. Peritoneal Dialysis Int 8:98, 1988
28. Rottembourg J, Brouard R, Issad B, et al: Prevention of peritonitis by "Y" connectors without disinfectant: prospective randomized two years study. Peritoneal Dialysis Bull 6: suppl., S64, 1986
29. Durnell TA, Smallwood SA, Sluder BA, et al: "Flush before fill" technique to reduce tubing change associated peritonitis. Peritoneal Dialysis Bull 6: suppl., S5, 1986
30. Nobl WC, Sommerville D: Microbiology of the Human Skin. WB Saunders, Philadelphia, 1974
31. Donald CM, Eastway A, McMillan M, et al: Peritonitis in CAPD with a disconnect system. Peritoneal Dialysis Bull 7:suppl., S25, 1987
32. Pappalardo G, Tanner F, Roussianos D, Pannatier A: Efficacy and stability of two chlorine-containing antiseptics. Drugs Exp Clin Res 12:905, 1986
33. Werner HP: Disinfectant in dialysis: dangers, drawbacks and disinformation. Nephron 49:1, 1988
34. Mackow RC, Argy WP, Winchester JF, et al: Sclerosis encapsulating peritonitis in rats induced by long term intraperitoneal administration of antisepsis. Proceedings of the IV International Symposium on Peritoneal Dialysis, Venice, 1987 (in press)
35. Buoncristiani U, Bianchi P, Clementi F, et al: Uso intraperitoneale di disinfettanti. p. 167. In Lamperi S, Cappelli G, Carozzi S, (eds): Dialisi Peritoneale. Atti del III Convegno Nazionale. Wichtig Editore, Milano, 1985
36. Savazzi GM, Bocchi B, Rustichelli R, et al: L'irrigazione lavaggio di cavità ascessualizzate intra o retroperitoneali con clorossidante elettrolitico. Minerva Chir 42:1365, 1987
37. Pappalardo G, Tanner F: Evaluation of a disinfectant in accordance with Swiss standard. Drugs Exper Clin Res 9:109, 1983
38. Buoncristiani U, Cozzari M, Quintaliani G, Carobi C: Abatement of exogenous peritonitis risk using the Perugia CAPD system. Dialysis Transplant 12:14, 1983
39. Oreopoulos DG, Khanna R, Williams P, Vas SI: Continuous ambulatory peritoneal dialysis, 1981. Nephron 30:293, 1982
40. Maiorca R, Cantaluppi A, Cancarini GC, et al: Prospective controlled trial of a Y-connector and disinfectant to prevent peritonitis in continuous ambulatory peritoneal dialysis. Lancet 2:642, 1983
41. Maiorca R, Cancarini GC, Manili L, et al: Y-connector with Amuchina in the prevention of peritonitis. p. 185. In La Greca G, Chiaramonte S, Fabris A, et al (eds): Peritoneal Dialysis. Wichtig Editore, Milano, 1986
42. Maiorca R, Cancarini GC, Colombrita D, et al: Further experience with Y-system in continuous ambulatory peritoneal dialysis. p. 172. In Khanna R, Nolph KD, Prowant B, et al (eds): Advances in Continuous Ambulatory Peritoneal Dialysis 1986. Peritoneal Dialysis Bulletin, Toronto, 1986
43. Maiorca R, Cancarini GC, Manili L, Camerini C: Effectiveness of an in-line disinfection and wash-out (Y-system) in reducing peritonitis rates in CAPD. A

long term experience. p. 176. In Khanna R, Nolph KD, Prowant B, et al (eds): Advances in Continuous Ambulatory Peritoneal Dialysis 1986. Peritoneal Dialysis Bulletin, Toronto, 1986

44. Maiorca R, Cancarini GC, Brasa S, et al: Y-system with disinfectant in the prevention of peritonitis in CAPD. Contrib Nephrol 57:178, 1987
45. Maiorca R, Cancarini GC, Manili L, et al: CAPD is a first class treatment: results of an eight-year experience with a comparison of patient and method survival in CAPD and hemodialysis. Clin Nephrol 30:suppl. 1, S3, 1988
46. Cantaluppi A, Scalamogna A, Guerra L, et al: Peritonitis prevention in CAPD: efficacy of a Y-connector and disinfectant. p. 198. In Maher JF, Winchester JF (eds): Frontiers in Peritoneal Dialysis. Field, Rich and Associates, New York, 1986
47. Cantaluppi A, Scalamogna A, Castelnovo C, Graziani G: Long-term efficacy of a Y-connector and disinfectant to prevent peritonitis in continuous ambulatory peritoneal dialysis. p. 182. In Khanna R, Nolph KD, Prowant B, et al (eds): Advances in Continuous Ambulatory Peritoneal Dialysis 1986. Peritoneal Dialysis Bulletin, Toronto, 1986
48. Scalamogna A, Castelnovo C, Crepaldi M, et al: Peritonitis on CAPD: 8-year experience in one center. Peritoneal Dialysis Int 8:99, 1988
49. Scalamogna A, Castelnovo C, Crepaldi M, et al: Incidence of peritonitis in diabetic patients on CAPD: intraperitoneal versus subcutaneous insulin therapy. Peritoneal Dialysis Bull 6: suppl., S18, 1986
50. Tarchini R, Segoloni GP, Gentile MG, et al: Long term results of CAPD in Italy: a report from the Italian CAPD Study Group. Clin Nephrol 30: suppl. 1, S68, 1988
51. Lupo A, Tarchini R, Segoloni GP, et al: Italian multicenter study on CAPD: 7 years' experience. p. 101. In Khanna R, Nolph KD, Prowant B, et al (eds): Advances in Continuous Ambulatory Peritoneal Dialysis 1988. Peritoneal Dialysis Bulletin, Toronto, 1988
52. Dozio B, Bonforte G, Scanzini R, et al: Peritonitis in CAPD: experience with the "Y" set. Peritoneal Dialysis Bull 7: suppl., S25, 1987
53. Catizone L, Gagliardini R, Zucchelli P: Incidenza della peritonite nella CAPD con set a Y: confronto con la CAPD con set standard e con la IPD. p. 159. In Lamperi S, Cappelli G, Carozzi S (eds): Dialisi peritoneale. Atti del III Convegno nazionale 1985. Wichtig Editore, Milano, 1985
54. Mileto G, Pellegrino E, Consolo F: CAPD in Sicily: decrease in peritonitis rate with the use of the Perugia system. Peritoneal Dialysis Bull 3:161, 1983
55. Buoncristiani U, Carobi C, Cozzari M, Di Paolo N: Clinical application of a miniaturized variant of the Perugia CAPD connection system. p. 193. In Maher JF, Winchester JF (eds): Frontiers in Peritoneal Dialysis. Field, Rich and Associates, New York, 1986
56. Buoncristiani U, Quintaliani G, Cozzari M, Carobi C: Current status of the Y set. p. 165. In Khanna R, Nolph KD, Prowant B, et al (eds): Advances in Continuous Ambulatory Peritoneal Dialysis 1986. Peritoneal Dialysis Bulletin, Toronto, 1986
57. Reynolds J: "O" set a disconnect system for CAPD. Peritoneal Dialysis Bull 6: suppl., S16, 1986
58. Elie M, Slingeneyer A, Laroche B, Mion C: The Y-aseptocap connector for CAPD. Results of a preliminary clinical trial. Peritoneal Dialysis Bull 7: suppl, S28, 1987

59. Diaz-Buxo JA, Walshe JJ, Flanigan M: Multicenter experience with Y-set CAPD system (Freedom set ™). Peritoneal Dialysis Bull 7: suppl., S23, 1987

60. Canadian CAPD Clinical Trials Group: Randomized clinical trial comparing peritonitis rates among new CAPD patients using the Y set disinfectant system to standard systems. Kidney Int 35:268, 1989 (abstr.)

61. Gentile MG, Fellin G, Redaelli L, et al: Multicenter study on peritonitis risk factors in CAPD. Report of the Italian CAPD Study Group. p. 138. In Khanna R, Nolph KD, Prowant B, et al (eds): Advances in Continuous Ambulatory Peritoneal Dialysis 1986. Peritoneal Dialysis Bulletin, Toronto, 1986

62. Gentile MG, Fellin G, Luciani L, et al: Studio multicentrico sui fattori di rischio della peritonite in CAPD. p. 265. In Lamperi S, Cappelli G, Carozzi S (eds): Dialisi Peritoneale. Atti del III Convegno Nazionale. Wichtig Editore, Milano, 1985

63. Fellin G, Gentile MG, Cancarini G, et al: Peritonitis in CAPD: role for patient and staff. Report of the Italian CAPD Study Group. Peritoneal Dialysis Int 8:78, 1988

64. Scalamogna A, Viglino G, Colombo A, et al: Controlled randomized trial between two Y-devices. Peritoneal Dialysis Int 8:99, 1988

Appendix

The following are the instructions we give during the training of patients using the Y-system (with the Y Solution Transfer Set). All of the principal steps are illustrated by drawings given to the patient.

PREPARATIONS FOR BAG EXCHANGE

Room

The bag exchanges must be performed in a room that is

Clean
Well-lit
With doors and windows closed
Without drafts
Without animals or plants
Equipped with a wash-basin, if possible

Worktable

Worktable requirements are as follows.

It must be in a comfortable and convenient position
The surface must be smooth and washable and must be cleared and disinfected every day
The needed items must be properly arranged to reduce the number of motions and the risk of accidental touch contamination
It must be away from radiators, ventilators, stoves, air conditioning

Clothes

Clothes to avoid include

Clothes that hamper movement
Clothes with frills or long or wide sleeves, etc.
Clothes with belts, ties, or shawls with fluttering extremities

Hair

Long hair must be kept out of the way.

BAG EXCHANGE

Collect Everything Necessary

1. Place the new bag, chosen according to scheduled glucose concentration and previously warmed, on the working desk
2. Place two graduated cylinders
3. Put on mask and cuff
4. Wash your hands
5. Remove the plastic covering and check the bag for
    a. Glucose concentration
    b. Lack of damage
    c. Expiration date
    d. Clarity of solution
    e. Temperature
    f. Caps on injection and outlet ports
6. Put the blue clamp on the outlet tube of the bag
7. Check the worktable for
    a. The container of 50 percent Amukin for the spike cap and screw plug (first container)
    b. The brown glass container with 50 percent Amukin to fill the Y-set (second container)
    c. Fifty percent Amukin spray
    d. Container of alcohol disinfectant for clamps and forceps
    e. Gauze and adhesive tape
    f. Waste tray
8. Check the Y-set
    a. Is it full of disinfectant and without leaks or breaks?
    b. Are the spike cap and the screw plug seated?
    c. Is the spike solidly joined to the lines?
9. Take off the tape (or the clamp) from the spike cap
10. Wash your hands carefully

Pay attention! From now on, you must avoid touching any object not strictly necessary for bag exchange.

Connecting Lines

During the following steps there is the highest risk of contamination. Take care!

1. Put the spike under the bag on the same side as the waste tray and the first container of 50 percent Amukin.
2. Place the blue clamp correctly on the outlet tube of the bag and take off the protective port covering. Spray 50 percent Amukin in and around the outlet port.
3. Take the inlet line. Give great attention so that the lines do not touch the outlet port. Remove the cap from the spike over the waste tray, pour the

Amukin in the cap into the waste tray and put the cap into the first Amukin container.

4. Hold the blue clamp on the outlet tube of the bag and, gently rotating, insert the spike into the outlet port of the new bag.

5. Attach the end of the outlet line to the first graduated cylinder with adhesive tape, remove the screw plug, and put the plug into the first Amukin container.

6. Suspend the new bag.

The steps with greatest risk of contamination are finished.

There must now be outflow of Amukin and dialysate and then inflow of dialysate and Amukin. It is very important to avoid:

Amukin entering the peritoneal cavity
Lifting the cylinder, causing a backflow of potentially contaminated dialysate from the end of the outlet line toward the peritoneum

Remember, the steps are in the following order:

1.	*Remove*	*Amukin*	from the lines.
2.	*Remove*	*dialysate*	from the peritoneal cavity
3.	*Fill*	peritoneal cavity	with fresh *dialysis fluid.*
4.	*Fill*	lines	with *Amukin.*

These steps are carried out as follows.

1. *Remove Amukin* from the lines (the roller clamp is still closed!)
   a. Take the blue clamp off the bag outlet port. Let 200 ml of fresh solution wash out Amukin into the first cylinder, then place and close blue clamp on the inlet tube of the Y-connector.
   b. Shift the outlet line from the first cylinder to the second.

2. *Remove the dialysate.*
   a. Open the roller clamp.
   b. Check flow rate, color and clarity, and volume.

3. *Fill* the peritoneal cavity with *dialysis fluid.*
   a. Shift the blue clamp from the inlet line to the outlet line, allowing the fresh dialysate to flow into the peritoneal cavity.

4. *Fill* the lines with *Amukin*
   Close the roller clamp!
   a. Place the empty bag on the worktable.
   b. Shift the outlet line from the second cylinder to the first cylinder.
   c. Fill the spike cap with Amukin.
   d. Take the spike off the outlet tube and put it into the first Amukin container.
   e. Open the blue clamp on the outlet line and, using the line as a siphon, wash fresh dialysate out and fill the line with Amukin (approximately 100 ml). Take care that air does not enter the lines. Close the clamp.

f. Put the spike into its cap filled with Amukin.

g. Spray the end of the outlet line with 50 percent Amukin and screw in the plug.

9

Bone and Mineral Metabolism in Continuous Ambulatory Peritoneal Dialysis

James A. Delmez

INTRODUCTION

Over the past 10 years, there have been many advances in the understanding of the effects of continuous ambulatory peritoneal dialysis (CAPD) on uremic bone and mineral metabolism. This, in turn, has led to improved

191

strategies directed toward the prevention, diagnosis, and treatment of these potential derangements. It should be noted, however, that this progress has occurred in concert with the expansion in knowledge of renal osteodystrophy. The term "renal osteodystrophy" encompasses a number of histologic bone lesions: osteitis fibrosa, osteomalacia, mixed lesions, and "adynamic" changes. Osteitis fibrosa results from high serum levels of parathyroid hormone (PTH) causing high rates of bone resorption and formation. Typical features seen on bone biopsy specimens are increased numbers of osteoclasts and osteoblasts, excess amounts of woven osteoid, fibrosis, and rapid bone turnover.[1] The pathogenesis of excessive PTH secretion is complex. Hypocalcemia is a potent stimulus for PTH secretion. In severe renal failure, hyperphosphatemia, impaired gastrointestinal absorption of calcium, and skeletal resistance to the biologic effect of PTH lead to hypocalcemia. It is clear, however, that hypocalcemia cannot be the sole cause of hyperparathyroidism. For example, it is possible to maintain normocalcemia or hypercalcemia in dogs rendered uremic if dietary calcium supplements are provided. Despite this, secondary hyperparathyroidism occurs.[2] It is likely that the mechanism for this observation is the relative resistance of the parathyroid gland in uremia to the suppressant effects of calcium.[3] Thus, higher levels of serum calcium are necessary to inhibit PTH secretion in chronic renal failure than in the non-uremic state. This resistance may be due in part to the low levels of $1,25\text{-}(OH)_2$ vitamin D usually observed with severe renal failure. This potent vitamin D metabolite has been recently shown to suppress PTH secretion[4–7] by decreasing the gene transcription of preproparathyroid hormone mRNA.[8,9] Furthermore, the parathyroid gland in uremia demonstrates decreased number of receptors for $1,25\text{-}(OH)_2$ vitamin D.[10–12] This phenomenon could conceivably present yet another mechanism promoting PTH secretion in chronic renal failure. It has also been observed that phosphorus restriction in dogs with advanced renal failure can prevent the development of secondary hyperparathyroidism in the absence of changes in the levels of $1,25\text{-}(OH)_2$ vitamin D.[13] It is thus possible that phosphorus in the uremic state could perhaps directly modulate the secretion of PTH. Finally, high levels of PTH may result in part from impaired degradation of the hormone by the liver and kidneys.[14]

The other end of the histologic spectrum of renal osteodystrophy is that of osteomalacia. The hallmarks of this form of bone disease are excess unmineralized bone collagen (osteoid) due to a defective mineralization and slow bone turnover.[1] Patients with osteomalacia usually have relatively low levels of PTH and a predilection to develop hypercalcemia.[15] It is likely that aluminum accumulation is the cause in the majority of cases. The sources of aluminum are either dialysate contaminated with the metal (epidemic form) or the ingestion of aluminum-containing phosphorus binders (sporadic form).[16,17] Impaired mineralization of bone may result from the direct toxic effects of aluminum on osteoblast function and number and/or impaired secretion of PTH due to its accumulation within the gland.[18,19]

"Adynamic" renal osteodystrophy refers to that bone histology demonstrating low rates of bone formation but normal amounts of osteoid.[20] Aluminum staining along the mineralization front is common. It is likely that if left untreated, this lesion will eventually evolve into osteomalacia. However, there are some patients with this lesion who have no evidence of aluminum intoxication.[21] Preliminary studies suggest that low plasma levels of insulin-like growth factor I is associated with the defective mineralization process.[22]

"Mixed" renal osteodystrophy refers to the histologic picture where elements of both osteitis fibrosa and osteomalacia are seen on bone biopsy.[1] The lesion is most commonly observed in patients who have osteitis fibrosa but are developing aluminum-induced osteomalacia, or in whom osteomalacia is being treated with deferoxamine with the resultant emergence of osteitis fibrosa.[23]

The general principles of the pathogenesis and treatment of renal osteodystrophy are the same in chronic hemodialysis and in CAPD patients. Nonetheless, there are several unique features of CAPD that deserve attention. The purpose of this chapter is to review the effects of CAPD on calcium, phosphorus, magnesium, vitamin D, PTH, and aluminum metabolism. In addition, the published series studying the short-term changes in bone histomorphometry during CAPD will be analyzed. Finally, approaches that optimize mineral metabolism during CAPD will be discussed.

CALCIUM

The current concentration of calcium in standard peritoneal dialysis dialysate is 3.50 mEq/L (7.0 mg/dl). The upper limit of normal for serum ionized calcium is usually 2.50 mEq/L (5.0 mg/dl). Assuming little calcium binding by protein in the dialysate, one would expect a net influx of calcium from the dialysate to the patient. There is, however, wide disparity in the literature concerning calcium fluxes during CAPD. Parker and Nolph[24] reported a net calcium influx of 300 mg/d and a net gain of 84 ± 18 mg/d was reported by Blumenkrantz et al.[25] In neither study were the patients' ionized calcium values measured. We[26] have shown a daily net calcium removal of 77 ± 23 mg during periods of hypercalcemia (ionized calcium, more than 5.0 mg/dl) and a net uptake of 48 ± 13 mg when patients were hypocalcemic (ionized calcium, less than 4.4 mg/dl). Thus, the ionized calcium levels play a major role in determining the direction and amount of calcium mass transfer. In addition, ultrafiltration volume plays a role in determining calcium mass transfer. For example, when ionized calcium levels were maintained at the upper limits of normal (4.9 ± 0.1 mg/dl) with calcium supplements, we noted a net influx of 9.8 mg with each 1.5 percent dextrose solution, but removal of 21 mg with each 4.25 percent dextrose exchange. This resulted in a positive calcium daily mass transfer of 9.9 mg. Kurtz et al.[27] reported similar findings. A third factor affecting calcium mass transfer in CAPD is the concentration of calcium in the dialysate. Calderaro et al.[28] noted a negative balance of 50 ± 9 mg/d using a dialysate calcium of 3 mEq/L. We[29] found that patients not taking calcium supplements with ionized calcium levels of 4.72 ± 0.09 mg/dl had a net uptake of 37 ± 17 mg/d with the standard 3.5 mEq/L calcium dialysate. The net uptake more than doubled to 84 ± 6 mg/d with the use of a dialysate solution containing calcium in a concentration of 4.0 mEq/L. A dialysate calcium concentration of 2.5 mEq/L is currently available, but no formal studies of calcium mass transfer with this solution have been performed. It is estimated that approximately 50 to 75 mg of calcium would be removed per day if the ionized calcium was maintained in the normal range.

Although knowledge of calcium mass transfer from dialysate is important, it provides little information about total-body calcium balance during CAPD. Blumenkrantz et al.[25] evaluated this important issue in short-term (2 to 4 weeks) studies on a metabolic ward. They found a positive calcium balance of 122 ± 51 mg/d on a 1.0 g/kg/d protein diet. This increased to 198 ± 194 mg/d with 1.4 g/kg protein diet. Although there was considerable variability, the net calcium absorption by the bowel varied directly with the dietary calcium intake. The latter ranged from 500 to 2,000 mg/d. Regression analysis revealed that the relation of the amount of calcium absorbed relative to calcium intake is comparable to, or perhaps higher than, that determined for nondialyzed uremic patients. Presumably, this phenomenon is the result of vitamin D-independent mechanisms affecting calcium absorption.[30]

PHOSPHORUS

A 1.2 to 1.5 g/kg protein diet has been recommended in order to maintain a positive nitrogen balance.[31] Despite elimination of dietary protein with a high phosphorus content, this recommendation leads to an obligate ingestion of at least 900 mg of phosphorus per day. Assuming a 70 percent gastrointestinal absorption of phosphorus, dialysate removal of phosphorus would not be sufficient to maintain normal phosphorus levels. For example, we were only able to remove 308 ± 22 mg/d of phosphorus when the mean phosphorus level of the patients was 5.2 ± 0.4 mg/dl.[26] As expected, the total amount removed correlated with the serum phosphorus level. In balance studies, Blumenkrantz et al.[25] noted a net positive phosphorus balance of 708 ± 152 mg/d while patients were ingesting a 1.4 g/kg protein diet. This positive phosphorus balance occurred despite the concomitant administration of 7.8 ± 1.0 g/d of aluminum hydroxide gels. The net gastrointestinal absorption of phosphorus directly correlated with the dietary intake.

MAGNESIUM

The original concentration of magnesium in the dialysate was 1.5 mEq/L (1.8 mg/dl). This led to a positive net magnesium balance. Blumenkrantz et al.[25] determined that the net intestinal absorption of magnesium ranged from 74 to 200 mg/d. The amount absorbed weakly correlated with the dietary magnesium intake. The quantity of magnesium removed in the dialysate was 46 ± 7.5 mg/d, a figure which is close to our findings of 31 ± 15 mg/d.[26] Serum magnesium levels are usually high when using dialysate containing 1.5 mEq/L of magnesium, but the long-term consequences of this are unknown. However, Meema et al.[32] have recently evaluated the development of arterial calcifications in CAPD patients treated with dialysate containing 1.5 mEq/L of magnesium. Interestingly, they found lower magnesium levels in patients developing progressive arterial calcification compared with those in whom calcification was not progressive. They postulated that hypermagnesemia may be a factor in inhibiting the calcification process.

By lowering the dialysate magnesium to 0.5 mEq/L, Shah et al.[33] were able to reduce magnesium levels to normal (2.2 ± 0.1 mg/dl). This was associated with a net daily magnesium removal of 66 ± 8 mg/d. Following 2 weeks of CAPD with a magnesium-free dialysate, the serum magnesium levels decreased further to 1.9 ± mg/dl as the daily magnesium removal increased to 83 ± 7 mg/dl. Nolph et al.[34] also observed the normalization of serum magnesium levels with the use of dialysate containing 0.5 mEq/L of this cation. Thus, magnesium dialysate mass transfer, like that of calcium, is dependent on the serum and dialysate concentrations of the cation as well as on dialysate volume.

VITAMIN D

Patients with nephrotic syndrome and normal renal function have low levels of 25-OH vitamin D.[35] Because patients on CAPD lose a comparable amount of protein into the dialysate per day, one would expect that levels of this metabolite would also be low. Unfortunately, the data is conflicting. We[26] found normal levels after 6 months of CAPD in patients not receiving vitamin D supplements and no tendency for the levels to decrease with time. Moreover, the serum levels of vitamin D-binding protein (molecular weight, 57,000 daltons) were higher in CAPD patients than in those treated with chronic hemodialysis. These higher serum levels occurred despite a daily removal of 6.2 ± 2 mg of this protein into the dialysate. Kurtz et al.[27] also could not find changes in 25-OH vitamin D values during 6 to 12 months of CAPD. However, several other groups reported low levels of 25-OH vitamin D. Gokal et al.[36] noted a decline in 25-OH vitamin D to subnormal levels after 2 or more months of CAPD. At least four other groups of investigators[37-40] also reported low levels of this metabolite during CAPD. A possible explanation for these discrepancies may be variability in the amount of sunlight exposure in the study populations. For example, Cassidy et al.[41] found a seasonal variation in the levels of 25-OH vitamin D. Only one of 21 patients had low values during the summer compared with six of 21 patients during the winter. Although it is clear that 25-OH vitamin D and vitamin D-binding protein are lost into the dialysate, it is likely that patients can maintain normal 25-OH vitamin D levels if there is adequate substrate availability. In support of this concept were the high levels of 25-OH vitamin D reported by Calderaro et al.[28] in CAPD patients receiving 50,000 U/wk of vitamin D_3.

Serum 1,25-$(OH)_2$ vitamin D levels are low in severe renal failure due to a reduction in renal mass.[42-44] Recent evidence, however, suggests that there may be a significant extrarenal production of this potent metabolite in renal failure. Barbour et al.[45] reported a case of an anephric hemodialysis patient with sarcoidosis who had normal levels of 1,25-$(OH)_2$ vitamin D. Several in vitro studies have clearly shown that the activated macrophage has the capacity to 1-hydroxylate 25-OH vitamin D.[46,47] Dusso et al.[48] recently administered oral 25-OH vitamin D to chronic hemodialysis patients and to uremic dogs. A marked increase in 1,25-$(OH)_2$ vitamin D levels into the normal range was noted. This occurred even in patients with prior nephrectomies. No changes were seen in normal controls. In this light, the preliminary findings of Hayes et al.[49] are of interest. They found that peritoneal macrophages, following a recent episode of peritonitis, were capable of synthesizing 1,25-$(OH)_2$ vitamin D. No production of 1,25-$(OH)_2$ vitamin D by peritoneal macrophages in the resting nonactivated state was noted. The physiologic significance of these findings is unknown. Shany et al.[50] reported undetectable serum levels of 1,25-$(OH)_2$ vitamin D in four patients treated with CAPD. Following 1 month's treatment with 2 μg/d of 1 α-OH vitamin D, the serum levels of 1,25-$(OH)_2$ vitamin D increased to values comparable to those of six chronic hemodialysis patients ingesting only 0.25 to 0.5 μg/d. The investigators postulated that because of dialysate losses of 1,25-$(OH)_2$ vitamin D, CAPD patients may require higher doses of this metabolite compared with hemodialysis patients. Closer inspection of the data, however, reveals that approximately 5 ng/d of 1,25-$(OH)_2$ vitamin D was lost in the dialysate compared with the 250 to 500 ng ingested per day. Even assuming incomplete absorption or conversion of the metabolite to its active form, the amount of 1,25-$(OH)_2$ vitamin D reemoved would be quite small in relation to the production rate. In view of the finding of Goodman et al.[51] that the serum half-life of 1,25-$(OH)_2$ vitamin D was the same in normal controls and in patients treated with peritoneal dialysis, it would seem unnecessary to routinely increase the dosage in order to compensate for dialysate losses.

Recently, there has been increasing interest in the effects of 24,25-$(OH)_2$ vitamin D on mineral metabolism. Hodsman et al.[52] noted an improvement in bone mineralization in some patients treated with a combination of 24,25-$(OH)_2$ vitamin D and 1,25-$(OH)_2$ vitamin D. This effect was not noted with therapy consisting of 1,25-$(OH)_2$ vitamin D as a single agent. Rubinger et al.[53] showed that simultaneous treatment with 24,25-$(OH)_2$ vitamin D and 1,25-$(OH)_2$ vitamin D in rats with renal failure led to lower bone resorption rates and less hypercalcemia compared with 1,25-$(OH)_2$ vitamin D alone. Shany et al.[54] reported low plasma levels of 24,25-$(OH)_2$ vitamin D in 16 CAPD patients. Treatment of four patients with 2 μg/d of 1α-OH vitamin D_3 led to near normal 1,25-$(OH)_2$ vitamin D levels and normal 24,25-$(OH)_2$

vitamin D concentrations. The clinical significance of these findings remains to be determined.

PARATHYROID HORMONE

The majority of PTH (molecular weight, 9,500 daltons) circulates in the form of biologically inactive carboxy-terminal fragments (molecular weight, approximately 5,000 daltons) in patients with renal failure.[14,55] We found that CAPD removed substantial quantities of this hormone.[26] Polyacrylamide gel electrophoresis of the dialysate showed a pattern similar to that seen in serum. Hence, most of the immunoreactive PTH (iPTH) removed during CAPD is comprised of carboxy-terminal fragments. The clearance of iPTH was 1.56 ± 0.75 ml/min and correlated with the clearance of inulin, a substance of similar molecular weight. Therefore CAPD, unlike hemodialysis, affords an avenue for removal of iPTH and the levels may decrease if secretion is controlled. Unfortunately, interpreting studies reporting the effects of CAPD on iPTH levels is extremely difficult. Calcium and phosphorus control, as well as the use of vitamin D preparations, vary from center to center. In addition, different PTH radioimmunoassays recognize different portions of the molecule and have their own unique binding specificities. Predictably, the reports conflict. Gokal et al.[36] for example, found that PTH levels decreased to the normal range in 30 of 40 patients after approximately 1 year of CAPD; 11 of these patients were treated with 1 α-OH vitamin D. Zucchelli et al.[40] compared 17 patients treated with CAPD for 7 to 30 months to 19 patients treated with hemodialysis for a comparable period; none of these patients received vitamin D. They found a significant decline in iPTH levels in patients on CAPD compared with those on hemodialysis. Unfortunately, there were no measurements of ionized calcium concentrations and it is unclear if the two groups had comparable calcium and phosphorus control. Kurtz et al.[27] on the other hand, report a subset of five patients on CAPD who developed secondary hyperparathyroidism during CAPD. These patients demonstrated high initial values of iPTH which continued to increase irrespective of serum calcium concentrations. This has also been our experience. In summary, if calcium and phosphorus balance can be optimally controlled, iPTH levels tend to decrease or remain within acceptable limits. However, in the remaining 20 to 30 percent or so of patients, more aggressive medical or surgical therapy may be needed.

Obviously, the simplest way to suppress PTH secretion is to increase ionized calcium levels via increased oral calcium and/or vitamin D supplements. Alternatively, one could attempt to increase dialysate mass transfer by increasing the concentration of calcium in the dialysate solution. Another possibility would be to administer intraperitoneal 1,25-$(OH)_2$ vitamin D_3. We became interested in this latter possibility because of previous work performed at our institution with intravenous (IV) 1,25-$(OH)_2$ vitamin D.[56] Twenty patients undergoing hemodialysis received IV 1,25-$(OH)_2$ vitamin D (0.5 to 4.0 μg) following each dialysis. A 70 percent decrease in iPTH levels was noted. The decline was partly due to increased calcium levels. In addition, there was a 20 percent decrement in iPTH concentrations before changes in ionized calcium levels. When the percent of baseline values were plotted against the increase in ionized calcium levels, the regression line intercepted the ordinate at 80 percent of the original value. This finding suggested that IV 1,25-(OH)$_2$ vitamin D may directly suppress PTH secretion. Recent studies using calcium infusions suggest that the mechanism may in part be due to increased sensitivity to the gland to ambient calcium levels.[57] We therefore sought to determine if PTH suppression could be achieved by either increasing calcium mass transfer with a high dialysate calcium (4 mEq/L) or by administrating intraperitoneal 1,25-(OH)$_2$ vitamin D in patients undergoing CAPD.[29] Eleven patients were dialyzed for 2 months with standard calcium dialysate (3.5 mEq/L), followed by 2 months with 4.0 mEq/L calcium dialysate and then 3 months with nocturnal dwells containing intraperitoneal 1,25-(OH)$_2$ vitamin D. Ionized calcium and total calcium did not change with the higher dialysate calcium; however, both increased significantly with the use of intraperitoneal 1,25-(OH)$_2$ vitamin D. Phosphorus levels did not change. High dialysate calcium led to a small but significant decrease in iPTH levels to 84 $\pm$ 5.5 percent of control values. With intraperitoneal 1,25-(OH)$_2$ vitamin D, however, there was a more profound decrease to 54 $\pm$ 8 percent of initial levels. Serum 1,25-(OH)$_2$ vitamin D levels increased from undetectable values to 47.7 $\pm$ 7.2 pg/dl. We then studied the kinetics of intraperitoneal 1,25-(OH)$_2$ vitamin D absorption. Following the instillation of 2 μg of 1,25-(OH)$_2$ vitamin D, peak levels were observed at 2 to 4 hours and remained elevated for at least 8 hours. These kinetics more closely parallel those of oral 1,25-(OH)$_2$ vitamin D than IV 1,25-(OH)$_2$ vitamin D. When the percentage of control iPTH values versus increases in the ionized calcium was plotted, a highly significant reciprocal relationship was determined, with the y-intercept approaching 100 percent of control values. These findings suggest that the major, if not sole, effect of intraperitoneal 1,25-(OH)$_2$ vitamin D in suppressing PTH secretion is due to increases in ionized calcium concentrations. Thus, increasing calcium mass transfer leads to only a modest decline in iPTH levels, whereas intraperitoneal 1,25-(OH)$_2$ vitamin D causes a rather dramatic decrease. It should be pointed out that significant amounts of 1,25-(OH)$_2$ vitamin D bind to dialysate bags.[58] Hence, the sterol should be administered immediately before an exchange. Whether intraperitoneal administration is superior to oral 1,25-(OH)$_2$ vitamin D or calcium carbonate remains to be determind. Salusky et al.[59] reported the effects of "high-dose" oral 1,25-(OH)$_2$ vitamin D in 16 children undergoing CAPD. Using dosages that averaged 0.61 μg/d, the serum calcium levels increased from 9.9 $\pm$ 0.9 mg/dl (SD) to 11.0 $\pm$ 0.06 mg/dl. This was associated with a concomitant decrease in iPTH by approximately 40 percent after 11 to 29 months. Aside from transient hypercalcemia, the regimen was well-tolerated.

ALUMINUM

Aluminum-related bone disease has been well-described in patients on long-term hemodialysis. It has also been described in patients on CAPD. It is doubtful that dialysate contaminated with aluminum currently plays a significant role. Hercz et al.[60] found aluminum levels of less than 6 μg/L in both Dianeal and Impersol solutions. In studying 19 patients on peritoneal dialysis with aluminum intoxication, these investigators noted a net removal of 200 to 400 μg/d. How does this compare with aluminum removal during standard hemodialysis? Milliner et al.[61] studied aluminum removal during hemodialysis in patients with roughly the same aluminum levels as those described by Hercz et al. and found a net removal of 200 ± 300 μg per treatment. Therefore, on a weekly basis, approximately twice as much aluminum is removed with peritoneal dialysis compared with hemodialysis. It is likely, nonetheless, that long-term ingestion of aluminum-containing phosphorus binders during CAPD would cause aluminum accumulation in a fashion similar to that described in hemodialysis patients. In support of this contention are the findings of Rottenbourg et al.,[62] who noted increasing serum aluminum levels in CAPD patients ingesting aluminum-containing phosphorus binders, and stable levels in those never receiving these compounds. Similar results were reported by Salusky et al.[63] Mactier et al.[64] found a positive correlation between serum aluminum levels and total intake of aluminum after starting CAPD, aluminum intake in the previous 6 months, and duration of CAPD. Salusky et al.[21] noted higher bone aluminum content and staining in pediatric patients receiving aluminum-containing gels for phosphorus binding than in those prescribed calcium carbonate.

Assuming that aluminum-related bone disease may become a problem if peritoneal dialysis patients are treated for long periods with aluminum-containing phosphorus binders, questions arise concerning its diagnosis and treatment. For example, Milliner et al.[15] found that a plasma aluminum level of greater than 200 μg/L was often associated with aluminum-related bone disease in chronic hemodialysis patients. Unfortunately, baseline Al levels were not particularly sensitive (sensitivity, 43 percent). Following an intravenous infusion of deferoxamine, most patients with aluminum-related bone disease had increments of greater than 200 μg/L. A good correlation could be found with the amount of trabecular bone aluminum and the increment in aluminum levels 24 hours after the chelation challenge. These findings could not be confirmed by Malluche et al.[65] in hemodialysis patients or by Salusky et al.[21] in pediatric patients treated with peritoneal dialysis. No comparable studies have been performed in adult patients on peritoneal dialysis. However, Hercz et al.[60] showed that the intraperitoneal administration of deferoxamine in aluminum-overloaded CAPD patients achieved increments in aluminum levels that were comparable to those following intravenous infusions. The amount of aluminum removed increased sixfold from baseline to $1,379 \pm 33.7$ $\mu g/d$ following intraperitoneal administration of 2 g of deferoxamine. These removal rates were comparable to those measured after intravenous administration of deferoxamine. Similar results have been reported by Molitoris et al.,[66] who found that the aluminum removal rates remained substantial for at least 4 days following deferoxamine. In view of reports of fatal rhizopus infections in chronic hemodialysis patients undergoing chelation therapy,[67] it would probably be wise to limit deferoxamine treatments to a once weekly regimen during CAPD. It should also be noted that there is little data concerning the long-term effects of intraperitoneal deferoxamine on the peritoneal membrane function and structure.

BONE HISTOLOGY

The results of several studies using serial bone biopsies are summarized in Table 9-1. Gokal et al.[36] studied bone histology in 20 patients around the time of initiation of CAPD and approximately 1 year later. Five patients were treated with 1α-OH vitamin D and all received between 1.5 to 3.0 g of $CaCO_3$ per day. The vast majority of subjects had either an improvement or no change in the degree of osteitis fibrosa. One patient developed osteomalacia following a parathyroidectomy. Zucchelli et al.[40] compared the changes in bone histology in 17 patients treated with CAPD with those of 19 receiving maintenance hemodialysis. After a little more than a year of follow-up, those patients on CAPD demonstrated a decrease in both percentage of bone volume and active formation surface. These changes were statistically greater than in patients treated with hemodialysis. There were no changes in the amount of osteoid during treatment with CAPD. These investigators concluded that CAPD may lead to osteopenia in the absence of worsening osteomalacia or osteitis fibrosa. These findings were not confirmed by Shusterman et al.,[68] who found that CAPD in six patients led to an improvement in osteomalacia but no change in the degree of osteitis fibrosa. It is of note that Zucchelli et al.[40] did not administer vitamin D to their patients, whereas $1,25\text{-}(OH)_2$ vitamin D was used in the study of Shusterman et al. Buccianti et al.[38] felt that all parameters of bone histology deteriorated in seven patients.

Table 9-1. A Summary of the Results of Studies Reporting Serial Changes in Bone Histomorphology During Treatment With Continuous Ambulatory Peritoneal Dialysis

Reference	Vitamin D	Osteitis Fibrosa	Osteomalacia
Gokal et al.[36]	$1 \alpha\text{-}(OH)D_3$ (some)	Improved	No development
Zucchelli et al.[40]	No	No change[a]	No change
Shusterman et al.[68]	$1,25\text{-}(OH)_2D_3$	No change	Improved
Buccianti et al.[38]	No	Worse	Worse
Loschiavo et al.[69]	No	Persistence	Persistence
Delmez et al.[70]	No	Variable	Improved

[a] Absolute cancellous bone volume declined.

Loschiavo et al.[69] reported the results of serial bone biopsies in 14 patients who did not receive aluminum-containing phosphorus binders or vitamin D. They found no healing of osteomalacia in five patients after 1 year. Quantitative assessment of the biopsy results was not provided. We recently reported the results of serial bone biopsies of 12 patients treated with CAPD.[70] All patients received calcium carbonate and aluminum-containing phosphorus binders, but no vitamin D preparations. We found no significant changes in indices of osteitis fibrosa. This no doubt reflected the variable effects of CAPD on iPTH levels during the study period. On the other hand, there was a good correlation between iPTH concentrations and fibrotic surface. The most impressive finding was a decline in the amount of osteoid. Of the eight patients with an increased total osteoid surface at the start of CAPD, seven demonstrated improvement after 12 months. These changes were not associated with changes in bone aluminum staining. The quantity of osteoid is a reflection of the relative rates of synthesis and mineralization. In order to determine if the decline in unmineralized matrix was due to enhanced mineralization or decreased osteoid production, time-spaced courses of tetracycline as morphologic markers of rates of mineralization were used. We found that the mineralization lag time decreased in the seven of eight patients in whom it was initially elevated. In other words, the bone mineralization rate improved. This suggests that, in general, CAPD has a beneficial effect on calcification of the uremic bone.

STRATEGIES IN OPTIMIZING MINERAL METABOLISM IN CONTINUOUS AMBULATORY PERITONEAL DIALYSIS PATIENTS

The therapeutic goals in optimizing mineral metabolism in CAPD are control of iPTH and phosphorus levels while avoiding toxic levels of calcium and magnesium. In order to avoid aluminum accumulation, the use of aluminum-containing phosphorus binders should be minimized. Phosphorus restriction, within the confines of a high protein diet, is clearly of paramount importance. The use of non-aluminum-containing phosphorus binders should also be considered. We[71] and others[72-75] have shown $CaCO_3$ to be an effective phosphorus binder in chronic hemodialysis patients. In our experience, it allowed the discontinuation of all aluminum-containing phosphorus binders in over half of the study patients. In those patients with a high dietary phosphorus intake, large doses (up to 12 g/d) of $CaCO_3$ were required. This frequently resulted in hypercalcemia. There are fewer reports of the use of $CaCO_3$ in CAPD patients. Salusky et al.[76] administered $CaCO_3$ (mean dose, 5.1 g/d) to 15 children on dialysis. Thirteen were treated with peritoneal dialysis. They noted good control of serum phosphorus levels, but mild hypercalcemia was a frequent event. It is of note that all of these patients also received $1,25\text{-}(OH)_2$ vitamin D. We have also found $CaCO_3$ to be useful in adults treated with CAPD.[77] Unfortunately, three of 14 patients developed moderately severe hypercalcemia (ionized calcium, greater than 5.5 mg/dl), necessitating the use of aluminum-containing phosphorus binders. When hypercalcemia develops in a patient on chronic hemodialysis, it is relatively simple to decrease the concentration of calcium in the dialysate and restart $CaCO_3$ when the hypercalcemia resolves.[78] With the availability of a dialysate for peritoneal dialysis containing 2.5 mEq/L calcium, it would similarly appear reasonable to switch to the lower concentration of dialysate calcium in CAPD patients. It should be emphasized that a source of concern over the long-term use of oral $CaCO_3$ therapy in CAPD is the development of metastatic calcifications. Ramirez et al.[79] studied chronic hemodialysis patients given a single standard meal along with placebo or 1,500 mg (75 mEq) of calcium in the form of $CaCO_3$. The net phosphorus absorption decreased from 79 percent to 65 percent with $CaCO_3$. The percentage of calcium absorbed, however, increased to 28 percent. Although it is hazardous to extrapolate single-dose studies to long-term effects, 28 percent calcium absorption in a patient ingesting 3.0 g elemental calcium per day results in 840 mg calcium being absorbed. Even if patients were to dialyze with a dialysate free of calcium, they would be in positive calcium balance. Of note, however, is the recent data by Renaud et al.,[80] who were unable to correlate the dose of $CaCO_3$ used for phosphorus binding in hemodialysis patients and the progression of vascular calcinosis after 3 years of treatment. Calcium citrate has been advocated as an effective phosphorus binding in chronic hemodialysis patients.[81] However, citrate markedly enhances the absorption of aluminum,[82] possibly via the opening of the tight junctions of the bowel.[83] Hence, the use of calcium citrate is absolutely contraindicated in those patients ingesting aluminum-containing phosphorus binders or medications containing aluminum (such as sucralfate). Another salt, calcium acetate, has recently been reported[84] to bind phosphorus more effectively than calcium carbonate (22 percent absorption versus 40 percent, respectively) in hemodialysis patients. If the preliminary data is confirmed, the potential advantage of controlling phosphorus with less oral elemental calcium is obvious.

Magnesium salts have also been advocated as effective phosphorus binders in CAPD. Jennings et al.[85] treated seven patients with magnesium hydroxide and aluminum hydroxide in the form of Maalox II and dialysate low in magnesium (0.5 mEq/L). In six of seven patients, the magnesium hydroxide dose was limited by gastrointestinal side effects. Shah et al.[33] however, reported successful control of phosphorus levels with the use of magnesium-containing phosphorus binders and a magnesium-free dialysate. Despite an additional oral magnesium load of 0.28 to 3.0 g/d, the mean serum magnesium levels remained normal (2.5 ± 0.2 mg/dl), due partly to an increase in daily dialysate magnesium removal rates to 128 ± 17 mg/d. The amount of aluminum ingested decreased by 22 to 75 percent in this 12-week study. Hence, magnesium-containing phosphorus binders prescribed in concert with dialysate low in magnesium may be efficacious in CAPD. However, long-term studies of efficacy and safety are necessary before routine use of magnesium is advised.

A novel approach to controlling phosphorus levels in CAPD patients is that of binding phorphorus in the dialysate fluid. McGary et al.[86] found that the polycation, polyethylenimine, more than doubled phosphorus clearance in vitro. Unfortunately, this polymer also caused marked morphologic distortion of the visceral peritoneal mesothelium in rats. Further research on a nontoxic polycation would appear to be warranted.

SPECIFIC THERAPEUTIC RECOMMENDATIONS

As knowledge of the pathophysiology of renal osteodystrophy expands, it is anticipated that improved therapy will also evolve. Here I will discuss helpful guidelines in the prevention and treatment of renal osteodystrophy. The initial thrust should be dietary instruction that restrict dietary phosphorus as much as possible within the limits of a 1.2 g/kg/d protein diet. If this maneuver alone is successful in normalizing phosphorus levels, there should be concern that the dietary protein intake is inadequate (assuming little urinary phosphorus excretion). Nonetheless, in the presence of normal phosphorus levels, the next effort should be directed toward increasing the serum ionized calcium levels toward the upper limits of normal in order to suppress PTH secretion. If the PTH levels are mildly or moderately elevated, calcium carbonate given at bedtime in the fasting state may suffice in increasing the calcium levels and preventing hypophosphatemia. If the PTH levels are markedly elevated, oral $1,25\text{-}(OH)_2$ vitamin D should be administered, with careful monitoring of calcium and phosphorus levels. The latter may increase due to increased phosphorus absorption. If the phosphorus levels are not controlled with diet alone, calcium carbonate should be prescribed with meals in amounts proportional to the usual dietary phosphorus content of each meal. If hypercalcemia develops, it would seem advisable to decrease the dialysate calcium concentration from 3.5 mEq/L to 2.5 mEq/L. If hypercalcemia persists in the presence of severe unrelenting secondary hyperparathyroidism and in the absence of other possible causes, a partial parathyroidectomy should be considered. If hypercalcemia and hyperphosphatemia coexist during calcium carbonate therapy, aluminum-containing phosphorus binders may be judiciously added to the regimen. One should bear in mind, however, that those patients with diabetes and/or low levels of PTH are at high risk for the development of aluminum-induced osteomalacia. Alternatively, lowering the dialysate magnesium to 0.5 mEq/L and adding magnesium-containing phosphorus binders may be efficacious. Careful monitoring of magnesium levels is mandatory in this situation. Some patients maintain low ionized calcium concentrations and well-controlled phosphorus levels despite calcium carbonate therapy. The therapy should, in part, be determined by the degree of hyperparathyroidism. In those patients with moderate or severe osteitis fibrosa, treatment with $1,25\text{-}(OH)_2$ vitamin D would be appropriate. With mild hyperparathyroidism, further intervention may not be necessary. If the patient demonstrates low serum levels of 25-OH vitamin D or lives in an area where the substrate availability for its synthesis is low, an empiric trial of low-dose vitamin D may be considered.

Hopefully, with less reliance on aluminum-containing phosphorus binders, the nephrologist will rarely be faced with the problem of treating patients with aluminum intoxication. At this time, guidelines for management of this condition are poorly defined. In view of the potential severe (albeit rare) complications of deferoxamine treatment, it is my bias to treat asymptomatic patients solely by the elimination of exogenous aluminum loads. Patients with presumed aluminum-induced symptomatic disease ideally should have the diagnosis confirmed with a bone biopsy. If positive, treatment with deferoxamine is indicated. The optimal dose, route, and frequency of deferoxamine therapy is unclear. Assuming the complication rate is roughly a function of exposure to the drug, a dose of 0.5 to 1.0 g given weekly via the subcutaneous or intraperitoneal route may suffice.

The above recommendations serve only as guidelines. Renal osteodystrophy is not a static process. Some patients may display improvement, whereas others deteriorate. A major consideration in the "decision-making tree" of therapy is the trend over time.

FUTURE CONSIDERATIONS

Although a 2.5-mEq/L concentration of calcium in the dialysate is now available, further reductions may be advantageous in those patients in whom high doses of oral calcium carbonate induce hypercalcemia. Alternatively, if the potential benefits of calcium acetate are confirmed in long-term studies, it may not be necessary to lower the dialysate calcium levels beyond 2.5 mEq/L. Studies to determine if the combination of $24,25\text{-}(OH)_2$ and $1,25\text{-}(OH)_2$ vitamin D decreases PTH levels and lessens the risk for the development of hypercalcemia are needed. Finally, great interest has arisen concerning synthetic analogues of vitamin D which may directly suppress PTH secretion without inducing hypercalcemia. These derivatives have the potential to allow the routine co-administration of calcium-containing phosphorus binders and compounds that directly suppress the secretion of PTH.

ACKNOWLEDGMENTS

I wish to thank Eduardo Slatopolsky, M.D. and David Windus, M.D. for reviewing the manuscript, and Donna Morgan for excellent help in its preparation.

REFERENCES

1. Coburn JW, Slatopolsky E: Vitamin D, parathyroid hormone, and renal osteodystrophy. p. 1657. In Brenner BM, Rector FC, Jr. (eds): The Kidney. 3rd Ed. WB, Saunders, Philadelphia, 1986

2. Lopez-Hilker S, Galceran T, Chan Y-L, et al: Hypocalcemia may not be essential for the development of secondary hyperparathyroidism in chronic renal failure. J Clin Invest 78:1097, 1986
3. Brown EM, Wilson RE, Eastman RC, et al: Abnormal regulation of parathyroid hormone release by calcium in secondary hyperparathyroidism due to chronic renal failure. J Clin Endocrinol Metab 54:172, 1982
4. Au WYW, Bukowski A: Inhibition of parathyroid hormone secretion by vitamin D metabolites in organ cultures of rat parathyroids. Fed Proc 35:530, 1976
5. Brumbaugh PF, Hughes MR, Hausler MR: Cytoplasmic and nuclear binding components for 1,25-dihydroxyvitamin D_3 in chick parathyroid glands. Proc Natl Acad Sci USA 72:4871, 1975
6. Chan YL, McKay C, Dye E, Slatopolsky E: The effect of 1,25-dihydroxychole-calciferol on parathyroid hormone secretion by monolayer cultures of bovine parathyroid cells. Calcif Tissue Int 38:27, 1986
7. Chertow BD, Baylink DJ, Wergedal JE, et al: Decrease in serum immunoreactive parathyroid hormone in rats and in parathyroid hormone secretion in vitro by 1,25-dihydroxycholecalciferol. J Clin Invest 56:668, 1975
8. Russell J, Lettieri D, Sherwood LM: Suppression by $1,25(OH)_2D_3$ of transcription of the parathyroid hormone gene. Endocrinology 119:2864, 1986
9. Silver J, Russell J, Sherwood LM: Regulation by vitamin D metabolites of messenger RNA for pre-proparathyroid hormone in isolated bovine parathyroid cells. Proc Nat Acad Sci USA 82:4270, 1985
10. Brown A, Dusso A, Lopez-Hilker S, et al: $1,25-(OH)_2D$ receptors are decreased in parathyroid glands from chronically uremic dogs. Kidney Int 35:19, 1989
11. Korkor AB: Reduced binding of [3H]1,25-dihydroxyvitamin D_3 in patients with renal failure. N Engl J Med 316:1573, 1987
12. Merke J, Hugel U, Zlotkowski A, et al: Diminished parathyroid $1,25(OH)_2D_3$ receptors in experimental uremia. Kidney Int 32:350, 1987
13. Lopez-Hilker S, Dusso A, Rapp N, et al: On the mechanism of the prevention of secondary hyperparathyroidism by phosphate restriction. Kidney Int 29:164, 1986 (abstr.)
14. Hruska KA, Kopelman R, Rutherford WE, et al: Metabolism of immunoreactive parathyroid hormone in the dog: the role of the kidney and the effects of chronic renal disease. J Clin Invest 56:39, 1975
15. Milliner DS, Nebeker HG, Ott SM, et al: Use of the deferoxamine infusion test in the diagnosis of aluminum-related osteodystrophy. Ann Intern Med 101:775, 1984
16. Ott SM, Maloney NA, Coburn JW, et al: The prevalence of bone aluminum deposition in renal osteodystrophy and its relation to the response to calcitriol therapy. N Engl J Med 307:709, 1982
17. Pierides AM, Edwards WG, Cullum UX, et al: Hemodialysis encephalopathy with osteomalacia fractures and muscle weakness. Kidney Int 18:115, 1980
18. Morrissey J, Rothstein M, Mayor G, Slatopolsky E: Suppression of parathyroid hormone secretion by aluminum. Kidney Int 23:699, 1983
19. Talwar HS, Reddi AH, Menczel J, et al: Influence of aluminum on mineralization during matrix-induced bone development. Kidney Int 29:1038, 1986
20. Andress DL, Maloney NA, Endres DB, Sherrard DJ: Aluminum-associated bone disease in chronic renal failure: high prevalence in a long-term dialysis population. J Bone Mineral Res 1:391, 1986
21. Salusky IB, Coburn JW, Brill J, et al: Bone disease in pediatric patients undergoing dialysis with CAPD or CCPD. Kidney Int 33:975, 1988

22. Andress DL, Pandian MR, Endres DB, et al: Elevated plasma insulin-like growth factor I correlates with bone formation in uremic hyperparathyroidism. Kidney Int 35:376, 1989 (abstr.)

23. Sherrard DJ, Ott SM, Maloney NA, et al: Renal osteodystrophy. Semin Nephrol 6:56, 1986

24. Parker A, Nolph KD: Magnesium and calcium mass transfer during continuous ambulatory peritoneal dialysis. Trans Am Soc Artif Internal Organs 26:194, 1980

25. Blumenkrantz MJ, Kopple JD, Moran JD, Coburn JW: Metabolic balance studies and dietary protein requirements in patients undergoing continuous ambulatory peritoneal dialysis. Kidney Int 21:849, 1982

26. Delmez JA, Slatopolsky E, Martin KJ, et al: Minerals, vitamin D and parathyroid hormone in continuous ambulatory peritoneal dialysis. Kidney Int 21:862, 1982

27. Kurtz SB, McCarthy JT, Kumar R: Hypercalcemia in continuous ambulatory peritoneal dialysis patients: observations on parameters of calcium metabolism. p. 467. In Gahl GM, Kessel M, Nolph KD (eds): Advances in Peritoneal Dialysis. Excerpta Medica, Amsterdam, 1981

28. Calderaro V, Oreopoulos DG, Meema HE, et al: The evolution of renal osteodystrophy in patients undergoing continuous ambulatory peritoneal dialysis. Proc Eur Dialysis Transplant Assoc 17:533, 1980

29. Delmez JA, Dougan CS, Gearing BK, et al: The effects of intraperitoneal calcitriol on calcium and parathyroid hormone. Kidney Int 31:795, 1987

30. Sheikh MS, Ramirez A, Emmett M, et al: Role of vitamin D-dependent and vitamin D-independent mechanisms in absorption of food calcium. J Clin Invest 81:126, 1988

31. Blumenkrantz MJ, Salusky IB, Schmidt RW: Managing the nutritional concerns of the patient undergoing peritoneal dialysis. p. 345. In Nolph KD (ed): Peritoneal Dialysis. 2nd Ed. Martinus Nijhoff Publishing, Boston, 1985

32. Meema HE, Oreopoulous DG, Rapoport A: Serum magnesium level and arterial calcification in end-stage renal disease. Kidney Int 32:388, 1987

33. Shah GM, Winer RL, Catler RE, et al: Effects of magnesium-free dialysate on magnesium metabolism during continuous ambulatory peritoneal dialysis. Am J Kidney Dis 10:268, 1987

34. Nolph KD, Prowant B, Serkes KD, et al: Multicenter evaluation of a new peritoneal dialysis solution with a high lactate and a low magnesium concentration. Peritoneal Dialysis Bull 3:63, 1983

35. Goldstein DA, Haldimann B, Sherman D, et al: Vitamin D metabolites and calcium metabolism in patients with nephrotic syndrome and normal renal function. J Clin Endocrinol Metab 52:116, 1981

36. Gokal R, Ramos JM, Ellis HA, et al: Histological renal osteodystrophy, and 25 hydroxycholecalciferol and aluminum levels in patients on continuous ambulatory peritoneal dialysis. Kidney Int 23:15, 1983

37. Alon U, Shany S, Chaimovitz C: Losses of 25-hydroxyvitamin D in peritoneal fluid: possible mechanism for bone disease in uremic patients treated with chronic ambulatory peritoneal dialysis. Min Electrolyte Metab 9:82, 1983

38. Buccianti G, Bianchi ML, Valenti G: Progress of renal osteodystrophy during continuous ambulatory peritoneal dialysis. Clin Nephrol 6:279, 1984

39. Tielemans C, Aubry C, Dratwa M: The effects of continuous ambulatory peritoneal dialysis on renal osteodystrophy. p. 454. In Gahl GM, Kessel M, Nolph KD (eds): Advances in Peritoneal Dialysis. Excerpta Medica, Amsterdam, 1981

40. Zucchelli P, Catizone L, Casanova S, et al: Renal osteodystrophy in CAPD patients. Miner Electrolyte Metab 10:316, 1984
41. Cassidy MJD, Own JP, Ellis HA, et al: Renal osteodystrophy and metastatic calcification in long-term continuous ambulatory peritoneal dialysis. Q J Med 213:29, 1985
42. Cheung AK, Manolagas SC, Catherwood BC, et al: Determinants of serum 1,25(OH)$_2$D$_3$ levels in renal disease. Kidney Int 24:104, 1983
43. Mason RS, Lissner D, Wilkinson M, Posen S: Vitamin D metabolites and their relationship to azotaemic osteodystrophy. Clin Endocrinol 13:375, 1980
44. Slatopolsky E, Grey ND, Adams J, et al: The pathogenesis of secondary hyperparathyroidism in early renal failure. p. 1209. In Norman AW (ed): Fourth International Workshop of Vitamin D. de Gruyter, Berlin, 1979
45. Barbour GL, Coburn JW, Slatopolsky E, et al: Hypercalcemia in an anephric patient with sarcoidosis: evidence for extra-renal generation of 1,25-dihydroxyvitamin D. N Engl J Med 305:440, 1981
46. Reichel H, Koeffler HP, Bishop JE, Norman AW: 25-Hydroxyvitamin D$_3$ metabolism by lipopolysacchride-stimulated normal human macrophages. J Clin Endocrinol Metabol 64:1, 1987
47. Reichel H, Koeffler HP, Barbers R, Norman AW: Regulation of 1,25-dihydroxyvitamin D$_3$ production by cultured alveolar macrophages from normal human donors and from patients with pulmonary sarcoidosis. J Clin Endocrinol Metab 65:1201, 1987
48. Dusso A, Lopez-Hilker S, Rapp N, Slatopolsky E: Extra-renal production of calcitriol in chronic renal failure. Kidney Int 34:368, 1988
49. Hayes ME, O'Donoghue DJ, Ballardie FW, Mawer EB: Peritonitis induces the synthesis of 1 α,25-dihydroxyvitamin D$_3$ in macrophages from CAPD patients. FEBS Lett 220:307, 1987
50. Shany S, Rapoport J, Goligorsky M, et al: Losses of 1,25- and 24,25-dihydroxycholecalciferol in the peritoneal fluid of patients treated with continuous ambulatory peritoneal dialysis. Nephron 36:111, 1984
51. Goodman WG, Salusky IB, Horst R, et al: Intravenous calcitriol: plasma kinetics and acute effect on serum PTH in normal and dialyzed subjects. Kidney Int 33:339, 1988 (abstr)
52. Hodsman AB, Wong EGC, Sherrard DJ, et al: Preliminary trials with 24,25-dihydroxyvitamin D$_3$ in dialysis osteomalacia. Am J Med 74:407, 1983
53. Rubinger D, Moscovitz A, Popovtzer MM, et al: 24,25(OH)$_2$D$_3$ in combination with 1,25(OH)$_2$D$_3$ ameliorates renal osteodystrophy in rats with chronic renal failure. Kidney Int 35:379, 1989 (abstr)
54. Shany S, Rapoport J, Zuili I, et al: Enhancement of 24,25-dihydroxyvitamin D levels in patients treated with continuous ambulatory peritoneal dialysis. Nephron 42:141, 1986
55. Martin KJ, Hruska KA, Freitag JJ, et al: The peripheral metabolism of parathyroid hormone. N Engl J Med 301:1092, 1979
56. Slatopolsky E, Weerts C, Thielan J, et al: Marked suppression of secondary hyperparathyroidism by intravenous administration of 1,25-dihydroxycholecalciferol in uremic patients. J Clin Invest 74:2136, 1984
57. Delmez JA, Tindira C, Groom P, et al: Parathyroid hormone suppression by intravenous 1,25(OH)$_2$D: a role for increased sensitivity to calcium. J Clin Invest 83:1349, 1989
58. Salusky IB, Adams JS, Horst R, et al: Enhanced calcitriol delivery after intraperitoneal administration. Kidney Int 35:276, 1989 (abstr.)

59. Salusky IB, Fine RN, Kangarloo H, et al: "High-dose" calcitriol for control of renal osteodystrophy in children on CAPD. Kidney Int 32:89, 1987

60. Hercz G, Salusky IB, Norris KC, et al: Aluminum removal by peritoneal dialysis: intravenous vs. intraperitoneal deferoxamine. Kidney Int 39:944, 1986

61. Milliner DS, Hercz G, Miller JH, et al: Clearance of aluminum by hemodialysis: effect of desferrioxamine. Kidney Int 29:S-100, 1986

62. Rottenbourg J, Gallego JL, Jaudon M, et al: Serum concentration and peritoneal transfer of aluminum during treatment by continuous ambulatory peritoneal dialysis. Kidney Int 25:919, 1984

63. Salusky IB, Coburn JW, Paunier L, et al: Role of aluminum hydroxide in raising serum aluminum levels in children undergoing continuous ambulatory peritoneal dialysis. J Pediatr 105:717, 1984

64. Mactier RA, Nolph KD, Khanna R, Twardowski Z: Risk factors for hyperaluminemia in continuous ambulatory peritoneal dialysis. Peritoneal Dialysis Bull 6:188, 1986

65. Malluche HH, Smith AJ, Abreo K, Faugere MC: The use of deferoxamine in the management of aluminum accumulation in bone in patients with renal failure. N Engl J Med 311:140, 1984

66. Molitoris BA, Alfrey PS, Millern NL, et al: Efficacy of intramuscular and intraperitoneal deferoxamine for aluminum chelation. Kidney Int 31:986, 1987

67. Windus DW, Stokes TJ, Julian BA, Fenves AZ: Fatal rhizopus infections in hemodialysis patients receiving deferoxamine. Ann Intern Med 107:678, 1987

68. Shusterman NH, Wasserstein MG, Audet P, et al: Controlled study of renal osteodystrophy in patients undergoing dialysis. Improved response to continuous ambulatory peritoneal dialysis compared with hemodialysis. Am J Med 82:1148, 1987

69. Loschiavo C, Fabris A, Adami S, et al: Effects of continuous ambulatory peritoneal dialysis on renal osteodystrophy. Peritoneal Dialysis Bull 5:53, 1985

70. Delmez JA, Fallon MD, Bergfeld MA, et al: Continuous ambulatory peritoneal dialysis and bone. Kidney Int 30:379, 1986

71. Slatopolsky E, Weerts C, Lopez-Hilker S, et al: Calcium carbonate as a phosphate binder in patients with chronic renal failure undergoing dialysis. N Engl J Med 315:157, 1986

72. Clarkson EM, McDonald SJ, de Wardener HE: The effect of a high intake of calcium carbonate in normal subjects and patients with chronic renal failure. Clin Sci 30:425, 1966

73. Makoff DL, Gordon A, Franklin SS, et al: Chronic calcium carbonate therapy in uremia. Arch Intern Med 123:15, 1969

74. Meyrier A, Marsac J, Richet G: The influence of a high calcium carbonate intake on bone disease in patients undergoing hemodialysis. Kidney Int 4:146, 1973

75. Moriniere P, Roussel A, Tahiri Y, et al: Substitution of aluminum hydroxide by high doses of calcium carbonate in patients on chronic hemodialysis: disappearance of hyperaluminaemia and equal control of hyperparathyroidism. Proc Dialysis Transplant Assoc 19:7484, 1982

76. Salusky IB, Coburn JW, Foley J, et al: Effect of oral calcium carbonate on control of serum phosphorus and changes in plasma aluminum levels after discontinuation of aluminum-containing gels in children receiving dialysis. J Pediatr 105:767, 1984

77. Delmez JA, Gearing BK: Renal osteodystrophy and aluminum bone disease in CAPD patients. p. 38. In Khanna R, Nolph KD, Prowant B, et al (eds): Ad-

vances in Continuous Ambulatory Peritoneal Dialysis. Peritoneal Dialysis Bulletin, Toronto, 1987

78. Mactier RA, VanStone J, Cox A, et al: Calcium carbonate is an effective phosphate binder when dialysate calcium concentration is adjusted to control hypercalcemia. Clin Nephrol 28:222, 1987

79. Ramirez JA, Emmett M, White MG, et al: The absorption of dietary phosphorus and calcium in hemodialysis patients. Kidney Int 30:753, 1986

80. Renaud H, Atik A, Herve M, et al: Evaluation of vascular calcinosis risk factors in patients on chronic hemodialysis: lack of influence of calcium carbonate. Nephron 48:28, 1988

81. Cushner HM, Copley JB, Lindberg JS, Foulks CJ: Calcium citrate, a nonaluminum-containing phosphate-binding agent for treatment of CRF. Kidney Int 33:95, 1988

82. Mischel MG, Salusky IB, Goodman WG, Coburn JW: Calcium citrate markedly augments aluminum absorption in man. Kidney Int 35:399, 1989 (abstr.)

83. Froment DH, Molitaris BA: Mechanism of enhanced gastrointestinal absorption of aluminum by citrate. Kidney Int 35:398, 1989 (abstr)

84. Mai MA, Emmett M, Sheikh MS, et al: Calcium acetate, an effective binder of dietary phosphorus in patients with chronic renal failure. Kidney Int 35:384, 1989 (abstr.)

85. Jennings AE, Bodvarsson M, Galicka-Piskorska G, et al: Use of magnesium hydroxide and low magnesium dialysate does not permit reduction of aluminum hydroxide during continuous ambulatory peritoneal dialysis. Am J Kidney Dis 8:192, 1986

86. McGary TJ, Nolph KD, Moore HL, Kartinos NJ: Polycation as an alternative osmotic agent and phosphate binder in peritoneal dialysis. Uremia Invest 8:79, 1984–85

Peritoneal Dialysis in Diabetic End-Stage Renal Disease Patients

10

Ramesh Khanna

INTRODUCTION

According to the USA U.S. Continuous Ambulatory Peritoneal Dialysis (CAPD) Registry survey, diabetes is the leading cause (26 percent) of end-stage renal disease (ESRD) among the 23,634 surveyed CAPD patients.[1] As recently as the 1960s, diabetics with ESRD were denied renal replacement therapy because of the relatively poorer outcomes of such therapies in such patients. Owing to the technical advances in hemodialysis and the advent of CAPD in the late 1970s, there has been a remarkable change in the prognosis and survival of diabetics with end-stage kidney disease requiring dialysis. Despite the improved prognosis, diabetics as a group are still considered to have a poorer prognosis than patients with other types of primary renal disease on dialysis, mainly because of the high morbidity and mortality related to cardiovascular complications. Nevertheless, in the last few years, survivals of more than 5 years for diabetic CAPD patients are being reported. The focus of this chapter will be the management of diabetic patients on CAPD, with an emphasis on their short- and long-term outcomes.

BENEFITS AND DRAWBACKS OF CONTINUOUS AMBULATORY PERITONEAL DIALYSIS

When patients with diabetic nephropathy approache the stage of requiring dialysis, they also usually have other target organ damage due to complications of diabetes and premature atherosclerosis. It is not uncommon to see all or some of the following complications in a diabetic patient: crippling coronary artery disease, peripheral vascular disease with ischemic complications, proliferative retinopathy, or cerebro-vascular disease. In addition, diabetic patients may have debilitating autonomic neuropathy with symptomatic orthostatic hypotension. These are difficult patients to care for on any form of dialysis. Any rapid fluctuations in the hemodynamic status of these patient are likely to precipitate acute coronary or cerebrovascular events. Creating a vascular access for hemodialysis in these patients with hardened arteries is a challenge to any vascular surgeon. Systemic heparinization required during hemodialysis is alleged to cause bleeding in the retinal tissue, which may be undergoing changes of neovascularization due to diabetes.

Experiences with CAPD in the past decade indicate that this form of dialysis therapy is ideally suited for such patients because it is a continous and slow therapy and is devoid of the rapid fluctuations in biochemical parameters and fluid status seen with the intermittent forms of dialysis therapy (Table 10-1). Not having to access a blood vessel and to give heparin are the additional medical benefits of CAPD. The ability to administer insulin during CAPD through the peritoneal route allegedly simulates the normal physiology of insulin uptake into the portal circulation once secreted by the pancreas. Preliminary evidences, which will be discussed later in this section, suggest that CAPD preserves residual renal function for a period longer than hemodialysis. Moreover, there are several social and economic benefits that may have impact on a patient's sense of well-being, such as the opportunity for home dialysis, no need to use machinery, a simple and flexible technique with a short training period, and the free mobility.

Table 10.1. Benefits of Continuous Ambulatory Peritoneal Dialysis

Medical	Social
No blood access required	Usually no partner required
No systemic anticoagulation necessary	No machine in the home
Steady ultrafiltration	Free mobility possible
Steady-state chemistry	Short training period
Low risk of life-threatening complications	Flexible dialysis schedule and location
Intraperitoneal insulin administration possible	
Preservation of renal function possible ?	
Cardiovascular system stability	

Despite the many attractive advantages of CAPD, some of its drawbacks are of significant consequence and therefore limit its application. Episodes of peritonitis related to CAPD, although not higher in incidence than in non-diabetic CAPD patients, are the major cause of morbidity and therapy failure. Long-term integrity of the peritoneum, a biologic membrane, has not been unequivocally established. Some of the social problems related to CAPD, such as the distorted body image and burn-out due to continuous therapy, may also limit its long-term use. Normalization of blood pressure in some diabetic patients with autonomic dysfunction and orthostatic hypotension may pose problems with maintaining fluid balance. Excessive weight gain and hyperlipidemia as a consequence of continuous glucose absorption in some patients can be causes for concern. During the past few years, advances in the field have enabled us to address some of the concerns expressed in this section and propose remedial measures to improve the risk benefit ratio of this therapy. These aspects will be discussed in detail more later in this chapter.

PERITONEAL ACCESS

Access to the peritoneal cavity is obtained through the use of either a Tenchkoff catheter or one of its modifications.[2,3] The techniques of catheter insertion, break-in procedure, and postoperative catheter care in diabetics are similar to nondiabetic patients and have been previously reported.[3] Infectious and noninfectious catheter complications and catheter survival rates are no different for diabetics compared with nondiabetic patients on peritoneal dialysis.[4] In an exhaustive survey of CAPD and continuous cyclic peritoneal dialysis (CCPD) patients with ESRD attributed to diabetes mellitus performed by the U.S. National Institutes of Health CAPD Registry, exit site and/or tunnel infection rates per patient-year by route of insulin administration were calculated.[1] Although differences in rates were small, diabetics never using insulin had the lowest rate of exit site/tunnel infection per patient-year (0.47), while patients using subcutaneous insulin reported the highest rate (0.65). The exit site/tunnel infection rate per patient-year for patients using intraperitonealy administered insulin (0.60) was similar to the rate reported for patients using a combination of subcutaneous and intraperitoneal insulin (0.54). Blind patients using subcutaneously administered insulin verses blind patients using intraperitoneal insulin reported similar rates per patient-year of exit site/tunnel infection. Catheter replacement rates per patient-year were similar for all patient groups (0.16 to 0.20).

DIALYSIS SCHEDULE AND TECHNIQUE

Intermittent peritoneal dialysis (IPD) for chronic renal failure was introduced by Boen et al.[5] Because of the benefits of peritoneal dialysis listed above, IPD was considered superior to hemodialysis in elderly diabetic ESRD patients living alone who had an unstable cardiovascular system. In the early 1970s IPD with an automatic peritoneal dialysis cycler providing 40 hours a week of dialysis, divided into two to three sittings, was the recommended scheme of peritoneal dialysis.[6] While on IPD blood sugar control was achieved with insulin administered both subcutaneously and intraperitonealy. The amount of insulin administered was adjusted to individual requirements. During the dialysis days, the patients were given the usual daily dose of insulin by subcutaneous injection and an additional amount of regular insulin was added to the dialysis solution until the last five exchanges of dialysis to cover for the glucose absorbed from the peritoneal cavity during the dialysis solution exchanges. Insulin was omitted from the last few exchanges to prevent postdialysis hypoglycemia. Insulin requirements were determined at the initiation of each patient's first few treatments. The amount of insulin required was directly proportional to the amount of glucose load instilled during dialysis to achieve ultrafiltration. It took up to 2 weeks after initiation of dialysis to determine the exact amount of insulin required by an individual patient. Once established, the insulin requirements did not generally change unless new complications were encountered. In these patients, retinopathy and neuropathy seemed to stabilize during the course of IPD treatment. Hemoglobin and hematocrit were maintained at satisfactory levels without blood transfusions. Compared with nondiabetic patients on IPD, these patients experienced a higher incidence of fibrin-clot formation in dialysis effluent and a higher incidence of peritonitis. The patients also experienced higher rates of arterial calcification and hypertension. The majority of the patients died from cardiac and cerebrovascular complications. Significant percentages of patients died suddenly at home, presumably due to a coronary event or from an electrolyte abnormality. The probability of patient survival at 1 and 2 years was 44 and 20 percent, respectively. Outcomes, of such therapies in centers with smaller numbers of patients were similar.[7-10] The main reason for the low survival rates may be related to inadequate dialysis since this IPD scheme, as advocated in the past, was only efficient enough to maintain symptom-free patients as long as they had small but significant amounts of residual renal function. It is common knowledge that the residual renal function in dialysis patients declines with time. Most patients were presumably underdialyzed and became more uremic with the cessation of residual renal function. Use of IPD has declined since the advent of CAPD in the mid-1970s. However, a variant of IPD (i.e., daily night-time IPD [NIPD] is now used in select patients who are unable to use CAPD.[11] During NIPD, the patient is confined to the bed and may sleep part of the time. In order to match the efficiency of CAPD, NIPD needs to be performed 10 to 12 hours a day using high dialysis flow rates. The total volume of dialysis solution used per treatment ranges from 8 to 20 L. Like IPD, the major benefit of NIPD is the lower incidence of complications related to high intra-abdominal pressure compared with CAPD. Because this is not as practical and is more expensive, NIPD has not been as popular as CAPD.

Tidal peritoneal dialysis (TPD) is a modification of the IPD technique in which only a portion of dialysate is drained after an initial fill of the peritoneal cavity and is replaced by fresh solution with each cycle, leaving the majority of dialysis solution in constant contact with the peritoneal membrane until the end of the dialysis session, when the fluid is drained as completely as possible.[11] Preliminary studies indicate that TPD is approximately 20 percent more efficient than NIPD at a dialysate flow rate of 3.25 to 3.5 L. During an 8-hour TPD session, ultrafiltration generation is higher, protein losses are similar, and phosphate clearances are lower than 24-hour CAPD for an equivalent glucose load.[11] It has been observed that 8- to 10-hour daily TPD regimen may provide adequate dialysis (area clearances and creatinine clearances per day similar to CAPD) to an anuric patient with average to low-average peritoneal membrane transport characteristics. This technique is still in an experimental stage and has the potential to be an alternative to CAPD in diabetic patients.

For all practical purposes, CCPD is a reversal of the CAPD schedule.[12] It uses multiple short cycles during the night with an automated cycler and a long day-time exchange while the patient is ambulatory. The essential parts of this technique consist of variable volumes of dialysis solution delivery for a prescribed dwell time with the aid of an automated cycler (three or four 2-L commercial dialysis solution infusions are generally administered during the night, each dwelling for 2 to 3 hours) and its drainage by gravity at the end of the dwell. An additional 2 L of dialysis solution is infused in the morning and is allowed to dwell intraperitoneally for the next 14 to 15 hours with the catheter capped. Hypertonic dialysis solution containing 2.5 to 4.25 percent dextrose is recommended for the day-time exchange in order to prevent significant absorption of the solution. Diaz-Buxo[12] observed that it is difficult to design a uniform method for intraperitoneal insulin administration for the blood glucose control in the CCPD patient due to the fact that during the day, when most of the dietary caloric load is consumed, there is only one peritoneal dialysis exchange, which remains intraperitoneally for 12 to 14 hours, and essentially no food is eaten during the night, when several dialysis exchanges are made. Nevertheless, Diaz-Buxo[12] claims that excellent glycemic control can be obtained in the majority of patients if time is spent to calculate the precise dose of insulin required and if a regular and predictable caloric intake is maintained wiht little day-to-day variation. He recommends that the insulin dose be appropriately divided among all the dialysis solution bags depending on the caloric load infusion. Such a distribution avoids sudden and massive infusions of insulin and consequent hypoglycemia or hyperglycemia. The average intraperitoneal insulin dose required for good control of glycemia has been approximately three times the predialysis total subcutaneous dose. In most cases, 50 percent of the intraperitoneal dose is used for the long dwell day-time exchange, with the remaining 50 percent equally divided among the nocturnal exchanges. For more detailed instructions, readers are advised to refer to the protocol recommended by Diaz-Buxo.[12] The 1-year patient survival for diabetic patients on CCPD is reported to be 76 percent.[12] The main indications for CCPD in diabetics include patient preference, young diabetics awaiting cadaver or living related renal transplantations, and older, blind, and dependent diabetics requiring partner support for the dialysis technique. The medical circumstances under which CCPD is recommended over CAPD are in those patients who have shown a tendency to develop complications that are related to the increased intra-abdominal pressure. Another group of patients who benefit from CCPD are those who complain of chronic low back pain on CAPD.

Continuous ambulatory peritoneal dialysis has established itself as a viable alternative to hemodialysis in the treatment of diabetic patients with ESRD. The standard CAPD technique has been previously reported.[13] In short, the technique consists of exchanging four 2-L dialysis solution bags per day using appropriate glucose concentration from the range available (0.5, 1.5, 2.5, and 4.25 g/dl) to achieve adequate ultrafiltration. The patients are taught to add insulin into the dialysis solution according to the protocol previously described.[13] The CAPD technique is usually modified to accommodate the handicapped diabetic patient's desire to self-perform dialysis at home. Visual impairment, peripheral vascular disease with amputation of a part of or an entire limb, and peripheral neuropathy with sensory and/or motor function impairment are some of the physical disabilities observed in these diabetic populations. Devices such as the ultraviolet box, [14] splicer,[15] Oreopoulos-Zellerman connector,[16] Y-system,[17] and injecta aid[18] are used with success in many patients. These devices have enabled a number of blind diabetics to self-perform CAPD. Although the published reports of usage of such devices are scarce, the anecdotal experiences of their usefulness are encouraging.

IS GLUCOSE AN IDEAL OSMOTIC AGENT FOR DIABETIC CAPD PATIENTS?

Glucose in an effective osmotic agent for inducing ultrafiltration during peritoneal dialysis. However, use of glucose has been associated with numerous metabolic undesirable effects (Table 10-2) which has led to the search of alternative osmotic agents. An average CAPD patient typically absorbs 100 to 150/dg of glucose during the course of CAPD therapy. This inevitably high amount of carbohydrate absorption presumably leads to undesirable metabolic problems, such as obesity, hypertriglyceridemia, and premature atherosclerosis. In addition, higher doses of insulin required to maintain the blood sugar at normal levels may cause hyperinsulinemia which has been shown in healthy persons to be a risk factor for coronary artery disease.[19,20] To obviate the undesirable metabolic consequences of glucose absorption, efforts have been made in the past to substitute glucose with alternative osmotic agents, such as xylitol,[21] amino acids,[22] gelatin,[23] polyglucose,[24] and glycerol.[25] However, none of the agents tried has been found to have the favorable profile of glucose. Either because of prohibitive cost, or an unacceptable toxicity profile, the use of these agents as osmotic agents has been limited. One to two percent amino-acid mixtures in the dialysis solution have been used effectively to induce ultrafiltration in nondiabetic CAPD patients.[22] Also, the absorbed aminoacids cause significant increases in the total body nitrogen and transferrin, reduce the inevitable glucose load, and lower serum triglyceride levels. Use of such mixtures in diabetic CAPD patients has the potential to reduce many of the undesirable effects of glucose. However, the high cost of amino-acids mixture is the major factor limiting its use. Glycerol-containing dialysis solution has been used successfully in diabetic CAPD patients. This agent was well-tolerated by the patients, was nontoxic to the peritoneal membrane, did not cause hepatotoxicity, and did not increase protein losses in the dialysate.[25] Blood sugar was easily controlled with insulin. Some patients did develop signs and symptoms of hyperosmolality. However, this agent showed no benefits over glucose because it delivered similar amounts of total caloric load and the problem with hyperlipidemia was unaltered. Thus, glucose remains the best osmotic agent for peritoneal dialysis.

To enhance ultrafiltration during peritoneal dialysis, a different approach of great promise is being tried. This approach makes use of non-osmotic

Table 10-2. Drawbacks of Glucose as an Osmotic Agent

Inevitable high amount of glucose absorption from the dialysis solution
Promotes obesity
Exaggerates pre-existing hypertriglyceridemia
Requires more insulin for blood glucose control
Hyperinsulinemia may promote atherosclerosis

agents to influence the ultrafiltration characteristics during the dialysis. Recent animal and human studies have shown that both oral and intraperitoneal administration of phosphatidylcholine,[26,27] a phospholipid surfactant that is normally secreted by the peritoneal mesothelial cells and functions as a membrane lubricant, results in enhanced ultrafiltration during exchanges with equivalent glucose loads. Its use allows the reduction of the amount of glucose load required by CAPD patients during the day to achieve adequate ultrafiltration. Its mechanisms of action is enhancing ultrafiltration are hypothesized to be due both to its surface active property[28] and to its ability to lower peritoneal cavity lymph flow.[27] To be able to achieve adequate ultrafiltration while using lower amounts of glucose as an osmotic load and without substituting an alternate osmotic agent is a very interesting advance, especially for CAPD daibetic patients.

EFFECTS OF INTRAPERITONEAL INSULIN

There are many similarities between the absorption kinetics of intraperitonealy administered insulin and the normal secretion of insulin by the islet cells (Table 10-3). Insulin release in a normal person is a complex coordinated interplay of food absorbed from the gut, gastrointestinal hormones, and other hormonal and neural stimuli. Pancreatic islets secrete insulin into the portal vein, and the liver removes 50 to 60 percent of the insulin presented to it. In the basal state, the portal to peripheral ratio of insulin is 3:1. Following bursts of secretion in response to glucose or amino acids, the portal to peripheral ratio may reach a value of 9:1. The insulin taken up by the liver inhibits hepatic glycogenolysis, gluconeogenesis, and ketogenesis, and facilitates glycogen and fatty acid synthesis.[29] The insulin secretory rate necessary to maintain normal basal concentrations of insulin is in the range of 0.25 to 1.5 U/h.[30] These basal rates of secretion are normally present in the intervals between meal ingestion. The significance of maintaining a basal level of insulin is emphasized by studies showing that programmed insulin infusion systems, which provide insulin in basal as well as premeal doses, are

Table 10-3. Similarities Between Intraperitoneal Insulin Administration and Physiologic Secretion of Insulin by the Islet Cells

Insulin Secretion by the Islet Cells	Intraperitoneal Insulin Administration
Secretion into portal circulation	Uptake by both portal and systemic circulation
Uptake by the liver during the first pass	Significant uptake by the liver during the first pass
Secretion in response to caloric intake	Insulin and glucose absorption occur simultaneously
Basal insulin level is maintained during the night	Basal insulin level can be maintained

far more effective in normalizing blood glucose concentrations in type 1 diabetes than are premeal insulin doses alone.[31] Because of the continuous therapy CAPD allows for maintenance of basal insulin levels in the blood. Insulin administered into the peritoneal cavity is absorbed by diffusion across the visceral peritoneum into the portal venous circulation and directly through the capsule of liver[32]; thus, it simulates physiologic insulin secretion more closely than systemic insulin therapy.[33] Intraperitoneal insulin also reaches the systemic circulation by convective transfer via the peritoneal cavity lymphatics.[34] Studies of insulin kinetics indicate rapid appearance of insulin in the serum after peritoneal instillation and a greater serum level of insulin when larger doses of insulin are instilled.[35,36] However, the amount of glucose required to maintain blood glucose during intraperitoneal insulin instillation decreased with higher insulin amounts, suggesting a plateau in intraperitoneal dose response. This phenomenon may suggest a significant trapping of insulin in the liver during its first pass, as is observed during normal insulin release from islet cells.

The absorption kinetics of intraperitoneal administration of regular insulin favors the control of glycemia throughout the dwell time and is most likely related to maintaining a basal level of insulin; intraperitoneal insulin is absorbed along with the obligatory glucose load from the dialysis solution, and insulin absorption is continuous until the end of the dwell. Peak insulin levels in the serum are observed 30 to 45 minutes after administration into an empty peritoneal cavity,[33] and are delayed until 90 to 120 minutes after administration, when insulin is added to the dialysis solution.[37] Approximately 50 percent of the insulin instilled into the peritoneal cavity is absorbed after an 8-hour dwell time.[38] Because of the similarities between the normal insulin secretion and the intraperitonealy administered insulin, intraperitoneal administration of insulin during CAPD appears to achieve a tighter control of blood sugar compared with other forms of insulin administration.

BLOOD SUGAR CONTROL DURING CONTINUOUS AMBULATORY PERITONEAL DIALYSIS

Insulin responsiveness and a patient's need for insulin depend on the type of diabetes and other variables. Therefore, it is futile to design a single blood sugar control method for peritoneal dialysis. Numerous approaches have been used for blood glucose control during CAPD (Table 10-4). The survey of the United States National Institutes of Health (NIH) CAPD Registry in patients with ESRD attributed to diabetic nephropathy found among five different treatment regimens for blood sugar control during CAPD therapy 499 surveyed patients; 86 percent of the surveyed patients were taking

Table 10-4. Different Methods of Blood Glucose Control During Continuous Ambulatory Peritoneal Dialysis

Intraperitoneal insulin
Subcutaneous insulin
Combination of intraperitoneal and subcutaneous insulin
Oral agents
Oral agents and insulin (intraperitoneal or subcutaneous)
Diet
Diet and oral agents

insulin with no oral agent, two percent were taking insulin with an oral hypoglycemic agent, for percent were on an oral agent only, six percent were on diet therapy alone, and the remaining two percent were on no specific therapy at all. Of the 434 patients taking insulin, 36 percent took subcutaneous injections, 54 percent administered insulin intraperitoneally, and ten percent used both routes for insulin administration. Although there are no studies to show a single regimen of insulin administration to be clearly superior CAPD, because of the similarities between absorption kinetics of normal insulin secretion and intraperitoneally administered insulin, the intraperitoneal route of administration, if feasible, should be the first choice when insulin therapy is indicated in CAPD patients.

Despite great interpatient variation in intraperitoneal insulin requirements of diabetic CAPD patients, the daily intraperitoneal insulin dose in a given patient is usually greater than twice the pre-CAPD daily subcutaneous dose.[38] At the initiation of CAPD, 150 percent of the pre-CAPD or 100 percent of the CAPD daily subcutaneous insulin dose can be safely divided among all four exchanges, with a reduced insulin dose added to the overnight dwell to avoid nocturnal hypoglycemia. Intraperitoneal insulin therapy must be individualized, and review of morning fasting and 2-hour postprandial and pre-exchange blood glucose results from the previous day allows stepwise changes in insulin to be added to each cycle until the desired blood glucose control is achieved. Each peritoneal dialysis exchange with intraperitoneal insulin should be performed before meals to promote peak insulin absorption at the time of food intake in order to minimize meal-related hyperglycemia. Strict aseptic technique using a long needle should be used to add insulin to the dialysis solution through the injection port. If blind diabetics are unable to use an Injecta-aid, a partner or nurse can premix insulin with the dialysis solution for up to 24 hours without any significant insulin adsorption to the plastic bags.[39] Increments of insulin are required for each additional hypertonic dialysis cycle incorporated into the daily routine. Intraperitoneal insulin requirements during episodes of peritonitis are widely believed to be increased, but hypoglycemia has recently been reported when the usual dose of intraperitoneal insulin was continued during peritonitis.[40] Blood glucose during peritonitis is likely to be determined by the relative importance of increased insulin absorption and reduced carbohydrate intake due to anorexia versus increased glucose absorption and the infection-related catabolic state. This emphasizes the need for close follow-up monitoring of blood glucose and subsequent modification of insulin dosage, especially during changes from the patient's routine treatments.

Intraperitoneal insulin therapy has been shown to better reduce the mean glucose level, meal-related hyperglycemia, and daily glucose fluctuations when compared with subcutaneous insulin. In diabetic CAPD patients, such treatment objectives as maintaining morning fasting glucose less than 140 mg/dl, post-meal hyperglycemia less than 200 mg/dl, and hemoglobin A_1C levels less than 9 percent have been achieved with intraperitoneal insulin administration. If care is not exercised, severe fatal hypoglycemia can be encountered with intraperitoneal insulin administration.[13] Insulin injected into the tubing and flushed into the peritoneal cavity with a small volume of dialysis solution reduces the total amount of insulin needed to normalize blood sugar compared with mixing insulin with the dialysis solution before infusion.[41,42] Not all patients can be maintained on intraperitoneal insulin because of individual patient variations, preferences, and insulin-receptor responsiveness. We have observed poor control of blood glucose in two CAPD diabetic patients despite very large doses (over 300 U) of intraperitoneal insulin. Subcutaneous multiple injections of insulin in these patients were effective in lowering blood glucose to acceptable levels. The reason for such refractoriness to intraperitoneal injection of insulin is not clear, but is believed to be due trapping of insulin in the mesenteric or omental lymphatics.[43] There are several published protocols of intraperitoneal insulin administration, with no clear advantage of one over the other.[44]

A wide variety of insulin preparations with relatively rapid action are available for subcutaneous injection. Despite the variety of preparations, their use alone or in combination, even with multiple daily injections, does not in any way reproduce the exquisite physiologic regulation of the blood sugar level observed in nondiabetic patients. This no doubt reflects the absence of finely regulated endogenous insulin secretion. The effectiveness of the subcutaneous injection for blood glucose control during CAPD was recently reported in 33 patients with adequate metabolic control; the glycosylated hemoglobin ranged between 9 and 12.[45]

CLINICAL RESULTS (SHORT-TERM AND LONG-TERM OUTCOMES)

The adequacy of patients on CAPD therapy appears to be good, as evidenced by hemoglobin levels of 8 to 10 g/dl without requiring blood transfusions, steady-state biochemical parameters, and normal blood pressures with or without medication. The 2-year cumulative survival rate on CAPD is significantly better than that achieved by intermittent peritoneal dialysis because of the better weekly solute clearances during CAPD and better control of blood pressure. However, the actuarial patient survivals for diabetics are lower than nondiabetics on CAPD. We previously reported that the 1- and 2-year cumulative survival rates for insulin-dependent diabetics on CAPD were 92 percent and 75 percent, respectively[46]; survival rates in age-matched nondiabetics at 1 and 2 years are reported to be similar. Non-insulin–dependent diabetics had similar cumulative survival rates of 90 percent and 75 percent at 1 and 2 years, respectively. Several centers in North America and Europe have reported similar encouraging short-term cumulative survival rates for diabetics on CAPD.[47–49] The outcome of treatment in non-insulin-dependent diabetics is poorer compared with insulin-dependent diabetics because as a group they are older, usually have severe ischemic heart disease, and generally have other associated medical problems.

During the early years of the use of CAPD, it was feared that long-term CAPD in diabetics was not feasible because of the diffuse microvascular disease. A lower solute and water clearance was predicted for diabetics compared with nondiabetics.[50] In addition, concerns due to membrane injury from high rates of peritonitis led most to predict a short life for the peritoneal membrane. A high dropout from the therapy after a short period was expected. Contrary to the earlier observations, a recent report based on peritoneal equilibration tests in a large group of CAPD patients presented similar peritoneal transport characteristics for both diabetics and nondiabetics.[51] Although experiences with long-term survival of diabetics on CAPD is very limited, diabetic patients who have been successfully managed on CAPD for more than 5 years are being reported.[52,53] Characteristically, the patients who survive longer tend to be free from associated cardiac disease and are nonsmokers. The actuarial survival rate was 44 percent at 5 years (26 patients at risk) in one of the series.[53] The United States CAPD Registry survey reported that of the 7,161 CAPD patients surveyed, 19 percent were on treatment for 3 years or more.[1] These long-term patients included a smaller percentage (18 percent) of patients with diabetes than the short-term cohorts (26 percent). Thus, it is becoming apparent that compared with nondiabetics, diabetic patients on CAPD may have lower technique and patient survival rates. This observation is significant because the average CAPD patient with diabetes is approximately 10 years younger than nondiabetic CAPD patients. However, diabetics tend to have significantly more cardiovascular complications than nondiabetics, which may explain the shorter survivals seen in diabetic CAPD patients. Compared with diabetic patients on hemodialysis, survival may not be very different, but we lack sufficient numbers of patients on long-term CAPD to make a meaningful comparison with hemodialysis. However, compared with nondiabetics on hemodialysis and diabetics after kidney transplant, the outcome of both hemodialysis and peritoneal dialysis in diabetics is poorer, mainly because of the steady progression of the associated cardiovascular complications.

PERITONITIS

Peritonitis related to CAPD is one of the major causes of morbidity in CAPD patients. The clinical manifestations and management of peritonitis in both diabetic and nondiabetic patients are similar. Over a decade of experience of managing diabetics with CAPD has indicated that these patients are not any more prone to infection with unusual microorganisms than nondiabetics.[54] Like nondiabetics, peritonitis in diabetics is caused predominantly by skin bacteria. Approximately 40 percent of bacterial peritonitis is due to *Staphylococcus epidermidis.* While this organism is a weak pathogen, in recent years it has been recognized with increasing frequency to be a cause of wound infections and endocarditis. *Epidermidis* does not produce potent toxins, and pathogenicity depends largely on its ability to initiate a pyogenic process. The clinical illness is usually mild and the disease responds will to antibiotic treatment. Other organisms isolated during episodes of peritonitis include *Staphylococcus aureus, Streptococcus viridans,* gram-negative enteric organisms, and, rarely, anaerobic organisms. A small fraction of peritonitis is caused by fungi. Insulin administration into the dialysis solution bag breaks the sterility of the system and could potentially contaminate the peritoneal cavity and cause peritonitis. However, clinical experience has shown that this is not a significant problem, The incidence of peritonitis in diabetics is not any different than that in nondiabetics on CAPD.[55] The U.S. NIH CAPD Registry surveyed peritonitis rates per patient-year by route of insulin administration and type of diabetes management.[1] Although the differences in the rates were not large, diabetics never using insulin had the highest rate of peritontis per patient-year (1.31), while patients using a combination of subcutaneous and intraperitoneal insulin experineced the lowest rate (0.93). The peritonitis rate per patient-year for patients using subcutaneously administered insulin (1.03) was similar to the rate reported for patients using intraperitoneal insulin (1.06). Blind patients using subcutaneously administered insulin versus blind patients using intraperitoneal insulin reported similar rates of peritonitis. The reason for relatively low peritonitis rates in patients using insulin is unclear; it has been suggested that insulin may have a bacteriocidal effect. The recent trend has been to use devices meant to facilitate exchange procedures or protect against peritoneal contamination, especially the Y-set system, the introduction of which has significantly lowered the incidence of peritonitis.[56]

Treatment of CAPD-related peritonitis, including the right selection of antibiotics and duration of treatment, the appropriate time for catheter removal, etc., is the same for diabetic and nondiabetic patients. Due to the enhanced absorption of glucose during peritonitis, hyperglycemia is observed frequently in diabetics, and insulin requirements may increase. However, some patients may experience hypoglycemia if they are unable to eat, and insulin administration is continued at the same dosage used before peritonitis. Close monitoring of blood glucose during the episode of peritonitis is essential to prevent either hypoglycemia or hyperglycemia. Due to increased protein losses during peritonitis, the patient's nutrition must be closely monitored during the acute phase, and parenteral nutrition should be considered in some patients. The outcome of peritonitis treatment is good generally. Most patients continue on CAPD after the peritonitis is cured. A small percentage (2 to 5 percent) will drop out of the CAPD program for a variety of reasons, including loss of membrane efficiency.

TECHNIQUE-RELATED COMPLICATIONS

Complications that are a direct result of increased intra-abdominal pressure, such as dialysate leaks, hernias, hemorrhoids, and a compromised cardiac pulmonary status, occur with the same frequency in diabetic and nondiabetic patients. As previously discussed peritoneal membrane function as assessed by the serum chemistries, in the absence of severe prolonged peritonitis, usually remains stable over many years. Transient loss of ultrafiltration during an episode of peritonitis is frequent, but full recovery is expected 1 to 2 weeks after successful treatment. Irreversible loss of ultrafiltration (as in nondiabetics) may occur in diabetic CAPD patients as a sequela of severe peritonitis or due to sclerosing peritonitis.[57–59] Although the exact etiology of sclerosing peritonitis has not been established, its occurrence (most prevalent in Europe) has been almost eliminated since the discontinuation of acetate in the dialysis solution.

Loss of proteins, amino acids, polypeptides, and vitamins in the dialysate contribute to the morbidity and slow rehabilitation of diabetic patients on CAPD. Such losses pose a special problem in those diabetics who may be wasted and malnourished because of poor food intake, vomiting, catabolic stresses, and intercurrent illness. Twenty-four hours of amino acid loss in the dialysate averages approximately 2.25g, with approximately 8 g/d of total proteins. In uncomplicated cases, dialysate daily protein losses correlate with serum protein concentration and body surface area. During peritonitis, the protein losses are excessive, and in association with inadequate food intake due to poor appetite or inability to eat, may produce severe hypoproteinemia, hypoalbuminemia, and hypoimmunoglobulinemia. Therefore, during peritonitis episodes that appear to be responding poorly, physicians should consider early parenteral nutrition.

Continuous absorption of glucose during CAPD may aggravate the preexisting hypertriglyceridemia which is frequently seen in both dialyzed and nondialyzed uremics.[60,61] Uremics have concentrations of high-density lipoproteins significantly lower than normal.[62] It has been observed that high-density lipoproteins are being lost in the dialysate during CAPD.[63] Obesity appears to occur in those who are premorbidly obese.

Most insulin-dependent diabetics have irreversible retinal lesions before they start dialysis, especially during the terminal phase of renal failure when hypertension tends to be severe. By the time the majority reach the stage of dialysis, ocular lesions ar far too advanced to expect any useful recovery. The common lesions seen at the time of initiating CAPD are background retinopathy, proliferative retinopathy, and vitreous hemorrhage. Retinal detachment may also be seen in some cases. Therefore, better preservation of ocular function depends on the more aggressive approach to blood pressure and glucose control during the predialysis phase. Retinal ischemia may be made worse by the rapid fluctuations in the intervascular volume during intermittent dialysis therapies. CAPD avoids many of the problems inherent in the intermittent forms of dialysis. To preserve a useful visual function, some patients may require vitrectomy. Stabilization or even improvement of ocular function in diabetic patients maintained on CAPD has been reported by several centers.[18,46,66-66]

Morbidity and mortality due to atherosclerotic heart disease and micro angiopathy remain the main cause of death among diabetics undergoing peritoneal dialysis. Small-vessel disease leading to ischemic gangrene of the extremties is a common eomplication of type I diabetes. Short-term experiences with CAPD in diabetics do not suggest that ischemic complications occur any more frequently in diabetics than in nondiabetic patients. In the only long-term experience reported, Zimmermann et al.[53] state that the incidence of ischemic and/or gangrenous complication was extremely low. The keys to preserving adequate circulation to the extremities include avoidance of smoking and hypotensive episodes and the maintainance of lipid regulation.

Blood pressure control during CAPD is relatively easy. In the majority of hypertensive patients, blood pressure normalizes within 6 months of initiating CAPD. [41,42,46] However, associated autonomic neuropathy with orthostatic hypotension makes blood pressure regulation extremely difficult in some patients because of intensified crippling orthostatic symptoms. Measures such as wearing elastic stockings during upright posture, maintaining a degree of overhydration, and administering salt tablets, mineralocorticoid, clonidine, or metaclopropamide singly or in combination may improve the patients symptoms.

Because of the numerous complications primarily due to diabetes, diabetic patients on CAPD tend to have increased morbidity and require more frequent hospitalization than nondiabetic patients. For type I and type II diabetics, the rate of hospitalization (33 days per patient-year of treatment) appears to be similar. Hospitalization due to causes directly related to the CAPD technique are decreasing. The rate of hospitalization for diabetics on CAPD is comparable to diabetics on hemodialysis.

Theoretically, CAPD may be associated with steady glomerular capillary pressure in the remaining functioning glomeruli without any fluctuations to high or low levels. This feature of CAPD may have a protective effect on a patient's residual renal function. A prospective study compared endogenous creatinine clearances in diabetic patients on CAPD and hemodialysis at the initiation of therapy, then serially over a period of 2 years.[42] There was a greater decline in the residual function in patients on hemodialysis (80 percent) compared with CAPD patients (25 percent). Another cross-sectional comparison study[67] of residual renal function in CAPD and hemodialysis patients found higher (2 ml/min) endogenous creatinine clearance in CAPD patients compared with hemodialysis patients (0.7 ml/min). If this observation is found to be a true phenomenon, one may theoretically recommend CAPD for the preservation of residual renal function. Preserving the residual renal function has clinical implications for the dialysis prescription and fluid, sodium, and potassium balance during dialysis treatment.

In summary, it is becoming apparent that with the proper selection of patients, diabetic patients can survive for long periods on CAPD. The morbidity and mortality observed on CAPD therapy is primarily related to associated risk factors, such as cardiovascular disease, atherosclerotic complications, and infection. The ability to administer intraperitoneal insulin during CAPD enables the simulation of normal insulin secretion by the islet cells. Patients on CAPD tend to retain residual renal function for a longer period of time. The incidence of peritonitis is decreasing, and this change may effect the CAPD drop-out rates.

REFERENCES

1. Lindblad AS, Novak JW, Nolph KD, et al: Final report of the National CAPD Registry. p 640. National Institute of Diabetes and Digestive and Kidney Diseases, Bethesda, 1988
2. Tenchkoff H, Schechter H: A bacteriologically safe peritoneal access device. Trans Am Soc Artif Internal Organs 14:181, 1968
3. Khanna R, Twardowski ZJ: Peritoneal dialysis access. p. 319. In Nolph KD (ed): Peritoneal Dialysis. Kluwer Academic Publishers, Dordrecht, The Netherlands, 1989
4. Ponce SP, Pierratos A, Izatt S, et al: Comparison of the survival and complications of three permanent peritoneal dialysis catheters. Peritoneal Dialysis Bull 2:82, 1982
5. Boen, ST, Mulinari AS, Dillard DH, Scribner BH: Periodic peritoneal dialysis in the management of chronic uremia. Trans Am Soc Artif Internal Organs 8:256, 1962
6. Katirtzoglou A, Izatt S, Oreopoulos DG: Chronic peritoneal dialysis in diabetics with end-stage renal failure. p. 317. In Friedman EA (ed): Diabetic Renal-Retinal Syndrome. Grune & Stratton, Orlando, FL, 1982
7. Blumenkrantz MJ, Shapiro DJ, Minura N, et al: Maintenance peritoneal dialysis as an alternative in the patients wiht diabetes mellitus and end-stage uremia. Kidney Int: 6 (suppl 1), S108, 1974
8. Quelhorst E, Schuenemann B, Mietzsch G, Jacob I: Hemo and peritoneal dialysis treatment of patients with diabetic nephropathy. A comparative study. Proc Eur Dialysis Transplant Assoc 15:205, 1978
9. Mion C, Slingeneyer A, Salem JL, et al: Home peritoneal dialysis in end stage diabetic nephropathy. J Dialysis 2:426, 1978
10. Warden GS, Maxwell JG, Stephen RL: The use of reciprocating peritoneal dialy-

sis with a subcutaneous peritoneal dialysis in end stage renal failure in dialbetes mellitus. J Surg Res 24:495, 1978

11. Twardowski ZJ: New approaches to peritoneal dialysis. p. 133. In Nolph KD (ed): Peritoneal Dialysis. Kluwer Academic Publishers, Dordrecht, The Netherlands, 1989

12. Diaz-Buxo JA: Continuous cyclic peritoneal dialysis. p. 169. In Nolph KD (ed): Peritoneal Dialysis. Kluwer Academic Publishers, Dordrecht, The Netherlands, 1989

13. Amair, P, Khanna R, Leibel B, et al: Continuous ambulatory peritoneal dialysis in diabetics with end-stage renal disease. N Eng J Med 306:625, 1982

14. Perras ST, Zappacosta AR: Reduction of peritonitis with patients' education and Travenol CAPD germicidal exchange system. Am Nephrol Nurses Assoc 13:219, 1986

15. Hamilton RW: The sterile connection device: a review of its development and status report—1986. p. 186 In Khanna R, Nolph KD, Prowant BF, et al (eds): Advances in Continuous Ambulatory Peritoneal Dialysis. Peritoneal Dialysis Bulletin, Toronto, 1986

16. Fenton SSA, Wu G, Bowman C, et al: The reduction in the peritonitis rate among high-risk CAPD patients with the use of the Oreopoulos-Zellerman connector. Trans Am Soc Artif Internal Organs 31:560, 1985

17. Buoncristiani U, Quintalinani G, Cozzari M, Carobi C: Current status of the Y-set. p. 165. In Khanna R, Nolph KD, Prowant BF, et al (eds): Advances in Continuous Ambulatory Peritoneal Dialysis. Peritoneal Dialysis Bulletin, Toronto, 1986

18. Flynn CT: The diabetics on CAPD. p. 321. In Friedman EA (ed): Diabetic Renal-Retinal Syndrome. Grune & Stratton, Orlando, Fl, 1982

19. Stout RW: Diabetes and atherosclerosis—the role of insulin. Diabetologia 16:141, 1979

20. Zavaroni A, Bonora E, Pagliara M, et al: Risk factor coronary artery disease in healthy persons with hyperinsulinemia and normal glucose tolerance. N Engl J Med 320:702, 1989

21. Bazzato G, Coli U, Landini S: Zylitol and low doses of insulin: new perspectives for diabetic uremic patients on CAPD. Peritoneal Dialysis Bull 2:161, 1982

22. Williams FP, Marliss EB, Anderson GH, et al: Amino acid absorption following intraperitoneal administration in CAPD patients. Peritoneal Dialysis Bull 2:124, 1982

23. Twardowski ZJ, Khanna R Nolph KD: Osmotic agents and utrafiltration in peritoneal dialysis. Nephron 42:93, 1986

24. The use of large molecular weight glucose polymer as an osmotic agent in CAPD. p. 7. In Khanna R, Nolph KD, Prowant B, et al (eds): Advances in Continuous Ambulatory Peritoneal Dialysis. Peritoneal Dialysis Bulletin, Toronto, 1986

25. Matthys E, Dolkart R, Lameire N: Extended use of a glycerol containing dialysate in the treatment of diabetic CAPD patients. Peritoneal Dialysis Bull 7:10, 1987

26. Di paolo N, Buoncristiani U, Capotondo L: Phosphatisylcholine and peritoneal transport during peritoneal dialysis. Nephron 44:365, 1986

27. Mactier RA, Khanna R, Twardowski ZJ, et al: Influence of phosphatidylcholine on lymphatic absorption during peritoneal dialysis in rat. Peritoneal Dialysis Int 8:179, 1988

28. Breborowicz A, Somblos K, Rodela H, et al: Mechanism of phosphatidylcholine action during peritoneal dialysis. Peritoneal Dialysis Int 7:6, 1987

29. Felig P, Wahren J: The liver as site of insulin and glucagon action in normal, diabetic and obese humans. Israel J Med Sci 11:528, 1975

30. Shafrir E, Bergman M, Felig P: Diabetes mellitus. p. 1043. In Felig P, Baxter JD, Broadus AE, et al (eds): Endocrinology and Metabolism. McGraw-Hill, New York, 1987

31. Tamborlane WV, Sherwin RS, Genel M, Felig P: Reduction to normal of plasma glucose in juvenile diabetes by subcutaneous administration of insulin with a protable pump. N Eng J Med 300: 573, 1979

32. Greenwood RH, Davies CJ, Senator GB, et al: The transport of peptide hormones across the peritoneal membrane in man. Clin Sci 57:28, 1979

33. Schade DS, Eaton RP: The peritoneum—a potential insulin delivery route for a mechanical pancreas. Diabetes Care 3:229, 1980

34. Rasio EA, Hampers CL, Soeldner JS, Cahill GF: Diffusion of glucose, insulin, insulin and Evans blue protein into thoracic duct lymph of man. J Clin Invest 46:903, 1967

35. Rubin J, Reed V, Adair C, et al: Effect of intraperitoneal insulin on solute kinetics in CAPD: insulin kinetics in CAPD. Am J Med Sci 291:81, 1986

36. Rubin J, Bell AH, Andrews M, et al: Intraperitoneal insulin-Adose response curve. Trans Am Soc Artif Internal Organs 35:17, 1989

37. Shapiro DJ, Blumenkrantz MJ, Levin SR, Coburn W: Absorption and action of insulin added to peritoneal dialysate in dogs. Nephron 23:174, 1979

38. Wideroe T, Smeby LC, Berg KJ, et al: Intraperitoneal insulin absorption during intermittent and continuous peritoneal dialysis. Kidney Int 23:22, 1983

39. Twardowski ZJ, Nolph KD, McGary TJ, Moore HL: Influence of temperature and time on insulin absorption to plastic bags. Am J Hosp Pharmacy 40:583, 1983

40. Henderson IS, Patterson KR, Leung ACT: Decreased intraperitoneal insulin requirements during peritonitis on continuous ambulatory peritoneal dialysis. Br Med J 290:1474, 1985

41. Rottembourg J, El Shahat Y, Agrafiotis A, et al: Continuous ambulatory peritoneal dialysis in insulin dependent diabetics: 40 months experience. Kidney Int 23:40, 1983

42. Rottembourg J, Issad B, Poignet JL, et al: Residual renal function and control of blood glucose levels in insulin-dependent diabetic patients treated by CAPD. p. 339. In Keen H, Legrain M (eds): Prevention and Treatment of Diabetic Nephropathy. MTP Press Ltd, Boston, 1983

43. Harrison NA, Rainford DJ: Intraperitoneal insulin and the malignant omentum syndrome. Nephrol Dial Transplant 3:103, 1988

44. Roscoe JM: Practices of insulin administration. Peritoneal Dialysis Bull 2:S27, 1982

45. Tzamaloukas AH, Rogers K, Ferguson BJ, et al: Management of diabetics on CAPD with subcutaneous insulin. p. 126. In Khanna, R, Nolph KD, Prowant BF, et al (eds): Advances in Peritoneal Dialysis. Peritoneal Dialysis Bulletin, Toronto, 1988

46. Khanna R, Wu G, Prowant B, et al: CAPD in diabetics with ESRD: a combined experience of two North American centers. p. 363. In Friedman EA, L'Esperance FA, Jr. (eds): Diabetic Renal-Retinal Syndrome. Grune & Stratton, Orlando Fl, 1986

47. Madden MA, Zimmerman SW, Simpson DP: CAPD in diabetes mellitus—the risks and benefits of intraperitoneal insulin. Am J Nephrol 2:133, 1982

48. Wing AF, Broyer M, Brunner FP, et al: Combined report on regular dialysis and transplantation in Eurpoe 1982. Proc Eur Dialysis Transplant Assoc ERA, 20:5, 1983

49. Williams C, University of Toronto Collaborative Dialysis Group: CAPD in Toronto—an overview. Peritoneal Dialysis Bull 35:2, 1983

50. Nolph KD, Stoltz M, Maher JF: Altered peritoneal permeability in patients with systemic vasculitis. Ann Intern Med 78:891, 1973

51. Twardowski ZJ, Nolph KD, Khanna R, et al: Peritoneal equilibration test. Peritoneal Dialysis Bull 7:138, 1987

52. Gilmore J, Wu G, Khanna R, Oreopoulos DG: Long term CAPD Peritoneal Dialysis Bull 5:112, 1985

53. Zimmerman SW, Johnson CA, O'Brien M: Survival of diabetic patients on continuous ambulatory peritoneal dialysis for over five years. Peritoneal Dialysis Bull 7:26, 1987

54. Vas SI: Peritonitis. p. 261. In Nolph KD (ed): Peritoneal Dialysis. Kluwer Academic Publishers, Dordrecht, The Netherlands, 1989

55. Nolph KD, Cutler SJ, Steinberg SM, et al: Special studies from the NIH USA CAPD Registry. Peritoneal Dialysis Bull 6:28, 1986

56. Rottembourg J, Brouard R, Issad B, et al: Prospective randomized study about Y connectors in CAPD patients. p 107. Khanna R, Nolph KD, Prowant, BF, (eds): Advances in Continuous Ambulatory Peritoneal Dialysis. Peritoneal Dialysis Bulletin, Toronto, 1987

57. Faller B, Marichal JD: Loss of ultrafiltration in CAPD. Clinical Data. p. 227. In Gahl G, Kessel M, Nolph KD (eds): Advances in Peritoneal Dialysis. Excerpta Medica, Amsterdam, 1981

58. Slingeneyer A, Mion C, Mourad G, et al: Progressive sclerozing peritonitis: a late and severe complication of maintenance peritoneal dialysis. Transactions Am Soc Artif Internal Organs 29:633, 1983

59. Rottembourg J, Brouard R, Issad B, et al: Role of acetate in loss of ultrafiltration during CAPD. p. 197. In Berlyne GM, Giovannetti S (eds): Contribution to Nephrology. S. Karger AG, Basel, 1987

60. Norbeck H: Lipid abnormalities in CAPD patients. p. 298. In Legrain M (ed): Continuous Ambulatory Peritoneal Dialysis. Excerpta Medica, Amsterdam, 1979

61. Khanna R, Brechenridge C, Roncari D, et al: Lipid abnormalities in patients undergoing continuous ambulatory peritoneal dialysis. Peritoneal Dialysis Bull 3:13, 1983

62. Norbeck H, Oro L, Carlson LA: Serum lipid and lipoprotein concentrations in chronic uremia. Acta Med Scand 200:487, 1976

63. Kagan A, Barkhayim Y, Schafer Z, Fainaru M: Low level of plasma HDL in CAPD patients may be due to HDL loss in dialysate. Peritoneal Dialysis Int 8:82, 1988 (abstr.)

64. Diaz-Buxo JA, Burgess WP, Greenman M, et al: Visual function in diabetic patients undergoing dialysis: comparison of peritoneal and hemodialysis. Int J Artif Organs 7:257, 1984

65. Kohner E, Chahal P: Retinopathy in diabetic nephropathy. p. 191. In Keen H, Legrain M (eds): Prevention and Treatment of Diabetic Nephropathy. MTP Press, Hingham, MA 1984

66. Rottembourg J, Bellio P, Maiga K, et al: Visual function, blood pressure and blood glucose in diabetic patients undergoing continuous ambulatory peritoneal dialysis. Proc Eur Transplant Assoc 21:330, 1984

67. Lysaght M, Pollock C, Schindaglm K, et al: The relevance of urea kinetic modeling to CAPD. Abstracts, ASAIO, 34:84, 1988

11

Pediatric CAPD/CCPD in the United States

A Review of the Experiences of the National CAPD Registry's Pediatric Patient Population for the Period of January 1, 1981 to August 31, 1986[*]

Steven R. Alexander
Anne S. Lindblad
Karl D. Nolph
Joel W. Novak

---

[*]The data contained in this chapter were presented in part at the 8th National CAPD Conference, Kansas City, MO, February 1988.

Anthropometric Data and Growth
Sexual Maturation
Termination of Continuous Ambulatory Peritoneal Dialysis/Continuous
Cyclic Peritoneal Dialysis

DISCUSSION

ACKNOWLEDGMENTS

INTRODUCTION

Continuous ambulatory peritoneal dialysis (CAPD) was first used to treat pediatric patients with end-stage renal disease (ESRD) as early as 1978,[1,2] but widespread use of CAPD in children in the United States did not begin until the summer of 1980, when dialysate in small plastic containers first became commercially available in this country.[3] By the end of 1986, CAPD and its mechanized cousin, continuous cycling peritoneal dialysis (CCPD), had both become popular therapies for children in dialysis programs throughout North America. The National CAPD Registry of the United States National Institutes of Health (NIH) began enrolling patients in 1981; by March 1982, the Registry contained data on 256 pediatric patients (aged less than 21 years at the time of registration), representing 5.3 percent of the Registry's population.[4] By August 31, 1986, the number of pediatric patients had increased to 962, accounting for 5.7 percent of the Registry's total population.[5]

The experiences of pediatric patients as a subgroup within the total CAPD Registry were first examined in a preliminary analysis of pediatric patient data contained in the January 1986 National CAPD Registry report.[6] The results of that analysis suggested that pediatric patients did not fare as well as adult patients, incurring increased risks for peritonitis, early hospitalization, and death while on CAPD/CCPD. However, small sample sizes precluded analysis by age group subcategories and weakened statistical inferences, and there was concern that specialized pediatric clinical centers and patients treated by pediatric nephrologists might have been underrepresented in the largely adult Registry. The large number of pediatric patients currently available for study provides an opportunity to perform a more complete analysis of the Registry's pediatric population.

In this chapter, we will first review data prospectively collected by the National CAPD Registry on a cohort of 658 pediatric patients enrolled between January 1, 1981, and August 31, 1986. We will also present the results of a retrospective special study, involving 485 of these patients, which was conducted during the latter half of 1986. Much of the data reported here may also be found in the 1987 report of the National CAPD Registry.[5] We have refined and expanded the data analyses contained in that 1987 report in an effort to provide a picture as complete as currently possible of the characteristics and experiences of a large number of children treated with CAPD/CCPD in the United States through the summer of 1986.

SUBJECTS AND METHODS

As of August 31, 1986 the National CAPD Registry contained data on 658 patients who were less than 21 years of age at the time of CAPD/CCPD initiation and who had had no prior CAPD/CCPD experience before being enrolled in the Registry. Another 304 patients who met age criteria were excluded from the analysis because of prior CAPD/CCPD experience at the time of enrollment or because of the absence of follow-up data after enrollment. Data on selected patient characteristics and on complications and outcomes of therapy were analyzed for the 658 study patients as a whole and by age group category. Age groups were assigned according to age of patients at first CAPD/CCPD exchange, as follows: less than 1 year, 1 to 4 years, 5 to 9 years, 10 to 14 years, and 15 to 20 years. Differences in patient characteristics among the age groups were tested using the χ^2 statistic.

Complication rates per patient-year were calculated using standard epidemiologic techniques. Probability distributions for various complications and outcomes were estimated using the methods of Kaplan and Meier,[7] and covariate contributions were assessed using Cox's proportional hazards model.[8] Data from the 658 pediatric patients were compared with data from 11,834 adult Registry patients (aged more than 21 years at first exchange; no prior CAPD/CCPD experience).

Additional information not routinely collected by the Registry was obtained on a large sample of pediatric Registry patients as part of a retrospective special study conducted during the last 6 months of 1986. To be eligible for the special study, patients had to have been less than 21 years of age at initiation of CAPD/CCPD, had to have had no prior CAPD/CCPD experience at time of registration, and had to have begun CAPD/CCPD after January 1, 1981 and before September 1, 1985. Questionnaires were distributed for all of the 485 patients who met eligibility criteria, and information was abstracted from hospital and clinic records by center personnel. Three hundred twenty (66 percent) of the 485 distributed questionnaires were completed: those 320 patients formed the cohort of the pediatric special study.

The special study requested data on primary renal disease diagnosis, selected anthropometric measures, sexual maturation, school attendance, the level of involvement of a pediatric nephrologist in the care of the patient, and the reasons for discontinuation of CAPD/CCPD. The requested anthropometric data included height, weight, triceps skinfold thickness, midarm circumference, and head circumference (for children less than 3 years of age) recorded at initiation of CAPD/CCPD and on completion of 12 months of uninterrupted peritoneal dialysis. Only children who were less than 19 years of age at initiation of CAPD/CCPD were included in the anthropometric data analysis.

Measurements of height and weight were compared with the 50th percentile values for normal American children of comparable chronologic age and sex[9] and were expressed as Z scores calculated in the usual manner[10]:

$$Z \text{ score} = \frac{(\text{individual measurement}) - (\text{50th percentile normal})}{1 \text{ standard deviation from 50th percentile normal}}$$

Baseline and 1-year Z scores as well as paired differences were tested using the t test. The changes in Z scores for height and weight over 1 year of observation (the 1-year "Δ Z score") were calculated for each patient. Growth was assessed by evaluating the observed change in Z scores over time. Negative values for Δ Z scores reflect subnormal growth; positive Δ Z scores reflect above-normal growth (i.e., "catch-up growth"). The Kruskal-Wallis test was used to identify differences in mean Δ Z scores between age groups.[11]

Measurements of head circumference, midarm circumference, and triceps skinfold thickness at baseline and after 1 year of CAPD/CCPD were compared with normal 50th percentile values for American children of comparable chronologic age and sex.[9,12] Clinics were asked to assess sexual maturation using the puberty staging methods of Marshall and Tanner.[13,14] Onset of puberty was defined as occurring when Tanner stage 2 was reached in pubic hair or genital development.

RESULTS OF THE PROSPECTIVE ANALYSIS

Selected Patient Characteristics

Patient characteristics by age group are presented in Table 11-1. Pediatric patients were more likely than adult patients to be treated with CCPD or a combination of CAPD and CCPD than with CAPD alone ($P < .001$). Males predominated in the younger age groups (aged less than 10 years), while females accounted for more of the patients 15 to 20 years of age ($P < .01$). White patients made up 72 percent of pediatric patients compared with 77 percent of adults ($P < .01$). Five percent of patients followed by the Registry (35 of 658) had begun CAPD/CCPD during the first year of life. Fifty percent of patients received other forms of renal replacement therapy (e.g., hemodialysis, intermittent peritoneal dialysis, or primary renal transplantation) before beginning CAPD/CCPD. However, 74 percent of patients less than 1 year of age were placed on CAPD/CCPD as their first therapy for ESRD.

Complications

Complication rates per patient-year and the probability of experiencing a first event by 1 year of therapy are presented in Table 11-2. Episodes or events per patient-year of peritonitis (1.5 per patient-year), exit site and tunnel infections (0.8 per patient-year), and catheter replacement (0.4 per patient-year) were slightly higher for children compared with adults. The probabilities of a pediatric patient experiencing a first episode of peritonitis or exit site and tunnel infection at 1 year were 65 percent and 40 percent, respectively, which were higher than the comparable probabilities for the adult cohort of 59 percent and 30 percent, respectively. The probability of having at least one catheter replaced within the first year of treatment for pediatric patients was almost twice that for adults (30 percent versus 18 percent, respectively).

Estimates of total days hospitalized per patient-year and days hospitalized

Table 11-1. Selected Patient Characteristics

| Characteristic | Age (yr) at First CAPD/CCPD Exchange | | | | | Total Registry, Pediatrics (n = 658) | Total Registry, Adults, (n = 11,834) |
	<1 (n = 35)	1–4 (n = 77)	5–9 (n = 115)	10–14 (n = 191)	15–20 (n = 240)		
CAPD only (%)	83	80	80	82	89	89	95
Male (%)	63	61	58	52	43	52	55
White (%)	66	73	77	70	71	72	77
Prior ESRD therapy (%)	26	36	38	55	59	50	56

Table 11-2. Complication Rates[a] and 1-Year Probabilities of First Event (95% CI) by Age at CAPD/CCPD Initiation

Age Group (yr)	N	Peritonitis		Exit Site and Tunnel Infections		Catheter Replacement	
		Rate	Probability (CI)	Rate	Probability (CI)	Rate	Probability (CI)
<1	35	1.7	.63 (.37,.83)	.3	.24 (.9,.51)	.4	.22 (.8,.48)
1–4	77	1.5	.59 (.39,.77)	.7	.30 (.17,.49)	.7	.20 (.5,.53)
5–9	115	1.4	.61 (.55,.74)	.7	.43 (.28,.59)	.4	.42 (.25,.56)
10–14	191	1.6	.67 (.57,.77)	.8	.41 (.30,.54)	.4	.24 (.14,.38)
15–20	240	1.4	.67 (.57,.75)	.9	.42 (.33,.51)	.4	.24 (.25,.45)
Total Registry, pediatrics	658	1.5	.65 (.59,.70)	.8	.40 (.34,.46)	.4	.30 (.24,.35)
Total Registry, adults	11,834	1.3	.59 (.57,.60)	.6	.30 (.29,.32)	.3	.18 (.17,.19)

[a] Episodes and events per patient-year.
Abbreviation: CI, confidence interval.

for CAPD/CCPD-related causes are shown by age group in Fig. 11-1. Note that the lowest rates were reported for patients in the 15 to 20-year-old age group. This cohort was estimated to have been hospitalized for a total of 16.1 days per patient-year for all causes and 6.5 days per patient-year for CAPD/CCPD-related causes. Overall, pediatric patients were estimated to have been hospitalized for 21.3 days per patient-year, 9.2 days of which were for CAPD/CCPD-related causes.

Death, Transplantation, and Transfer to Another Modality

Probabilities of terminating CAPD/CCPD due to death, transfer to another dialysis modality, or transplantation are shown in Table 11-3. The probability of dying while on CAPD/CCPD at 1 year was substantially lower for pediatric patients when compared with adults (6 percent versus 17 percent, respectively). However, the highest 1-year death probability (22 percent) was observed among infants who began CAPD/CCPD during the first year of life. The small sample size in this age group resulted in a large, 95 percent confidence interval width.

The important role of transplantation in the care of children treated with peritoneal dialysis in the United States is also reflected in the data shown in

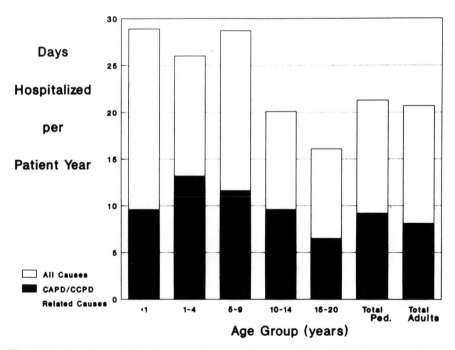

Fig. 11-1. Days hospitalized per patient-year by age at first CAPD/CCPD exchange for all causes and for CAPD/CCPD-related causes.

Table 11-3. 1-Year Outcome Probabilities (95% CI) by Age at First CAPD/CCPD Exchange

| Outcome | Age Group (yr) | | | | | | Total Registry, Pediatrics (n = 658) | Total Registry, Adults (n = 11,834) |
	<1 (n = 35)	1–4 (n = 77)	5–9 (n = 115)	10–14 (n = 191)	15–20 (n = 240)			
Death while on CAPD/CCPD	.22 (.06, .52)	.12 (.05, .28)	.06 (.01, .32)	.03 (.01, .07)	.03 (.01, .10)		.06 (.04, .10)	.17 (.16, .18)
Transfer to hemodialysis, intermittent peritoneal dialysis, or off dialysis	.05 (.01, .42)	.12 (.03, .33)	.09 (.04, .20)	.16 (.10, .25)	.24 (.16, .29)		.16 (.13, .21)	.20 (.19, .21)
Transplantation	.17 (.06, .39)	.27 (.16, .42)	.31 (.21, .43)	.32 (.24, .42)	.23 (.17, .29)		.27 (.23, .32)	.09 (.08, .10)

Abbreviation: CI, confidence interval.

Table 11-3. The probability that a pediatric patient will have received a kidney transplant by the end of 1 year of CAPD/CCPD was 27 percent overall. Even very young infants, less than 1 year of age at initiation of CAPD/CCPD, had a 17 percent probability of receiving a transplant during the first year of peritoneal dialysis.

Pediatric patients had a lower 1-year probability of transfer either to an alternative dialysis modality or off dialysis as compared with adults (16 percent versus 20 percent; see Table 11-3), but this difference was not statistically significant. Younger children (less than 10 years of age) had a significantly lower probability of transferring to another dialysis modality or off dialysis when compared with older children (10 to 20 years of age) or with adults ($P = 0.02$).

Considering transplanted patients as "lost to follow-up" and patient death or transfer to another dialysis modality as "technique failures," a 12-month actuarial technique survival rate of 81 percent was calculated for the entire pediatric patient cohort. When only patients who began CAPD/CCPD before the age of 15 were included in these calculations, a 12-month actuarial technique survival rate of 87 percent was obtained.

Complications and Outcome Measures as a Function of Center Pediatric Experience

One hundred seventy of the participating centers that joined the Registry before December 1, 1985, had registered at least one pediatric patient by August 31, 1986. The distribution of the 658 pediatric patients among these 170 centers is displayed in Fig. 11-2. Ninety-one percent of 170 centers registered fewer than 11 pediatric patients (Fig. 11-2a), accounting for 58 percent of the Registry's pediatric population (Fig 11-2b). Twenty-seven percent of the pediatric population was being followed in the seven centers that had registered more than 20 pediatric patients (Fig. 11-2b). Using a Cox proportional hazards model, a reduced risk of developing first peritonitis was found for children treated at centers that had registered more than 10 pediatric patients (relative risk = .80). That risk was even lower for patients treated at the most experienced pediatric centers (more than 20 pediatric patients; relative risk = .68). Differences in pediatric experience did not affect the probabilities of exit site and tunnel infections, catheter replacements, death, transfer, or transplantation.

RESULTS OF THE SPECIAL STUDY

Primary Renal Disease

Table 11-4 summarizes primary renal disease diagnoses reported for 273 of the 320 patients included in the study. Primary disease type frequencies were widely distributed over the 29 categories offered on the questionnaire;

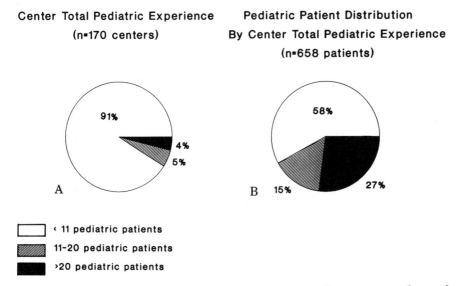

Fig. 11-2. Pediatric CAPD/CCPD patient distribution.(**A**) Centers grouped according to center total pediatric experience. (n = 170 centers.) (**B**) Pediatric patient distribution by center total pediatric experience. (n = 658 patients.)

Table 11-4. Primary Renal Disease Diagnosis

Disease Type	Percent (n = 273)
Aplastic/hypoplastic/dysplastic kidney(s)	15
Chronic glomerulonephritis	12
Focal glomerulosclerosis	9
Pyelonephritis/interstitial nephritis due to congenital obstructive uropathy with or without vesico-ureteric reflux	6
Obstructive uropathy	5
Rapidly progressive glomerulonephritis	5
Hemolytic uremic syndrome	4
Systemic immunologic disease with renal involvement	4
Cystinosis	3
Medullary cystic disease/juvenile nephronophthisis	3
Pyelonephritis/interstitial nephritis due to vesico-ureteric reflux without obstruction	2
Hypertensive renal disease	2
Syndrome of agenesis of abdominal musculature	2
Diabetic glomerulosclerosis	1
Polycystic kidney disease	1
Hereditary nephritis	1
Chronic pyelonephritis; nephrosclerosis	1
Other	6
Unknown	15

only disease types reported for three or more patients are listed separately in Table 11-4. Aplastic/hypoplastic/dysplastic kidney(s) was the most frequently reported primary diagnosis, accounting for 15 percent of the patients studied. Obstructive uropathy, another congenital urologic condition in pediatric patients, was responsible for an additional 11 percent of the total. Chronic glomerulonephritis and focal glomerulosclerosis were diagnosed in 12 percent and 9 percent of the study children, respectively.

Transplantation

Twenty-one percent of the special study patients received a renal transplant within 12 months of starting CAPD/CCPD. Another 28 percent were actively pursuing renal transplantation (25 percent cadaver, 3 percent live donor), although one third of the children on cadaver transplant waiting lists had high plasma reactive antibody titers (i.e., greater than 50 percent). A total of 58 (18 percent) of the special study patients had no active plans for transplantation at the time of the survey, 45 of whom cited "the wishes of the patient and/or family" as the reason transplantation was not being pursued. Medical complications were considered as prohibiting transplantation in six children, three of whom were noted to have nonfunctioning bladders. Another seven children were not pursuing transplantation due to recent allograft failure.

Pediatric Nephrologist Involvement

The role of pediatric nephrologists in the care of 307 of the special study patients is summarized in Figs. 11-3 and 11-4. Pediatric nephrologists served as the primary attending nephrologists for 66 percent of the children surveyed (Fig. 11-3). Pediatric nephrology consultation, defined as seeing the child and/or reviewing medical records at least annually, was reported for 15 percent of patients; 19 percent had no pediatric nephrologist involved in their CAPD/CCPD treatment. When the data were analyzed according to patient age group (Fig. 11-4), pediatric nephrologist involvement was found to decline with increasing patient age. Pediatric nephrologists were listed as the primary renal physicians for 89 percent of children under 5 years of age, compared with 44 percent of patients 15 to 20 years of age ($P < 0.05$). Almost 10 percent of children under 10 years of age had no pediatric nephrologist involved in their CAPD/CCPD therapy.

School Attendance

Information on school attendance was received for 174 children. Eighty percent of the children 5 to 18 years of age were reported to be attending school on a full-time basis. Only two of 174 children were receiving homebound tutoring in lieu of regular school attendance. Fourteen percent of

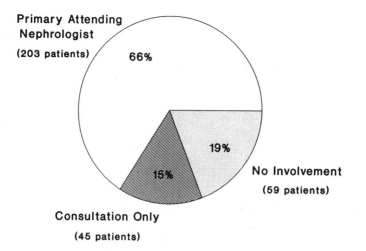

Fig. 11-3. Pediatric nephrologist involvement in the care of children treated with CAPD/CCPD in the United States (age , < 21 years at first CAPD/CCPD exchange).

adolescents (15 to 18 years of age) had dropped out of school; only two school-age children were reported to be medically incapable of receiving at least part-time schooling.

Anthropometric Data and Growth

Measures of height, weight, head circumference (only in children less than 3 years of age), triceps skinfold thickness, and midarm circumference were obtained at the time of CAPD/CCPD initiation and following 1 year of

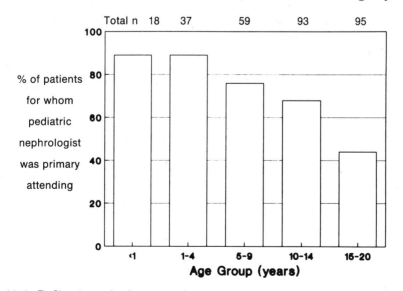

Fig. 11-4. Pediatric nephrologist involvement as primary attending nephrologist in the care of U.S. children by age at first CAPD/CCPD exchange.

uninterrupted peritoneal dialysis. Adequate data were available for analysis as follows: height, 145 patients (81 males and 64 females); weight, 170 patients (92 males and 78 females); head circumference, 14 patients (nine males and five females); triceps skinfold thickness, 61 patients (35 males and 26 females); and midarm circumference, 54 patients (29 males and 25 females).

Patients were grouped by age as follows: 0 to 4 years, 5 to 9 years, 10 to 14 years, and 15 to 18 years. Mean Z scores calculated for heights and weights at CAPD/CCPD initiation and after 1 year of therapy by sex and age group are listed in Table 11-5. Mean Δ Z for height and weight after 1 year of CAPD/CCPD calculated for males and females are shown in Table 11-6. Mean 1-year Δ Z scores for height for males and females 0 to 4 years of age were -0.89 and -1.22, respectively. Mean 1-year Δ Z scores for height for older patients of both sexes were near 0, and thus substantially better than those observed in patients younger than 5 years of age at onset of CAPD/CCPD (Table 11-6).

Head circumference, midarm circumference, and triceps skinfold thickness at baseline and after 1 year of therapy are plotted for individual patients against the normal 50th percentile values in Fig. 11-5, 11-6, and 11-7. Small sample sizes precluded statistical analysis of the data on these anthropometric parameters by age group. However, consistently poor growth in head circumference was observed among the nine children depicted in Fig. 11-5.

Sexual Maturation

Assessments of sexual maturation were available for 146 of the surveyed patients. Sixty-seven percent (10 of 15) boys aged 10 to 12 years at the time of sexual maturation assessment had not yet reached onset of puberty. By 16

Table 11-5. Mean Z Scores and Standard Errors for Height and Weight at Initiation of CAPD/CCPD and After 1 Year of Treatment by Sex and Age Group

| | Age Group (yr) | | | | | | | |
| | 0–4 | | 5–9 | | 10–14 | | 15–18 | |
	Z	SE	Z	SE	Z	SE	Z	SE
Height								
Females								
Initial	−2.59	.48	−3.02	.45	−2.36	.44	−2.65	.62
1 Year	−3.77	.67	−3.92	.54	−2.22	.46	−3.00	.52
Males								
Initial	−2.01	.46	−2.50	.44	−2.74	.34	−1.96	.68
1 Year	−2.90	.61	−2.63	.42	−2.75	.31	−2.48	.55
Weight								
Females								
Initial	−1.94	.53	−1.95	.34	−1.20	.28	−1.40	.35
1 Year	−2.50	.67	−2.44	.35	−1.60	.27	−1.68	.28
Males								
Initial	−1.50	.45	−1.10	.34	−1.15	.40	− .93	.51
1 Year	−1.90	.62	−1.34	.32	−1.63	.26	−1.66	.40

Table 11-6. Mean 1-Year ΔZ Scores for Height and
Weight by Patient Sex and Age Group

Measurement	Age Group (yr)			
	0–4	5–9	10–14	15–18
Height				
Males (n = 81)	−.89[a]	−.06	−.10	−.11
Females (n = 64)	−1.22	−.08	−.16	−.09
Weight				
Males (n = 92)	−.24	−.15	−.36	−.58
Females (n = 78)	−.39	−.20	−.24	−.13

[a] $P = 0.02$ compared with older age groups of males.

years of age, all boys had progressed to at least Tanner stage 3, and 78
percent were considered fully mature. Similar observations were recorded in
girls 10 to 12 years of age, 65 percent of whom had not reached Tanner stage 2
when assessed. Median age of menarche was 15 (normal = 12.8 years[13]); 34
percent (15/44) of girls 12 years of age and older had reached menarche.

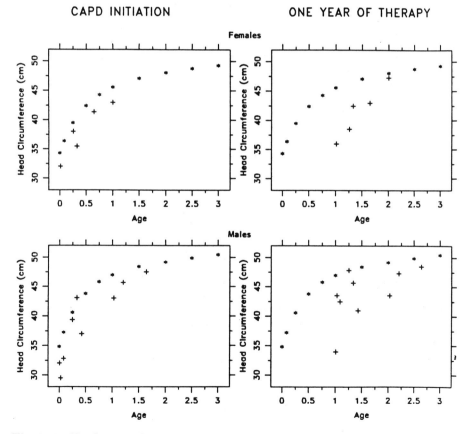

Fig. 11-5. Head circumference at CAPD/CCPD initiation and after 1 year of peritoneal dialysis for individual study patients (+), with 50th percentile normal reference
values (*).

CAPD INITIATION   ONE YEAR OF THERAPY

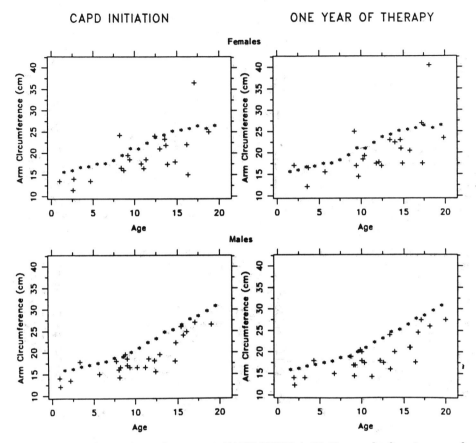

Fig. 11-6. Midarm circumference at CAPD/CCPD initiation and after 1 year of peritoneal dialysis for individual study patients (+), with 50th percentile normal reference values (∗).

Termination of CAPD/CCPD

Nearly two thirds (204/320) of the special study patients had terminated CAPD/CCPD by September 1, 1986. The status of these patients immediately following CAPD/CCPD termination was as follows: transplantation, 137 patients (67 percent); in-center hemodialysis, 36 patients (18 percent); death, 14 patients (7 percent); reutrn of kidney function, six patients (3 percent); home hemodialysis, three patients (1 percent); medical management, two patients (1 percent); in-center intermittent peritoneal dialysis, two patients (1 percent); and not reported, four patients (2 percent). Terminal cancer was the reason two children were transferred off CAPD to medical management.

Centers were asked to report all contributing causes of the termination of CAPD/CCPD and to select one primary reason for each patient. Transplan-

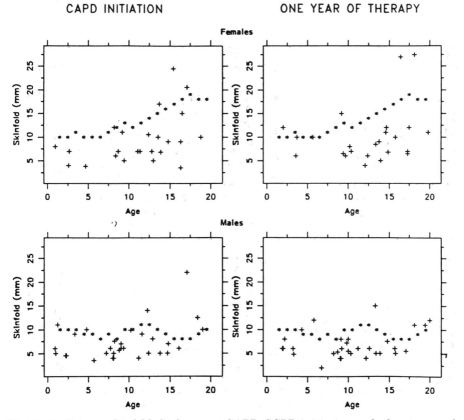

Fig. 11-7. Triceps skinfold thickness at CAPD/CCPD initiation and after 1 year of peritoneal dialysis for individual study patients (+), with 50th percentile normal reference values (*).

tation was the most frequently cited reason for leaving CAPD/CCPD (67 percent). Of the 67 patients who were not transplanted, 14 died, six had return of renal function, and 47 terminated CAPD/CCPD in favor of an alternative dialysis modality. Table 11-7 summarizes primary and contributing causes of termination of CAPD/CCPD reported for these 47 patients. Excessive peritonitis was listed as the primary reason for termination of CAPD/CCPD in 21 percent of cases (10/47) and as a contributing reason in another 62 percent of cases (29/47). Exit site and tunnel infections were primary causes of CAPD/CCPD termination in 9 percent of cases (4/47) and contributing causes in 38 percent (18/47). Catheter failures due to leaks and other malfunctions were primary causes in 10 percent of cases (5/47) and contributed to CAPD/CCPD failure in another 34 percent (16/47). Of the seven patients whose primary reason for leaving CAPD was listed as "inability to cope," five also noted CAPD/CCPD-related complications as contributing causes.

Table 11-7. Reasons for Termination of CAPD/CCPD (n = 47)[a]

Reason	Primary[b]	(%)	Contributing[c]	(%)
Excessive peritonitis	10	(21)	29	(62)
Patient/family choice; inability to cope	7	(15)	15	(32)
Catheter malfunctions	5	(11)	16	(34)
Exit site and tunnel infections	4	(9)	18	(38)
Inadequate ultrafiltration	3	(6)	8	(17)
Inadequate solute clearance	3	(6)	4	(8)
Excessive hospitalizations for CAPD-related complications	2	(4)	14	(31)
Hospitalization for other than CAPD-related complications	2	(4)	1	(2)
Hernia	0		1	(2)
Visual/manual impairment	0		1	(2)
Other (medical)	6	(13)	7	(15)
Other (nonmedical)	3	(6)	7	(15)
Not stated	2	(4)	0	
Socioeconomic reasons	0		0	

[a] Excludes transplantation (n = 137), death (n = 14), and return of renal function (n = 6).

[b] One primary reason was specified for each patient.

[c] All contributing reasons cited for all patients.

DISCUSSION

The 1976 discovery of CAPD by Popovich et al.[15] was greeted with enthusiasm by pediatric nephrologists in North America and Western Europe.[16] Compared with hemodialysis, CAPD appeared to offer several distinct advantages for pediatric ESRD patients: near steady-state biochemical and fluid control, no dysequilibrium syndrome, greatly reduced dietary restrictions, freedom from repeated dialysis needle punctures, and, perhaps most important, the opportunity to routinely receive dialysis in the home. With CAPD, it also became possible to offer chronic dialysis treatment to infants less than 1 year of age,[17] a patient group that was previously not considered suitable for renal replacement therapy.[18,19] It was suggested early on that CAPD might become the dialysis modality of choice for infants and young children awaiting renal transplantation.[3,20]

Initial reports from several large pediatric dialysis programs documented that CAPD was an acceptable alternative to hemodialysis for children of any age.[21-27] Subsequent reports have remained generally favorable, further encouraging the steady growth of CAPD and CCPD in pediatric dialysis centers in the United States, Canada, and Europe. Data from the European Dialysis and Transplant Association (EDTA) Registry show that the percentage of children beginning renal replacement therapy whose first method of treatment was CAPD increased from 8.3 percent of 436 children in 1980 to 17.7 percent of 492 children who began dialysis in 1984.[28] The total contribution of CAPD to pediatric dialysis in the 32 member countries of the EDTA (calculated as the percentage of total patient-months of dialysis therapy per year) increased from less than 4 percent in 1980 to 17.6 percent in 1984.[28] In some countries, the contribution of CAPD has been much greater. For example, in the United Kingdom, Switzerland, and Sweden, CAPD accounted for more than 50 percent of all chronic dialysis therapy received by children in 1984.[29] On December 31, 1985, 16 percent of the total EDTA pediatric dialysis patient population (279/1,729 patients) were receiving CAPD.[30]

A more dramatic trend toward CAPD has been seen in recent years in Canada and the United States. Since 1983, peritoneal dialysis (CAPD or CCPD) has been the initial renal replacement therapy for over 60 percent of pediatric ESRD patients in Canada.[31] Of all children receiving dialysis in Canada on December 31, 1986, 62 percent were on either CAPD or CCPD.[31]

Preliminary 1987 data from the United States Health Care Financing Administration on pediatric dialysis modalities are shown in Fig. 11-8. Fifty-three percent of the 684 children less than 15 years of age who were receiving dialysis in the United States on December 31, 1987, were being treated with

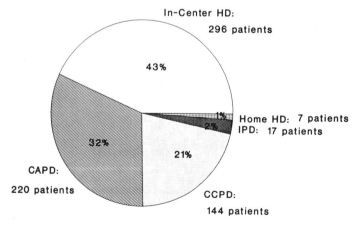

HD • Hemodialysis
IPD • Intermittent Peritoneal Dialysis

Fig. 11-8. Maintenance dialysis of the 684 U.S. children under 15 years of age who were receiving dialysis on December 31, 1987 by dialysis modality. (Courtesy of P. Eggers, Health Care Financing Administration)

either CAPD (220/684 patients) or CCPD (144/684 patients). (Eggers P: Personal communication, Health Care Financing Administration, 1989.)

Note that the Canadian and U.S. data are only indirectly comparable to that from the EDTA. Tabulation involved three different years. Moreover, the Canadian and U.S. patient totals included only children who had not yet reached their 15th birthday by December 31 of the year of tabulation, whereas the EDTA totals included all patients whose ESRD therapy began before their 15th birthdays, regardless of their ages on December 31, 1985. Presumably, a substantial number of patients over 15 years of age on December 31, 1985, were included in the EDTA totals. The mean age of the 1,309 pediatric patients receiving in-center hemodialysis in the member countries of the EDTA on December 31, 1985, was 15.3 years, compared with a mean age of only 11.0 years for the 279 EDTA pediatric CAPD patients.[30]

The present article contains data on 658 pediatric CAPD/CCPD patients treated in 170 different centers in the United States and represents the largest pediatric CAPD/CCPD experience reported to date. Participation by U.S. dialysis centers in the National CAPD Registry is voluntary and without monetary compensation. It is thus impossible to eliminate biases which might result from the effects of receiving treatment in a center that was motivated to participate in the National CAPD Registry and/or in the pediatric special study. While not statistically significant, the generally younger age of the 320 special study patients, compared with the 165 eligible patients for whom no data were received, may be a reflection of increased interest in a study of this type among more specialized pediatric centers.

It is difficult to determine the degree to which the 658 patients in this study reflect the total United States pediatric CAPD/CCPD patient population. When data from the United States Health Care Financing Administration (HCFA) covering the years 1981 to 1985 are compared with the National CAPD Registry's active patient totals for the same years, the Registry is seen to contain information on 45 to 55 per cent of the patients identified by HCFA as receiving CAPD or CCPD in the United States.[6] However, the Registry's *pediatric* population may not represent the same percentage of the total United States *pediatric* CAPD/CCPD population. From the limited available HCFA data on the ages of CAPD/CCPD patients in the United States, it has been estimated that only approximately 2.5 percent of the total U.S. CAPD/CCPD patient population is less than 21 years of age (Eggers P: Personal communication, Health Care Financing Administration, 1989). Since the Registry's pediatric patient population makes up approximately 4.5 percent of its total population, it is likely that the Registry has captrured a proportionately larger pediatric patient population compared with the United States as a whole.

Over 90 percent of the United States centers providing CAPD/CCPD to the children included in this report have a limited amount of pediatric experience. More than one half of the children studied were receiving treatment in centers with a total pediatric experience of less than 11 patients. Only 4 percent of the centers providing treatment to children had treated more than

20 such patients. It is not known if the small number of high-volume pediatric centers participating in the Registry accurately reflects the situation in the United States as a whole.

Despite the small number of high-volume specialized pediatric centers participating in the Registry, most of the children in this study were cared for by pediatric nephrologists. Sixty-six percent of the children studied listed a pediatric nephrologist as primary attending nephrologist and nearly 90 percent of children less than 5 years of age were followed primarily by a pediatric nephrologist. The possible influence of pediatric nephrologist involvement on complication rates and other outcome measures was not examined by this study.

The potential importance of a center's total experience with pediatric patients was suggested by the observation that peritonitis risk was inversely correlated with the total number of children treated in the center; the best results were obtained in centers that had treated more than 20 total pediatric patients. Other potentially important influences on a center's complication rates, such as the center's total patient experience (adult and pediatric) and staffing ratios, were not examined in this study.

Not surprisingly, excessive peritonitis emerged from this study as an important factor in nearly 75 percent of the decisions to terminate CAPD/CCPD for another dialysis modality. The EDTA has reported similar observations; 50 percent of the European children who abandoned CAPD for hemodialysis between 1981 and 1984 did so because of excessive peritonitis.[29]

The importance of renal transplantation as the preferred renal replacement therapy for children in the United States is clearly evident from this study. Within 12 months of initiating CAPD/CCPD, approximately one fourth of these children had received a renal transplant. Two thirds of the special study patients who terminated CAPD/CCPD did so to obtain a renal transplant. Recent reports describing renal transplantation in children receiving CAPD/CCPD have shown no significant differences in patient or graft survival rates when compared with children receiving hemodialysis.[32,33] No data have been obtained in the present study on the outcome of renal transplantation in the study patients.

The present report contains evidence that the major CAPD/CCPD complications (peritonitis, exit site and tunnel infection, and catheter failure) occur earlier and more often among pediatric patients compared with adults. However, this apparently does not result in a comparably high treatment failure rate, especially among younger children. Overall, the actuarial 12-month "technique survival" rate for pediatric patients in this study was 81 percent.

We were able to compare some of the findings from this study of U.S. children with data that are available from the EDTA on children treated with CAPD/CCPD in Europe. The EDTA pediatric patient population is restricted by convention to children who began renal replacement therapy before their 15th birthday. Clinical practice in the United States is somewhat different, with many pediatric ESRD programs caring for adolescent patients through ages 18 to 21 years. The 15- to 20-year-old age group included in the present report was excluded from comparisons with EDTA pediatric data.

The EDTA reported that during 1984 and 1985, peritonitis occurred in pediatric patients at a rate of 1.23 episodes per patient-year.[30] When the data on U.S. children contained in the present report were also limited to children less than 15 years of age at the time of first CAPD/CCPD exchange, we found a comparable peritonitis rate of 1.4 episodes per patient-year.

The "technique survival" rate among the patients in the U.S. study was somewhat greater than that previously reported by the EDTA, which used the same criteria for calculating technique survival as were used in the present study. For children under 15 years of age at first CAPD/CCPD exchange, the 12-month actuarial technique survival reported by the EDTA for the 1981 to 1984 period was 72 percent,[29] compared with a rate of 87 percent for U.S. children less than 15 years of age at first exchange. Statistical analysis of the observed differences in peritonitis and technique survival rates seen in European and U.S. pediatric CAPD/CCPD patients is not possible from the available information.

The present report provides information on the growth of a large number of U.S. children treated with CAPD/CCPD for 1 year. When expressed as the mean 1-year change in Z scores for height, linear growth was found to be substantially below normal for children who began CAPD/CCPD before 5 years of age. More encouraging was the observation that near normal linear growth occurred among older children, the best growth occurring in the 5 to 9-year-old age group. In no age group was "catchup" growth observed, a finding consistent with previous reports from single centers.[34-36]

It is also noteworthy that mean Z scores for height at the time of initiation of CAPD/CCPD demonstrated that most children began CAPD/CCPD two or more standard deviations below the mean for normal children of the same age and sex. In view of the apparent inabiltiy to obtain catch-up growth during CAPD/CCPD treatment, the results of this study suggest that attention should be given to the development of therapies that promote and protect normal growth during the period of chronic renal insufficiency which occurs before initiation of CAPD/CCPD.

While much remains unknown about the use of CAPD/CCPD in children in the United States, the experiences of the National CAPD Registry's pediatric population reported here offer some important insights. The mortality risk for children receiving CAPD/CCPD appears to be 6 percent overall, but may be several times greater for infants and very young children. Complications occur earlier and more often among pediatric CAPD/CCPD patients compared with adults, but this does not result in a comparably high treatment failure rate, perhaps because so many children in the United States receive a renal transplant relatively soon after beginning CAPD/CCPD. In fact, the success of CAPD/CCPD as a dialysis treatment that can be used in children for at least 1 year while awaiting renal transplantation is clearly evident from this study. This relatively short-term use of CAPD/CCPD in concert with renal transplantation appears to be a major treatment pattern among centers currently caring for pediatric CAPD/CCPD patients in the United States. Whether CAPD/CCPD can be as successfully used for longer periods by children who are not readily transplantable remains to be seen. Moreover, a full assessment of CAPD/CCPD as renal replacement therapy for children in the United States cannot be accomplished until comparable broadly based information on outcomes and experiences becomes available for U.S. children treated with alternative dialysis modalities and renal transplantation.

ACKNOWLEDGMENTS

We thank the staffs of the 467 dialysis centers participating in the National CAPD Registry, especially those center personnel who contributed to the pediatric special study. A complete list of participating centers is available.[37]

Special thanks to Paul W. Eggers, PhD, Chief, Program Evaluation Branch, Office of Research, Health Care Financing Administration for the data displayed in Fig. 11-8. Additional thanks go Mary Blanchett and Janell McQuinn for preparation of the manuscript.

This study was supported by NIH contracts NO1-AM-3-2244 and NO1-AM-3-2245 of the National Institute of Diabetes and Digestive and Kidney Diseases.

REFERENCES

1. Oreopoulos DG, Katirtzoglou A, Arbus G, et al: Dialysis and transplantation in young children. Br Med J 1:1628, 1979 (letter)
2. Balfe JW, Irwin MA: Continuous ambulatory peritoneal dialysis in pediatrics. p. 131. In M Legrain (ed): Continuous Ambulatory Peritoneal Dialysis. Excerpta Medica, Amsterdam, 1980
3. Alexander SR: Pediatric CAPD update, 1983. Peritoneal Dialysis Bull 3: (suppl) S15, 1983
4. National CAPD Registry: National CAPD Registry Report #83-1. National Institutes of Health. NIH, Bethesda, MD, April 15, 1983, p 2
5. National CAPD Registry: Report of the National CAPD Registry of the National Institutes of Health. NIH, Bethesda, MD, January, 1987, p 6/1
6. National CAPD Registry: Report of the National CAPD Registry of the National Institutes of Health. NIH, Bethesda, MD, January, 1986
7. Kaplan E, Meier P: Nonparametric estimation from incomplete observations. J Am Statistical Assoc 53:457, 1958
8. Cox DR: Regression models and life tables. J Statistics (Soc. B.) 34:187, 1972
9. National Center for Health Statistics: Growth curves for children. In Hamill PVV (ed): Vital and Health Statistics Series 11. Data from the National Health Survey #165 (DHEW publication #[PHS] 78-1650) DHEW, Washington, 1977

10. Potter DE, Broyer M, Chantler C, et al: Measurement of growth in children with renal insufficiency. Kidney Int 14:378, 1978

11. Lehmann EL, D'abrera HJM: Nonparametrics: Statistical Methods Based on Ranks. Holden-Day, San Francisco, 1975

12. Frisancho RA: New norms of upper limb fat and muscle areas for assessment of nutritional status. Am J Clin Nutr 34:2540, 1981

13. Marshall WA, Tanner JM: Variations in patterns of pubertal changes in girls. Arch Dis Childhood 44:291, 1969

14. Marshall WA, Tanner JM: Variations in patterns of pubertal changes in boys. Arch Dis Childhood 45:13, 1970

15. Popovich RP, Moncrief JW, Decherd JB, et al: The definition of a novel portable/wearable equilibrium peritoneal dialysis technique. Trans Am Soc Artif Internal Organs 5:64, 1976 (abstr)

16. Fine RN: Peritoneal dialysis update. J Pediatr 100:1, 1982

17. Alexander SR: CAPD in infants less than one year of age. p. 149. RN Fine, AB Gruskin (eds): End Stage Renal Disease in Children. WB Saunders, Philadelphia, 1984

18. Arbus GS, DeMaria JE, Galivango J, et al: The first 10 years of the dialysis-transplantation program at The Hospital for Sick Children, Toronto. 1: Predialysis and dialysis. Can Med Assoc J 122:655, 1980

19. Potter DE, Holliday MA, Piel CF, et al: Treatment of end-stage renal disease in children: a 15-year experience. Kidney Int 18:103, 1980

20. Fine RN: Choosing a dialysis therapy for children with end-stage renal disease. Am J Kidney Dis 4:249, 1984

21. Alexander SR, Tseng CH, Maksym KA, et al: Clinical parameters in continuous ambulatory peritoneal dialysis for infants and young children. p. 195. In JW Moncrief, RP Popovich (eds): CAPD Update. Masson Publishing USA, New York, 1981

22. Balfe JW, Vigneaux A, Williamson J, et al: The use of CAPD in the treatment of children with end-stage renal disease. Peritoneal Dialysis Bull 1:35, 1981

23. Eastham EJ, Kirplani H, Francis D, et al: Pediatric continuous ambulatory peritoneal dialysis. Arch Dis Childhood 57:677, 1982

24. Guillot M, Clermont M-J, Gagnadoux M-F, Broyer M: Nineteen months' experience with continuous ambulatory peritoneal dialysis in children: main clinical and biologic results. p. 203. In Gahl GM, Kessel M, Nolph KD (eds): Advances in Peritoneal Dialysis. Excerpta Medica, Amsterdam, 1981

25. Kohaut EC: Continuous ambulatory peritoneal dialysis: a preliminary pediatric experience. Am J Dis Children 135:270, 1981

26. Potter DE, McDaid TK, McHenry K, et al: Continuous ambulatory peritoneal dialysis (CAPD) in children. Trans Am Soc Artif Internal Organs 27:64, 1981

27. Salusky IB, Lucullo L, Nelson P, Fine RN: Continuous ambulatory peritoneal dialysis in children. Pediatr Clin North Am 29:1005, 1982

28. Rizzoni G, Broyer M, Brunner FP, et al: Combined report on regular dialysis and transplantation of children in Europe, 1985. Pro EDTA-ERA 23:65, 1985

29. Rizzoni G, Broyer M, Challah S, Selwood N: The use of peritoneal dialysis in Europe for treatment of children with end stage renal disease—EDTA Registry data. p. 1. In Fine RN (ed): Chronic Ambulatory Peritoneal Dialysis (CAPD) and Chronic Cycling Peritoneal Dialysis (CCPD) in Children. Martinus Nijhoff Publishing, Boston 1987

30. Golper TA, Geerlings W, Selwood NH, et al: Peritoneal dialysis results in the

EDTA Registry. p. 414. In Nolph KD (ed): Peritoneal Dialysis. 3rd Ed. S Karger AG, Dordrecht, 1989

31. Arbus GS: Pediatric patients in 1986. p. 89. In Posen GA (ed): Canadian Renal Failure Register, 1986 Report. Kidney Federation of Canada, Montreal, 1987

32. Leichter HE, Salusky IB, Ettenger RB, et al: Experience with renal transplantation in children undergoing peritoneal dialysis (CAPD/CCPD). Am J Kidney Dis 8:181, 1986

33. Stefanidis CJ, Balfe JW, Arbus GS, et al: Renal transplantation in children treated with continuous ambulatory peritoneal dialysis. Peritoneal Dialysis Bull 3:5, 1983

34. Fennell RS, Orak JK, Hudson T, et al: Growth in children with various therapies for end stage renal disease. Am J Dis Children 138:28, 1984

35. Potter DE: Comparison of CAPD and hemodialysis in children. p. 297. In Fine RN (ed): Chronic Ambulatroy Peritoneal Dialysis (CAPD) and Chronic Cycling Peritoneal Dialysis (CCPD) in Children. Martinus Nijhoff Publishing, Boston, 1987

36. Stefanidis CJ, Hewitt IK, Balfe JW: Growth in children receiving continuous ambulatory peritoneal dialysis. J Pediat 102:681, 1983

37. Lindblad AS, Novak JW, Nolph KD (eds): Continuous Ambulatory Peritoneal Dialysis in the U.S.A. Kluwer Academic Publishers, Dorchecht, 1989

Index

Page numbers followed by f denote figures; those followed by t denote tables.

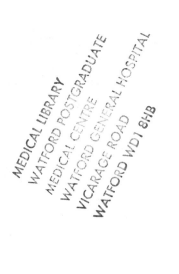